Survival Guide for the Beginning Speech–Language Clinician

Survival Guide
for the Beginning
Speech–Language Clinician

SECOND EDITION

Susan Moon Meyer

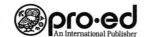
pro·ed
An International Publisher

8700 Shoal Creek Boulevard
Austin, Texas 78757-6897
800/897-3202   Fax 800/397-7633
www.proedinc.com

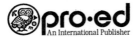
An International Publisher

© 2004 by PRO-ED, Inc.
8700 Shoal Creek Boulevard
Austin, Texas 78757-6897
800/897-3202   Fax 800/397-7633
www.proedinc.com

Notice: PRO-ED grants permission to the user of this book to make unlimited copies of Appendix 1.A (pp. 41–50) for teaching or clinical purposes. Duplication of this material for commercial use is prohibited.

Library of Congress Cataloging-in-Publication Data

Meyer, Susan Moon.
    Survival guide for the beginning speech–language clinician / Susan Moon Meyer.—2nd ed.
        p. ; cm.
    Includes bibliographical references and index.
    ISBN 0-89079-981-4 (soft cover : alk. paper)
    1. Speech therapy—Practice. 2. Speech therapy. I. Title.
    [DNLM: 1. Language Disorders—therapy. 2. Speech Disorders—therapy.
    3. Speech–Language Pathology—methods. WL 340.2 M613s 2004]
    RC428.5.M49 2004
    616.85'506—dc22

                                                                        2003066422

Art Director: Jason Crosier
Designer: Nancy McKinney-Point
This book is designed in Janson Text, Lucida Sans, Dom Casual, Kabel, and Trade Gothic.

Printed in the United States of America

2 3 4 5 6 7 8 9 10   08 07 06 05

To My Family

The most important commodity!

This book is dedicated to my husband
for his unending love, guidance, suggestions,
and support.

To our children
for their continuing love and challenge.
May they become best friends in my lifetime!

To the Student

Nothing is as moving as the expression of gratitude
expressed by a newly discharged child's gift of flowers
to the clinician. It symbolizes not the end of the process
but, for the client, the beginning of a new life.
This is the best reason to endure your arduous education
and clinical training—the opportunity to bring joy
and wonder to those who may have felt that their lives
would hold neither.

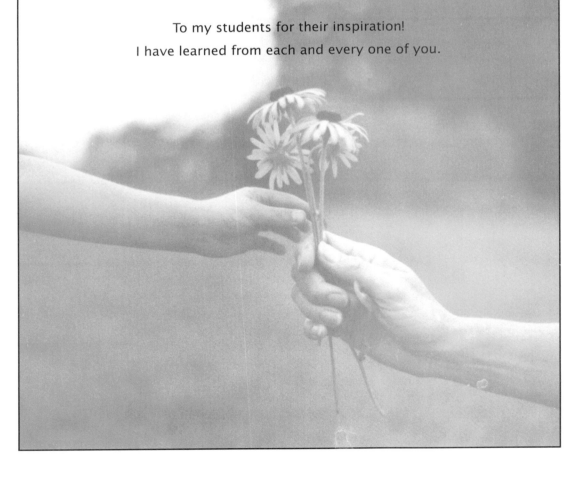

To my students for their inspiration!
I have learned from each and every one of you.

Contents

Preface ◄ xi ►

Introduction
Bridging the Gap—
Taking Your First Step Toward Obtaining Professional Status
◄ 1 ►

Needs for Different Levels of Introductory Clinical Functioning   2
How To Use This Book   6
Conclusion   7

Chapter 1
Behavioral Objectives:
Background
◄ 11 ►

Components of a Behavioral Objective   12
Samples of Well-Written Behavioral Objectives   22
Application and Importance of Behavioral Objectives   33
Appendix 1.A: Exercise: Identifying Components of Behavioral Objectives   41
Appendix 1.B: Answers: Identifying Components of Behavioral Objectives   51

Chapter 2
Behavioral Objectives:
Common Writing Problems
◄ 63 ►

Problem 1: Incorrect Format Following the Lead-In   63
Problem 2: Consistency   65
Problem 3: Performance Component   66
Problem 4: Condition Component   69
Problem 5: Criterion Component   71
Problem 6: Lack of Support or Harmony   74

Chapter 3
Evaluation and Progress Reports:
Organization and Content
◄ 79 ►

Substandard Evaluation   80
General Guidelines for Speech–Language Evaluation Reports   87
Progress Reports: Organization and Content   95

Chapter 4
Evaluation, Reevaluation, and Progress Reports:
Writing Reports That Shine
◄ 99 ►

Evaluation Reports   100
Reevaluation Reports   120
Progress Reports   128

Chapter 5
Progress Notes
◄ 141 ►

Background   141
Cumulative Progress Note Entries   143
Subjective-Objective-Assessment-Plan Format   156

Chapter 6
Taming the Paper Giant:
Assuring Accuracy and Accountability
◄ 165 ►

Paperwork Process and a System for Streamlining   167
Accountability   177
Important Advice   190

Chapter 7
Therapy Conferences
◄ 195 ►

Therapy Conference Reports   198
Conclusion   205

Chapter 8
Preparing for the Public Schools
◄ 207 ►

Brief Background 208
Required Paperwork 210
Conclusion 217
Appendix 8.A: Example of Progress Report Form 218
Appendix 8.B: Example of Language Arts Standards 219
Appendix 8.C: Example of Notice of Educational Evaluation/Reevaluation Plan 220
Appendix 8.D: Example of Prior Notice About Evaluation/Consent for Evaluation 223
Appendix 8.E: Example of Notice of Procedural Safeguards 225
Appendix 8.F: Example of Invitation to a Meeting of the Individualized Education Program (IEP) Team 232
Appendix 8.G: Example of Notice and Consent for Placement in Special Education Services 235
Appendix 8.H: Completed Example of Evaluation Report 237
Appendix 8.I: Example of a Completed Individualized Education Program 244
Appendix 8.J: Example of a Completed Notice of Recommended Educational Placement 256

Chapter 9
Beyond Basic Therapy
◄ 261 ►

Group Therapy 262
Play Therapy 267
Curriculum-Based Therapy 272

Chapter 10
Enhancing Performance
◄ 279 ►

Problem and Solution 1: Seating Arrangement 280
Problem and Solution 2: Reinforcement 282
Problem and Solution 3: Verbal Models 292
Problem and Solution 4: Loquaciousness 296
Problem and Solution 5: Smothering the Client 296
Problem and Solution 6: Fostering Dependency 297
Problem and Solution 7: Choice Constancy 299
Problem and Solution 8: Reading Sequence 300
Problem and Solution 9: Elicitation Techniques 301
Problem and Solution 10: Risky Questions 305
Problem and Solution 11: Appearing Foolish 306
Problem and Solution 12: Being Overpowering 308
Problem and Solution 13: Directions 308

Problem and Solution 14: Receptive Tasks 309

Problem and Solution 15: Head Nodding and
Forward Upper Body Movement 310

Problem and Solution 16: Habits That May Be Misinterpreted 312

Problem and Solution 17: The Game "Mirage" 313

Problem and Solution 18: Carry-Over 314

Problem and Solution 19: Too Much Work 318

Problem and Solution 20: Sign Language 319

Problem and Solution 21: Session Opening 321

Problem and Solution 22: Session Closing 321

Problem and Solution 23: Pause Time 323

Problem and Solution 24: Mirror Usage 323

Problem and Solution 25: Differentiating Sound from Letter 325

Problem and Solution 26: Singsong Voice 326

Chapter 11
Self-Evaluation
◀ 329 ▶

Initial Self-Evaluations 331

Six General Strategies 331

Self-Observation Techniques 332

Initial Focus: Benchmark Measurements 334

Later Focus: Fine-Tuning Clinical Competence 337

Additional Strategies To Facilitate Self-Evaluation 342

Student Self-Appraisal 343

Epilogue: The Basics Are Not Enough! ◀ 347 ▶

Glossary ◀ 351 ▶

Index ◀ 359 ▶

About the Author ◀ 368 ▶

Preface

Survival Guide for the Beginning Speech–Language Clinician, now in its second edition, is intended as a supplemental text to guide you when taking your first clinical steps toward a career as a speech–language pathologist. This book is useful to both undergraduate and graduate students undertaking their *very first* clinical experience. The goals of this book are (a) to provide a realistic, practical, and comprehensive overview of clinical problems that are often encountered by beginning clinicians; (b) to present solutions to those problems; and (c) to help prepare you for what you will experience along the way. This book does not focus on the numerous principles and theories that underlie various aspects of the clinical process because these are thoroughly covered in the classroom.

A secondary purpose of this book is to assist the newest segment of the profession—speech–language pathology assistants—as they journey through their training programs. Although speech–language pathology assistants differ from speech–language clinicians in terms of educational requirements and the scope of responsibilities, they still have to complete a fieldwork experience under the supervision of a speech–language pathologist certified by the American Speech-Language-Hearing Association. Having pointed this out, what follows is a discussion of what you will find in this book.

The introduction includes the rationale for writing this book. My former students' comments regarding feelings, attitudes, and perceptions toward the clinical practicum procedure are included to help you realize that your apprehensions are not unique. Three groups of students performing at different levels of the clinical process are identified, and the major clinical problem encountered by each group is addressed to show you how you will progress and what will be expected of you.

The importance of writing behavioral objectives is stressed in Chapter 1. The three components of a behavioral objective are discussed and examples pertinent to each component are presented. Relevant examples of various communication problems encountered in the profession of speech–language pathology are given. Opportunities are provided for you to identify the performance, condition, and criterion portions of objectives. The importance of understanding and writing behavioral objectives is discussed.

Chapter 2 is based on more than 30 years of my personal experience in reading, correcting, revising, rewriting, and approving behavioral objectives that were written by many hundreds of former beginning clinicians. Frequent problems in designing behavioral objectives are provided and discussed in an attempt to prevent you from doing the same.

The purpose of Chapter 3 is to make you aware of the necessity of writing well-written evaluations. First, a poorly written evaluation is presented and analyzed. Then general guidelines are provided for writing both professional-style evaluations and progress reports. Both organization and content are emphasized.

Chapter 4 contains samples of evaluations, reevaluations, and progress reports that are well written. You can experience the flow and style of professional writing by actively reading and rereading these samples. Additional guidelines for writing professional reports are provided.

Writing progress notes in a professional manner is the focus of Chapter 5. The information and examples provided are designed to stimulate your thinking and analytical skills and to help you write acceptable progress notes. Examples of both acceptable and problematic progress note entries are presented and discussed. Suggestions for improvement are provided when necessary. You will discover that progress notes are not ends in themselves, but should be scrutinized and used to help determine the flow and direction of the therapeutic program.

Chapter 6 addresses several attributes of clinical accountability that are important to beginning clinicians. The first involves the paperwork process. An efficient system for handling the voluminous amount of paperwork expected of you is described and a rationale is presented. Record keeping during therapy sessions is also a focus. Examples, problems, suggestions, and samples of record-keeping systems are presented and discussed. An emphasis is also placed on keeping track of clinical hours. The types of activities that should be recorded in clinical hours are discussed and presented in a check-sheet format.

From reading Chapter 7, beginning clinicians gain insight into the purpose of a therapy conference as well as areas that should be addressed. Examples of therapy conference reports are provided so beginning clinicians can get ideas pertaining to the information that should be included in these reports. This chapter resulted directly from beginning clinicians' input on a questionnaire asking what additional topics they would like addressed in the second edition of *Survival Guide for the Beginning Speech–Language Clinician.*

Preparing for the public schools is addressed in Chapter 8. A brief background of the laws that have an impact on the performance of school-based speech–language clinicians is provided. Paperwork unique to the public school systems and resulting from these laws is addressed. Examples are provided to help you appreciate the complex, but necessary, process of keeping accurate records.

Chapter 9 takes you beyond basic therapy. Group therapy is discussed, and the concept is contrasted with conducting therapy in a group setting. Non–goal-related and goal-related interaction within a group is discussed and examples are given. Play therapy is addressed, and things to include in a play therapy session are stated and demonstrated. Background information is provided on curriculum-based therapy, and examples depicting this type of therapy are included.

The purpose of Chapter 10 is to offer suggestions to make your therapeutic sessions run more smoothly and to enable you to perform more efficiently and effectively during the clinical process. The content of this chapter is based on frequently occurring problematic areas noted during observations of former beginning clinicians. By identifying problems, showing how they can interfere with the effectiveness of the therapeutic process, and providing solutions, I hope to help you avoid these common pitfalls. Helpful hints to enhance performance are presented and discussed. Some areas that are discussed are seating arrangement, reinforcement for therapy and testing, verbal models, smothering the client, fostering dependency, choice constancy, reading sequence, elicitation techniques, avoidance of being physically overpowering, receptive tasks, elimination of habits that may be misinterpreted, avoidance of game emphasis, carry-over, sign language, session opening and closing, pause time, and mirror usage.

The final chapter encourages you to consciously and continuously evaluate all aspects of your professional performance. Some simple techniques are presented to help you begin to evaluate your own clinical performance. Basic clinical behaviors that need to be addressed when evaluating your sessions are presented and discussed. Additionally, abstract and complex clinical behaviors are presented as you need to incorporate them into your self-evaluations. These are also the behaviors that will be evaluated by most of your supervisors.

It is important to underscore a few points. The names and addresses of clients have been changed to preserve their identity. The actual years in which various clinical events occurred are not given to prevent this book from immediately becoming obsolete. Although the word *beginning* does not always precede *clinician*, the intent is that nearly all references to the clinician in this book refer to the beginning clinician. When this is not true, the meaning should be obvious from the context. Initially an attempt was made to refer to a clinician as "he or she," or "him or her," as appropriate. Although socially correct, this usage is most often dropped in this book in favor of referring to clinicians as female and clients as male (except in some reports) because it made the text less awkward and because this better reflects the statistical reality of the profession. I hope this does not offend readers.

In this book, the recipients of speech–language services are referred to variably as clients, patients, students, or children. There is no precise way to differentiate among these terms. For purposes of this book, if a preschool child is receiving services, *child* is the referent used. If a school-aged person receives services, *student* is used. The term *client* is used to refer to a person receiving services in a private practice or agency setting. The term *patient* usually refers to someone receiving services in a hospital or other medical-related facility.

Perhaps other terms should be addressed now. Frequently students have asked me what the difference is between a speech–language pathologist and a speech–language clinician. Unfortunately, I have neither a good nor an accurate answer. I can simply comment on past practice. The terminology appears to be based on both educational level and employment setting. If one has a master's degree and a Certificate of Clinical Competence, the term *speech–language pathologist* seems to be used. However, if one is employed in the schools, regardless of educational level, the term *speech–language clinician* seems to be the frequently used term.

Another convention adopted in this book is to enclose sample documents within a border. Although this technique is not intended to fully "simulate" the document, it will serve to alert you to whether you are reading from a document or have returned to the text. (*Note:* Quick Checks and reviews are also boxed, but they will be obvious to you as you use them. Please *do use them* as they can alert you to topics you may need to review more thoroughly.)

The profession of speech–language pathology continues to benefit from the continuing evolution of information-based technology. Augmentative devices and computer software are readily available to assist with all aspects of the clinical process (administration, diagnosis, treatment, report writing, etc.). Although I ignore the great impact of this technology in this book, I believe that you will be better able to select and use available technology if you first experience the clinical process without the aid of computers and software. Experiencing the clinical process in this manner will enable you to better understand it, evaluate your needs, and ultimately be more knowledgeable of the technology you may require. You will better understand and appreciate the value of computers and software if first required to perform without the aid of this technology. For these reasons, the use of computer technology is not further addressed in this book. In a sense, being a good clinician rests on your shoulders and not in a keyboard or mouse.

My understanding of how you can be successful in speech–language pathology continues to grow. My intent is that this book will stimulate everyone (supervisors, former beginning clinicians, etc.) who uses it to explore additional ways to help future beginning clinicians have an easier, more enjoyable initial experience—an experience that not only ends, but also begins, with their delighting in their new clinical roles.

Acknowledgments

There are many people to whom I owe thanks. Sincere thanks go to all the students whom I have supervised. I have learned something from each and every one of you. Thank you for this opportunity. To Ellen Kwiatkowski, thank you for information, feedback, and support. To Rusty (Ronald) Miller, thanks for designing the new illustrations along with redesigning the old ones. Appreciation is expressed to the following speech–language clinicians for providing me with various "pieces" of the paperwork process: Kathy Arbogast, Kate Frantz,

Peggy Goll, Diane Harpster, April Rose, Michele Scesa, and Pam Smith. Thanks also to Tom Mullen and Kate Frantz for reading and providing substantive feedback on Chapter 8. Thanks are also extended to the fine professionals of PRO-ED. Their comments and expertise resulted in a better end result. Above all, a very special thank-you goes to my husband, John, and to our children, Chris and Scott, who were very supportive and endured my preoccupation with this book. John's numerous readings of this material and gentle suggestions were greatly appreciated. This work could not have been completed without his patience and knowledge while solving my numerous computer problems. For this, I am extremely and forever grateful.

Bridging the Gap— Taking Your First Step Toward Obtaining Professional Status

Needs for Different Levels of Introductory Clinical Functioning

Ideally, this book is intended for your use while you are a speech–language pathology student prior to entering your first clinical practicum experience. Although you can also use it while in your first clinical setting, reading it before then will enable you to get a head start on the clinical process. Depending on your program's curriculum, your first clinical experience may occur at the undergraduate or graduate level. Your status, undergraduate or graduate, does not have any bearing on using this book, which addresses clinical problems that cut across all skill levels. The book's focus is on helping you make steady progress while dealing with the persistent clinical problems that nearly all students encounter. These ongoing clinical problems may stand in your way of achieving clinical competence unless you understand and deal with them in a forthright and professional fashion.

The actual clinical problems that you encounter may differ depending on your place and your progress in the learning process. This variation can be compared to the different ways that a number of blind or partially sighted persons describe an elephant in the well-known parable. An individual's description can only be based on the part of the elephant that is under exploration and is influenced by the degree of visual challenge. Problems you encounter will vary according to your involvement in the learning discovery processes and your *understanding* of the problems you face.

In general, the nature of the clinical problems you may encounter could differ as you move through three stages: (a) when you are about to start the clinical experience, (b) when you become initially involved with the clinical experience, and (c) when you are actively involved in the clinical experience. Clinicians in Stage 3 will already have an initial evaluation in place (done either by self or another), will have had long-range and short-range objectives approved by their supervisors, and will be designing and executing therapy. Students in Stages 1 and 2 will need to realize that their work leads up to their own initial evaluation, and they must plan and learn accordingly.

Conceptually, the ideal case for your passage from the undergraduate classroom to the clinic (or from the graduate classroom to the clinic for graduate students without any previous clinical experience) can be represented by Figure I.1. This smooth transition, without overlaps, is rarely seen in practice, however, because movement across the three stages is not strictly sequential.

Figure I.2 better reflects the classroom-to-clinic passage that will be experienced by most of you. Most likely, you will not have acquired

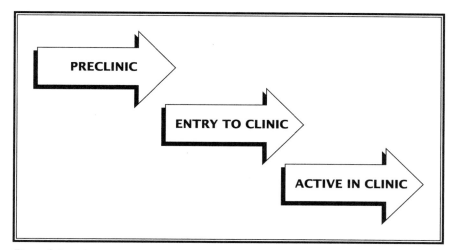

Figure I.1. The "ideal case" for students moving from classroom to clinic.

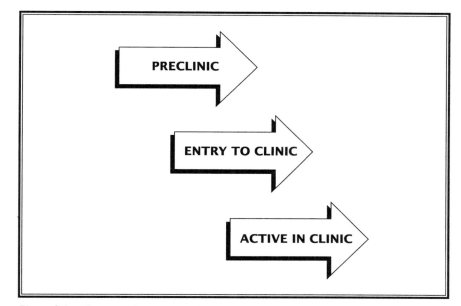

Figure I.2. The typical experience for students moving from classroom to clinic.

some behaviors or skills by the time you find you need them. Therefore, movement back and forth in a pendulum fashion is the rule rather
than the exception. Overlap in process, the need to learn what should
have been already acquired, or, in the worst case, the need to relearn
material, are represented in this figure. If you are a graduate student,
the model (and the problems at each stage) remains the same, but your
own expectations of your work and those of your supervisors and professors will be different from those of an undergraduate student.

Stage 1: Immediately Prior to Starting the Clinical Experience

Many students about to enter the first clinical experience have admitted to me that they were "scared to death" about their upcoming transition into the clinical practicum. This mind-set is counterproductive because this transition can be exhilarating and often can make or break a person's career. To better understand students' feelings, I once developed an entrance survey to be completed by students about to enter their first clinical practicum. The survey asked these students to write their feelings, attitudes, and perceptions of their upcoming experience. The anticipated impact of the impending professional experience was clarified after reviewing these data. In sum, the survey revealed that the students perceived a disjunction between the classroom and the clinic and also a discontinuity between the knowledge they *had* and the knowledge they *believed was needed* to perform successfully in the clinical situation. These students did not know how the clinic and the classroom were related or whether their knowledge base was sufficient.

On the basis of the survey results, I determined that the biggest problem for beginning students was the preponderance of negative self feelings. In their descriptions, words such as "anxious," "nervousness," "uneasy," "uncomfortable," "fright," "scared," "overwhelmed," "intense frustration," "apprehension," "paranoia," and "worried" were plentiful. Based on another study related to clinical education in speech–language pathology students, Chan, Carter, and McAllister (1994) wrote that

> anxiety appears to have an impact on the nature and quality of students' clinical learning experiences. Therefore, identification of both the level of anxiety experienced and the factors contributing significantly to the anxiety may facilitate constructive modification of the clinical learning experience. (p. 126)

I hope that this book will help reduce your anxiety by better preparing you for your initial clinical experience.

In addition, some of your predecessors felt that they were not academically prepared to undergo involvement with the clinical process, whereas others questioned their overall competence. In the survey, positive descriptors, although occasionally present, were infrequent. Therefore, it appears that it is necessary to bridge the gap between the classroom and the clinic in both an experiential and intellectual fashion in order to (a) help in the status change from students to professionals, (b) give guidance on how to help translate classroom materials into practical tools, and (c) build more self-confidence in students' academic preparation. If, in making these transitions, you do not have convenient access to your supervisor at times, you will need somewhere to turn for assistance. In such cases, let this book perform this surrogate function. You will find leafing through this entire book to be helpful, as it will enable you to prepare for what is ahead.

Stage 2: Becoming Involved with the Clinical Experience

Beginning clinical students frequently get bogged down with paperwork. My previous students repeatedly cited paperwork as being the number one problem encountered during this phase of their clinical process. Haynes and Hartman (1975) clearly addressed this problem in their assessment of the paperwork agony:

> In our training institutions, beginning speech clinicians are required to write several types of clinical reports (diagnostic, initial, progress, final, etc.). It has been the experience of the present authors, both as students and as supervisors, that these reports are a major source of conflict, negative emotion and student insecurity. Each quarter in universities across the country, there exists a massive ebb and flow of clinical reports between supervisors and student clinicians. The reports are submitted to the supervisors and then returned to the students with numerous multicolored criticisms. These flaws must then be corrected and the reports resubmitted to the supervisor for further scrutiny. So it goes, back and forth. In many cases, the report goes through this process so repeatedly that the finished product is almost totally written in installments by the supervisor. The reasons behind the supervisor's manifold revisions are not always clear to the burgeoning speech clinician; however, these students are assured that they will understand the rationale and substance of the corrections when they have had more experience with report writing. (p. 7)

If the ambiguity and confusion can be removed from the paperwork process, undue anxiety will be avoided and your time and energy can be better channeled, allowing you to be more productive. Further, by reducing some of the mystery of how you should approach various aspects of the paperwork process, you can develop more positive feelings about your performance earlier in the clinical experience, and ultimately achieve more success. An increase in the quality of your therapy is likely as you are freed from the burdens of paperwork. Help given in selected chapters of this book will be of special benefit for those who mistake filing forms as the "end" of therapy. Keep in mind that the first concern is to achieve therapeutic objectives; recording work in progress is for the sole purpose of keeping accurate records.

Stage 3: Being Actively Involved in the Clinical Experience

Students at Stage 3 are knowledgeable in terms of therapeutic techniques taught in the classroom, but not in the actual orchestration of the therapy session or therapeutic process, which is the major clinical problem for this group. Most of this orchestration is learned through actual experience, trial and error, and feedback from a supervisor's evaluations. However, if much of this information is presented, explained, and demonstrated *prior* to your being expected to conduct therapy, you will not be as frustrated as you struggle with understanding what a therapy session is all about. Clients will benefit because their sessions will flow more smoothly and therapy will be more effective and efficient. Supervisors will also benefit because their time can be spent helping you master the more important advanced aspects of the therapeutic process. Basically, you and your supervisors can become partners in your growth because you both can be "on the same page" (literally and figuratively).

How To Use This Book

You will use this book differently depending on which of the three groups best represents your status. Generally, because not all students experience the transition into the clinic in the same way, this book could not be strictly organized to fit the ideal type shown in Figure I.1. The best advice is for you to "graze" through the entire book, stopping now and then to "consume" what you feel is the most relevant material to you at that particular time and to write notes on what additional related information is included for your future reference. Later, this book will become a resource to assist you while navigating within your present or next stage. To assist in this process of exploration, the following comments apply.

The Stage 1 group, those of you about to start the clinical experience, should begin reading this book about 1 month prior to your actual involvement in a clinical practicum. Many students experience anxiety during this stage. By reading this book and obtaining information about the clinical process, as well as becoming knowledgeable about expectations of your work, anxiety levels should decline. The result is a more positive mind-set, which can only help you get started on the right foot. Remarkably, when you actively prepare for your clinical practicum, you develop a "stake" in the outcome. This softens the perceived disjunction between the classroom and clinic and between acquired knowledge and the knowledge you believe is needed.

The Stage 2 group, those of you getting involved with the clinical experience, should use this book to help you survive the voluminous amount of required paperwork. The system offered in Chapter 6 will help you to organize and manage the mountain of paper. At this point in your professional training, this book will likely be your constant companion as you write evaluations, lesson plans, and progress notes. This book will also be your source for information about maintaining records during therapy sessions. Nothing puts a chill on student enthusiasm as effectively as that first paperwork "snowstorm." To help you survive this phase, Chapters 1 through 6 will be particularly helpful.

This book will also be helpful to those of you at Stage 3, who are actively involved in the clinical experience. You will need help orchestrating therapy sessions as you come to terms with the therapeutic process. Therefore, you will find the chapter dealing with performance-enhancing therapy suggestions (Chapter 10) most helpful. Avoiding the problems presented and implementing the solutions provided in this chapter will help you function more effectively and efficiently. You will also find the information in Chapter 11 on self-evaluation pertinent to this level of functioning.

When using this book, you need to be aware of your performance proficiency. Functioning is cumulative. If you are in Stage 3 and are having difficulty writing behavioral objectives or evaluations, you will have to acquire these skills just as would a student in Stage 2. Chapters 1 and 2 will help you to brush up on behavioral objectives, and Chapters 3 and 4 will assist you with writing evaluations. Therefore, you will rely on this book to refresh and renew your performance skills. However, you need to realize that skills might *not* improve if you jump ahead and try to incorporate material or skills that are best left to higher levels of involvement in clinical functioning. Remember that trying to do too much too soon might lead to a failure to learn the basics and unnecessarily negate excellent performance by otherwise good students. Instead, this book should be used as a preview of what is expected as you mentally role-play your part as more advanced clinical students soon to be professionals. Those of you who want to succeed will do this anyway, but all of you will benefit by using mental role playing.

Conclusion

Cleanly and efficiently bridging the gap in knowledge between the classroom and the clinic is possible, although it cannot be done solely in the classroom or in the clinic. You can and should use the transition time between the two settings to better prepare yourself for your upcoming clinical experience. If you are provided with direction, you yourself can actively attempt to bridge this gap. Previously, it often appeared that students were expected to learn effective and efficient clinical performance through trial and error. However, a better approach is possible. It is far more logical and supportive of effective teaching techniques if these common *faux pas* are identified so they can be counteracted or prevented from occurring. There is no reason why *you* should make the same mistakes as yesterday's beginning clinicians. Therefore, if these clinical problem areas are identified and addressed, many of these inappropriate clinical behaviors will be eliminated and more effective clinical performance will result. This is the intent of this book: to be a tool that you can use to help yourself bridge the gap and take the first step toward achieving professional status. The end result should be that your clinical performance starts above and far surpasses that of those previous beginning clinicians who did not have access to this tool or of current beginning clinicians who chose to ignore this book.

Returning to the elephant parable, it is apparent that an adequate description of an elephant cannot be obtained through exploration of single or isolated parts. Likewise, with the clinical experience. To take those first steps toward achieving professional status, you need to integrate all parts of the clinical experience. It is necessary to have positive feelings toward the clinical experience, mastery as well as expedient execution of all parts of the paperwork process, and knowledge about, as well as appropriate application of, clinical information in the orchestration of therapy sessions.

If you are conscientious and try to prepare yourself for each step of the clinical process before actually taking that step, common clinical errors should be prevented. Therefore, your supervisor should not have to deal with minor aspects of the clinical process and will direct his or her energy toward helping you achieve a higher level of performance than was previously possible.

This introduction is a bridge between the book's stated intent described in the Preface and the much more specific content of Chapters 1 through 11. It is, therefore, quite short. I earnestly hope that your travels across your bridges to becoming a competent professional will also be short.

After reading this introduction, you should be able to

1. state 10 words describing feelings, attitudes, and/or perceptions frequently encountered in Stage 1, immediately prior to starting the clinical experience.

2. state the number one problem encountered at Stage 2, when first becoming involved with the clinical experience, and explain why that problem is not the goal of therapy.

3. state the major clinical problem in Stage 3, when actively involved in the clinical experience.

4. state the single most important way this book can be used in each of the three clinical stages.

References

Chan, J., Carter, S., & McAllister, L. (1994). Sources of anxiety related to clinical education in speech–language pathology students. In M. Bruce (Ed.), *Proceedings of The 1994 International & Interdisciplinary Conference on Clinical Supervision: Toward the 21st Century* (pp. 126–132). Houston, TX: University of Houston.

Haynes, W., & Hartman, D. (1975). The agony of report writing: A new look at an old problem. *The Journal of the National Student Speech and Hearing Association, 3,* 7–15.

Chapter 1

Behavioral Objectives: Background

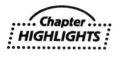

Chapter HIGHLIGHTS

- Background information on behavioral objectives
- Reasons for writing behavioral objectives
- Composition of behavioral objectives
- Construction of behavioral objectives
- Application of behavioral objectives
- Role of behavioral objectives in lesson plans

In 1984, Robert Mager wrote a book titled *Preparing Instructional Objectives*. Several years later, Donald Mowrer (1988) expanded Mager's ideas and applied them to speech–language pathology. Mager defined an objective as "a description of a performance you want learners to be able to exhibit before you consider them competent" (p. 5). Mowrer adopted a more research-oriented definition when he defined a behavioral objective as one that "is stated in terms of behaviors which can be observed and measured" (p. 148).

According to Mager (1984), objectives are important for three reasons. First, when objectives are not clearly defined, one does not have a good basis for selecting materials, content, or procedures (p. 5). In other words, if a clinician does not know where she is headed in terms of the remediation process, it is impossible to design or implement a therapy program to help a client succeed. Clinicians and clients alike function in a state of confusion if they do not know what the client is expected to accomplish as a result of the therapeutic process. Mager's second reason for clearly stating objectives is to determine later if they have been accomplished (p. 5). It is possible to formally or informally assess the client's success only if both the client and the clinician know the desired end result. In other words, if clinicians do not know what they are working toward, they will not know when the objective has been reached. A third reason for stating objectives is to enable the client to meaningfully participate (p. 6). A client cannot fully cooperate if the clinician has not informed him of the nature of the task and its goal.

As a beginning clinician, you need to write clear behavioral objectives as a step toward ensuring effective therapy. To write these objectives, you must look beyond the client's obvious problem(s) and analyze all data that have been collected during formal and informal assessments, synthesize those data, and formulate an informed opinion. Objectives are better when you have determined the client's current level of functioning and the level at which the client should be functioning. Doing so allows you to formulate the steps for enabling the client to move from where he is functioning to where he should be functioning. Objectives, therefore, must reflect the emphases of the therapy program or they will never become the base for any meaningful therapy program.

Components of a Behavioral Objective

For a behavioral objective to be meaningful, the primary reader (at first this will be your clinical supervisor) and the writer (in this case, you, the beginning clinician) must have identical interpretations of a client's performance. If these interpretations are not identical, the objective is not well written, and misinterpretation results. If the meaning is not clear, the objective needs to be revised to convey the correct intent. When your goal is to write meaningful behavioral objectives, you must include three components: performance, condition, and criterion.

Performance Component

Mager (1984) noted that an objective must state what a learner is expected to do or perform in order to demonstrate mastery of the objective. The little word *do* is the key here, because an objective cannot be complete without inclusion of the "doing" aspect. Mager suggested that, to check if the objective includes performance, the clinician should ask, "What is the learner DOING when demonstrating achievement of the objective?" (p. 25). To assess whether performance is addressed, Mowrer (1988) recommended asking, "Can I count it?" (p. 158). Mowrer wrote that one of the major pitfalls in writing the performance component of behavioral objectives is the use of ill-defined or vague verbs. Mager also cautioned against using "slippery" verbs, such as *know, understand,* and *appreciate,* which can be interpreted in many ways (p. 20). Others in the field (Wheeler & Fox, 1977) also have cautioned against using ambiguous action verbs, such as *demonstrate, perform,* and *select* (p. 26). You need to know that the performance portion of the behavioral objective is the "verb" component (Mowrer, 1988). Table 1.1 lists acceptable verbs for use in objectives.

Table 1.2 presents a list of verbs to be avoided. Because many supervisors in speech–language pathology accept the verb *use* (it is, after all, a natural aspect of performance), I recommend that you discuss its acceptability with your supervisor. Before you discuss it,

TABLE 1.1
Acceptable Verbs

build	match	repeat
compare	name	repeat orally
construct	place	say
contrast	point	smile
count	pour	sort
demand	press lever	state
diagram	put	tell what
draw	reach	walk
fold	read orally	write
label	recite	
list	remove	

Note. Words compiled from Mager (1984), Mowrer (1988), and Wheeler and Fox (1977).

TABLE 1.2
Verbs To Avoid

acknowledge	enjoy	make
acquaint	familiarize	plan
apply	feel	play
appreciate	give	realize
arrange	grasp the significance of	respond to
believe	have faith in	select
communicate	internalize	understand
demonstrate	know	use
develop	learn	
discover	like	

Note. Words compiled from Mager (1984), Mowrer (1988), and Wheeler and Fox (1977).

however, consider how or why the verb *use* can be both appropriate and inappropriate.

Overt and Covert Verbs

Mager (1984) differentiated between types of verbs used in behavioral objectives. According to him, *overt verbs* refer to performance that is directly observable through vision or audition. *Covert verbs* refer to performance that cannot be directly observed. This type of performance "is mental, invisible, cognitive or internal" (p. 43). Covert performance can only be detected if the client is asked to say or do something. Some examples of covert verbs are *discriminate, recall, identify,* and *solve.*

Covert performance can only be correctly stated in a behavioral objective if there is a direct way of determining whether the objective has been satisfied. Mager's rule is, "Whenever the performance stated in an objective is covert, add an indicator behavior to the objective" (1984, p. 44). Mager's (1984, p. 44) examples showing measurable indicator behaviors include "Be able to add numbers (write the solutions) written in binary notation" and "Be able to identify (underline or circle) misspelled words on a given page of news copy."

Wheeler and Fox (1977) listed action verbs that are not directly observable and that "should not be used when writing instructional objectives" (p. 27). A few examples of these action verbs are *recognize, infer, analyze,* and *know.* According to Mager (1984), however, these verbs can be used if an indicator behavior is included. Some of the verbs on Wheeler and Fox's list are shown in Table 1.3.

Performance Examples Common to Speech–Language Pathology

In this section, I address the performance portion of behavioral objectives by providing pertinent examples in areas that are frequently

TABLE 1.3

Action Verbs Requiring Indicators

analyze	deduce	realize fully
be aware	determine	recognize
be curious	discriminate	solve
become competent	distinguish	test
concentrate	generate	think
conclude	infer	think critically
create	perceive	wonder

Note. Data from Wheeler and Fox (1977). Examples of both overt and covert verbs can be found in the performance examples provided in this chapter. If the verbs listed in this table or similar verbs appear in the performance component, the verbs are covert and require that indicator behaviors be added.

emphasized with clinical populations. For ease of reference, examples are provided in the following order throughout this chapter: articulation, phonology, language, voice, fluency, pragmatics, problem behavior, phonological awareness, dysphagia, and augmentative and alternative communication.

Performance Examples 1: Articulation

correctly produce the /r/ phoneme
correctly imitate /s/
raise his tongue tip to the alveolar ridge
auditorily discriminate (by raising his hand) /s/ from /f/
correctly monitor (state if correct or not) production of the /l/ phoneme
correctly monitor (self-correct) production of the /s/ phoneme

Performance Examples 2: Phonology

close syllables
correctly imitate the consonant clusters /sk/, /sp/, and /st/
produce unstressed syllables
produce voiceless consonants
produce fricatives or affricates
produce liquids

Performance Examples 3: Language

name pictures spontaneously
identify (name) pictures expressively
identify (point to) pictures receptively
use present progressive tense correctly
use the pronouns *he* and *she* appropriately
use plurals correctly
use correct subject–verb agreement
follow directions
use the prepositions *in* and *on* correctly
use three-word utterances
ask questions
say complete sentences

Performance Examples 4: Voice

identify (raise hand) vocal abuses
explain laryngeal functioning
use appropriate pitch
produce easy onset of voice
produce appropriate oral resonance

Performance Examples 5: Fluency

identify (say "there") nonfluencies
read fluently
speak fluently
cancel stuttering episodes
identify (state) factors in his stuttering equation
use pullouts

Performance Examples 6: Pragmatics

request (by pointing or using eye gaze) an object
take turns
attend to (look at) the speaker
initiate a greeting
specify a topic
maintain a topic

Performance Examples 7: Problem Behavior

walk into the therapy room
sit without kicking
attend to (look at) a picture when directed
perform a task
follow directions

Performance Examples 8: Phonological Awareness

provide a rhyming word
clap once for each syllable in a word
clap once for each word in a sentence
correctly identify the beginning sound in a word
correctly blend the word
correctly state the sound letters make

Performance Examples 9: Dysphagia

masticate and transfer semisolids
protrude, elevate, and lateralize his tongue
tuck his chin
utilize a supraglottic swallow
swallow single-teaspoon presentations of a puree diet
swallow a nectar-consistency liquid

Performance Examples 10: Augmentative and Alternative Communication

use eye gaze to request an activity
request an object in his communication book

turn his communication device on
direct her older sister to dress a doll
make the clown dance
select appropriate greetings on his communication device

QUICK CHECK

You must critically examine your behavioral objectives to make certain you have included a performance component. Then check to see if the verb is overt or covert. If the verb is covert, a behavior indicator is needed. If the desired behavior is not immediately apparent, the objective is not written clearly. In this case, you need to rethink exactly what the client is supposed to do and then rewrite the objective until there is no ambiguity regarding the client's role.

Condition Component

The second component to be included in a well-written behavioral objective is the condition under which the performance is to be done. This is the condition that will be imposed on clients when they are demonstrating achievement of an objective. Mager (1984) stated that the definition of terminal behavior should be "detailed enough to be sure the desired performance would be recognized by another competent person, and detailed enough so that others understand your intent as YOU understand it" (p. 51). Mowrer (1988) stated,

> Conditions specify what you will provide to the individual in order to help him do the task, or they may describe what you will deny the learner. They can also pinpoint where the behavior will be performed, when it will be performed, and in whose presence it will be performed. (p. 160)

Mowrer (1988) further added that because conditions describe the situation in which the behavior is to be performed, the condition component comprises the "adjective" portion of the objective. The following are some examples of conditions as stated by Mager (1984, p. 50):

Given a problem of the following type ...
Given a list of ...
Given any reference of the learner's choice ...
Without the aid of references ...
Without the aid of a slide rule ...
Without the aid of tools ...

Mager (1984) provided the following four questions to use as a guide for identifying important aspects of target or terminal performances (p. 51):

1. What will the learner be allowed to use?
2. What will the learner be denied?
3. Under what conditions will you expect the desired performance to occur?
4. Are there any skills that you are specifically NOT trying to develop? Does the objective exclude such skills?

It is not obligatory for behavioral objectives to contain a condition aspect. If the objective is clearly stated without it, a condition is not necessary. If someone else's interpretation does not match yours, then further description is needed. Add as much description as necessary to clearly communicate the intent to others (Mager, 1984).

Condition Examples Common to Speech–Language Pathology

The following are examples of conditions included in behavioral objectives for areas that are frequently emphasized with clinical populations.

Condition Examples 1: Articulation

in all word positions
in isolation
with his mouth open at least 1 ½ inches
in consonant–vowel combinations
during spontaneous conversation
during reading
without a model

Condition Examples 2: Phonology

on spontaneously produced monosyllabic target words
without a pause between the two consonants
in bisyllabic words
when preceding vowels
of all appropriate contexts

Condition Examples 3: Language

in a child's dictionary
of common objects
given a field of three
while describing pictures
during conversation
in a structured situation
when telling a story

in less than 5 seconds
when describing spatial relations
without prompts
beginning with *how*
using the conjunction *and*

Condition Examples 4: Voice

when eight choices are presented
one session after the clinician's explanation
while producing /ɑ/
on the vowels /o/ and /i/
on vowel–consonant combinations
on vowels

Condition Examples 5: Fluency

consisting of prolongations lasting longer than 2 seconds
in front of his class
for 5 minutes
while talking on the telephone
the session after this discussion occurred
while speaking to the principal

Condition Examples 6: Pragmatics

which is out of reach
when a familiar joint action routine is initiated by a significant other
during communication episodes
upon seeing the clinician
during each therapy session
initiated by someone else

Condition Examples 7: Problem Behavior

without yanking the clinician's arm
after the removal of restraints
when a desirable toy is within reaching distance
without throwing a temper tantrum
within a 2-second period

Condition Examples 8: Phonological Awareness

when presented auditorily with a word
presented auditorily by the clinician
when given syllables auditorily
when presented visually

Condition Examples 9: Dysphagia

without pocketing in the buccal cavity

following auditory and visual cueing

before each swallow and maintaining this position during
the swallow

independently

using a double swallow

using single straw sips

Condition Examples 10: Augmentative
and Alternative Communication

given a field of two icons

by pointing to an icon

in less than 30 seconds

by pointing to picture symbols in the correct order

by activating the switch when requested

using scanning

QUICK CHECK

> If a condition component is needed in a particular behavioral objective, it must be written specifically to avoid misunderstanding. If the condition is not written specifically, a mismatch may occur between the intent of the writer (you) and the interpretation of the reader (your supervisor).

Criterion Component

The third component to be included in behavioral objectives is a criterion that states how well the learner is expected to perform. Mager (1984) defined *criterion* as "the standard by which performance is evaluated, the yardstick by which achievement of the objective is assessed" (p. 71). The criterion enables the clinician to determine whether the therapy techniques were successful in accomplishing the behavioral objectives. The desired criterion can be specified in several ways. According to Mowrer (1988), "the criterion resembles an 'adverb' statement in that it states how or when the objective is to be met. It could also be considered an adjective statement because often the criterion consists of a description of 'how many behaviors'" (p. 161). Mager (1984) stated that the criterion often is established by answering these questions (p. 78):

1. How well must a student be able to perform in order for practice to be the only requirement for improvement?

2. How competent must the student be in order to be ready for the next assignment (the next objective, the next course, the job itself)?

According to Mager (1984), a criterion is frequently stated in terms of speed, accuracy, or quality. In the speech–language pathology discipline, accuracy is frequently cited, speed is less frequently cited, and quality is rarely cited. A common way to describe performance relative to speed "is to describe a time limit within which a given performance must occur" (Mager, 1984, p. 74). An example cited by Mager is "four of five malfunctions must be located within ten minutes each" (1984, p. 75). Accuracy is another way to measure criterion. Some of Mager's examples are as follows (p. 79):

... and solutions must be accurate to the nearest whole number.

... with materials weighed accurately to the nearest gram.

... correct to at least three significant figures.

... with no more than two incorrect entries for every 10 pages of log.

... with the listening accurate enough so that no more than one request for repeated information is made for each customer contact.

Quality is another way to measure criterion. To communicate the desired quality of performance, the criterion needs to specify the amount of acceptable deviation from perfection or another standard (Mager, 1984, p. 83). One of Mager's examples is to "be able to adjust the PPI [round TV screen in a missile] range-marker to acceptable roundness…. [defined as] no more than one-eighth inch deviation from a standard template" (p. 83). As stated previously, quality criteria are rare in speech–language pathology.

Criterion Examples Common to Speech–Language Pathology

The following criterion examples are not divided into accuracy, speed, and quality because these types of criteria are not equally distributed across behavioral objectives written in speech–language pathology. Also, the examples are not grouped according to areas frequently emphasized with clinical populations because these examples are usually not specific to any particular area.

Criterion Examples

in 90% of his attempts

in 90% of all appropriate contexts

in 8 of 10 attempts
on 8 of 10 trials
for 20 of 25 pictures
with 90% agreement
with fewer than .5 stuttered words per minute
in 2 of the 3 weekly therapy sessions
for 25 minutes
5 new words
twice during a 10-minute time segment
3 consecutive
3 conversational turns
without signs of choking, coughing, or wet, gurgly vocal quality
without signs of aspiration
3 of 4

Although a criterion of 90% is usually used in speech–language pathology, in certain situations (for clients who are mentally challenged, extremely young, etc.), a criterion of 80% is common.

| |
| If a criterion is not specified, the objective is not complete. Without a criterion, it is not possible to determine whether an objective has been accomplished. |

Samples of Well-Written Behavioral Objectives

At this point, you should be able to state the three components of a behavioral objective, describe each component, divide an objective into the components, and give pertinent examples. You will now have an opportunity to check your mastery. This can be done in two ways. The first way involves looking at the following sample objectives and following the text. The second way involves skipping the 10 sets of sample objectives that follow and instead completing the exercise in Appendix 1.A. If the latter is your choice, please turn to Appendix 1.A at this time. (The answers to the exercise are in Appendix 1.B.) If you have selected the first option, the emphasis is placed on reviewing examples of behavioral objectives that include these three components. Behavioral objectives are grouped according to area of clinical emphasis. Although many lead-ins are available for behavioral objectives, the introductory phrase, "The client will" is understood for all examples in this section. If you have selected the first option, read on.

Sample Objectives 1: Articulation

The client will

[handwritten annotations: "do", "condition", "criterion"]

1. correctly produce the /r/ phoneme in all positions of words in 90% of his attempts.
2. correctly imitate /s/ in isolation in 8 of 10 attempts.
3. raise his tongue tip to the alveolar ridge with his mouth open at least 1½ inches on 8 of 10 trials.
4. auditorily discriminate (by raising his hand) /s/ from /f/ in consonant–vowel combinations in 90% of his attempts.
5. correctly monitor (state if correct or not) production of the /l/ phoneme during spontaneous conversation in 90% of his attempts.
6. correctly monitor (self-correct) 90% of the incorrect /s/ productions during reading.

If it is difficult for you to separate the above objectives into the components of performance, condition, and criterion, it would be wise to go back and review the pertinent sections before continuing. Every component included in the previous objectives has appeared earlier in this chapter.

The following numbers correspond to the behavioral objectives just listed. The performance aspect of each objective is as follows:

1. correctly produce the /r/ phoneme
2. correctly imitate /s/
3. raise his tongue tip to the alveolar ridge
4. auditorily discriminate (by raising his hand) /s/ from /f/
5. correctly monitor (state if correct or not) production of the /l/ phoneme
6. correctly monitor (self-correct) incorrect /s/ productions

The following conditions are present in the behavioral objectives:

1. in all positions of words
2. in isolation
3. with his mouth open at least 1½ inches
4. in consonant–vowel combinations
5. during spontaneous conversation
6. during reading

The criterion for each of the behavioral objectives is as follows:

1. in 90% of his attempts
2. in 8 of 10 attempts

3. on 8 of 10 trials
4. in 90% of his attempts
5. in 90% of his attempts
6. 90%

Sample Objectives 2: Phonology

The client will

1. close syllables on spontaneously produced monosyllabic target words in 90% of his attempts. (*Note:* This objective addresses the process deletion of final consonants.)
2. correctly imitate the consonant clusters /sk/, /sp/, and /st/ without a pause between the two consonants in 90% of his attempts. (*Note:* This objective addresses the process cluster reduction.)
3. produce unstressed syllables in bisyllabic words in 90% of his attempts. (*Note:* This objective addresses the process deletion of unstressed syllables.)
4. produce voiceless consonants when preceding vowels in 90% of the appropriate contexts. (*Note:* This objective addresses the process prevocalic voicing of consonants.)
5. produce fricatives or affricates in 90% of the appropriate contexts. (*Note:* This objective addresses the process stopping.)
6. produce liquids in 90% of the appropriate contexts. (*Note:* This objective addresses the process gliding.)

The numbers that follow correspond to the behavioral objectives just listed. The performance aspect of each objective is as follows:

1. close syllables
2. correctly imitate the consonant clusters /sk/, /sp/, and /st/
3. produce unstressed syllables
4. produce voiceless consonants
5. produce fricatives or affricates
6. produce liquids

The following conditions are present in the behavioral objectives:

1. on spontaneously produced monosyllabic target words
2. without a pause between the two consonants
3. in bisyllabic words
4. when preceding vowels
5. the appropriate contexts
6. the appropriate contexts

The criterion for each of the behavioral objectives is as follows:

1. in 90% of his attempts
2. in 90% of his attempts
3. in 90% of his attempts
4. in 90% of the appropriate contexts
5. 90%
6. 90%

Sample Objectives 3: Language

The client will

1. spontaneously name 20 of 25 pictures in a child's dictionary.
2. expressively identify (name) pictures of common objects in 90% of his attempts.
3. receptively identify (point to) pictures given in a field of three in 8 of 10 attempts.
4. correctly use present progressive tense while describing 20 of 25 pictures that are not visible to the clinician.
5. appropriately use the pronouns *he* and *she* during conversation in 90% of his attempts.
6. correctly use regular plurals in at least 90% of his attempts while telling a story.

The following performance aspects can be found in the behavioral objectives just listed:

1. spontaneously name pictures
2. expressively identify (name) pictures
3. receptively identify (point to) pictures
4. correctly use present progressive tense
5. appropriately use the pronouns *he* and *she*
6. correctly use regular plurals

The following conditions are included in the behavioral objectives:

1. in a child's dictionary
2. of common objects
3. given in a field of three
4. while describing pictures that are not visible to the clinician
5. during conversation
6. while telling a story

The criterion contained in each of the behavioral objectives is:

1. 20 of 25
2. in 90% of his attempts
3. in 8 of 10 attempts
4. 20 of 25
5. in 90% of his attempts
6. in at least 90% of his attempts

Sample Objectives 4: Voice

The client will

1. identify (raise hand) at least 7 of his vocal abuses when all possible abuses are stated.
2. explain 3 steps in laryngeal functioning one session after the clinician's explanation.
3. use appropriate pitch while producing /ɑ/ in 8 of 10 trials.
4. produce easy onset of voice on the vowels /o/ and /i/ in 90% of his attempts.
5. produce appropriate oral resonance on vowel–consonant combinations in 90% of his attempts.

The following performance aspects can be identified in the objectives just listed:

1. identify (raise hand) vocal abuses
2. explain steps in laryngeal functioning
3. use appropriate pitch
4. produce easy onset of voice
5. produce appropriate oral resonance

The following conditions are present in the behavioral objectives:

1. when all possible abuses are stated
2. one session after the clinician's explanation
3. while producing /ɑ/
4. on the vowels /o/ and /i/
5. on vowel–consonant combinations

The criterion for each of the behavioral objectives is as follows:

1. at least 7
2. 3

3. in 8 of 10 trials
4. in 90% of his attempts
5. in 90% of his attempts

Sample Objectives 5: Fluency

The client will

1. identify (say "there") 90% of his nonfluencies that consist of prolongations lasting longer than 2 seconds.
2. read in front of his class with fewer than .5 stuttered words per minute.
3. speak with fewer than .5 stuttered words per minute during 5 minutes of spontaneous conversation with the clinician.
4. cancel 90% of the stuttering episodes that occur while talking on the telephone.
5. identify (state) all factors in his stuttering equation one session after this discussion occurred.
6. use pullouts during all episodes of blocking while speaking to the principal for 5 minutes.

The following performance aspects are included in the behavioral objectives just listed:

1. identify (say "there") his nonfluencies
2. read
3. speak
4. cancel stuttering episodes
5. identify (state) factors in his stuttering equation
6. use pullouts during episodes of blocking

Conditions found in the behavioral objectives are as follows:

1. that consist of prolongations lasting longer than 2 seconds
2. in front of his class
3. during 5 minutes of spontaneous conversation with the clinician
4. that occur while talking on the telephone
5. one session after this discussion occurred
6. while speaking to the principal for 5 minutes

Note that confusion can result in interpreting the third and sixth behavioral objectives. Although numbers are frequently the criterion or part of the criteria, this is not always true. Therefore, you must exert caution. The phrase "5 minutes" in the third and sixth objectives is part of the condition component and not the criterion. The criterion contained in each of the behavioral objectives is as follows:

1. 90% of his nonfluencies
2. with fewer than .5 stuttered words per minute
3. with fewer than .5 stuttered words per minute
4. 90%
5. all (implies 100%)
6. all (implies 100%)

Sample Objectives 6: Pragmatics

The client will

1. request (by pointing or using eye gaze) an object that is out of reach twice during a 10-minute time segment.
2. take 3 consecutive turns when a familiar joint action routine is initiated by a significant other.
3. attend to (look at) the speaker during 2 of 3 communication episodes.
4. initiate a greeting upon seeing the clinician on 4 of 5 appropriate occasions.
5. specify a topic once during each therapy session.
6. maintain a topic initiated by someone else for 3 conversational turns.

The following performance aspects can be found in the behavioral objectives just listed:

1. request (by pointing or using eye gaze) an object
2. take turns
3. attend to (look at) the speaker
4. initiate a greeting
5. specify a topic
6. maintain a topic

The behavioral objectives include the following conditions:

1. that is out of reach
2. when a familiar joint action routine is initiated by a significant other
3. during communication episodes
4. upon seeing the clinician
5. during each therapy session
6. initiated by someone else

The following criteria are contained in the behavioral objectives:

1. twice during a 10-minute time segment
2. 3 consecutive
3. 2 of 3
4. on 4 of 5 appropriate occasions
5. once
6. for 3 conversational turns

Sample Objectives 7: Problem Behavior

The client will

1. walk into the therapy room without yanking the clinician's arm in 2 of the 3 weekly therapy sessions.
2. sit without kicking for 5 minutes after the removal of restraints (your hands on the client's knees).
3. attend to (look at) a picture for 2 minutes when a desirable toy is within reaching distance.
4. perform a specified task for 25 minutes without throwing a temper tantrum.
5. follow 8 of 10 directions within 2 seconds of the initial presentation.

The following performances can be identified in the behavioral objectives just listed:

1. walk into the therapy room
2. sit without kicking
3. attend to (look at) a picture
4. perform a specified task
5. follow directions

The following conditions can be identified in the behavioral objectives:

1. without yanking the clinician's arm
2. after the removal of restraints (your hands on the client's knees)
3. when a desirable toy is within reaching distance
4. without throwing a temper tantrum
5. within 2 seconds of the initial presentation

The following criteria are contained in the behavioral objectives:

1. in 2 of the 3 weekly therapy sessions
2. for 5 minutes

3. for 2 minutes
4. for 25 minutes
5. 8 of 10

Sample Objectives 8: Phonological Awareness

The client will

1. provide a rhyming word when presented auditorily with a word in 90% of his attempts.
2. clap once for each syllable in a word presented auditorily by the clinician in 90% of his attempts.
3. clap once for each word in a sentence presented auditorily by the clinician in 90% of his attempts.
4. correctly identify the beginning sound in a word presented auditorily by the clinician in 90% of his attempts.
5. correctly blend the word when given its syllables auditorily in 90% of his attempts.
6. correctly state the sounds that letters make when presented visually in 90% of his attempts.

The following performances can be identified in the behavioral objectives just listed:

1. provide a rhyming word
2. clap once for each syllable in a word
3. clap once for each word in a sentence
4. correctly identify the beginning sound in a word
5. correctly blend the word
6. correctly state the sounds that letters make

The following conditions can be identified in the behavioral objectives:

1. when presented auditorily with a word
2. presented auditorily by the clinician
3. presented auditorily by the clinician
4. presented auditorily by the clinician
5. when given its syllables auditorily
6. when presented visually

The following criteria are contained in the behavioral objectives:

1. in 90% of his attempts
2. in 90% of his attempts
3. in 90% of his attempts
4. in 90% of his attempts

5. in 90% of his attempts
6. in 90% of his attempts

Sample Objectives 9: Dysphagia

The client will

1. masticate and transfer semisolids without pocketing in the buccal cavity during 90% of his swallows.
2. protrude, elevate, and lateralize his tongue following auditory and visual cueing in 90% of his attempts.
3. tuck his chin before each swallow and maintain this position during the swallow in 90% of his attempts.
4. utilize a supraglottic swallow independently during 9 of 10 swallows.
5. swallow single-teaspoon presentations of a puree diet using a double swallow without signs of choking, coughing, or wet, gurgly vocal quality.
6. swallow a nectar-consistency liquid using single straw sips without signs of aspiration.

The following performances can be identified in the behavioral objectives just listed:

1. masticate and transfer semisolids
2. protrude, elevate, and lateralize his tongue
3. tuck his chin
4. utilize a supraglottic swallow
5. swallow single-teaspoon presentations of a puree diet
6. swallow a nectar-consistency liquid

The following conditions can be identified in the behavioral objectives:

1. without pocketing in the buccal cavity
2. following auditory and visual cueing
3. before each swallow and maintain this position during the swallow
4. independently
5. using a double swallow
6. using single straw sips

The following criteria are contained in the behavioral objectives:

1. during 90% of his swallows
2. in 90% of his attempts
3. in 90% of his attempts

4. during 9 of 10 swallows
5. without signs of choking, coughing, or wet, gurgly vocal quality
6. without signs of aspiration

Sample Objectives 10: Augmentative and Alternative Communication

The client will

1. use eye gaze to request an activity given a field of two icons in 90% of his attempts.
2. request an object by pointing to an icon in his communication book in 9 of 10 attempts.
3. turn on his communication device in less than 30 seconds in 3 consecutive trials.
4. direct his older sister to dress a doll by pointing to 3 of 4 picture symbols in the correct order.
5. make the clown dance by activating the switch when requested in 9 of 10 attempts.
6. select appropriate greetings on his communication device using scanning in 90% of his attempts.

The following performances can be identified in the behavioral objectives just listed:

1. use eye gaze to request an activity
2. request an object in his communication book
3. turn on his communication device
4. direct his older sister to dress a doll
5. make the clown dance
6. select appropriate greetings on his communication device

The following conditions can be identified in the behavioral objectives:

1. given a field of two icons
2. by pointing to an icon
3. in less than 30 seconds
4. by pointing to picture symbols in the correct order
5. by activating the switch when requested
6. using scanning

The following criteria are contained in the behavioral objectives:

1. in 90% of his attempts
2. in 9 of 10 attempts

3. in 3 consecutive trials
4. 3 of 4
5. in 9 of 10 attempts
6. in 90% of his attempts

Application and Importance of Behavioral Objectives

The ability to understand and write behavioral objectives has far-reaching ramifications in speech–language pathology. Mowrer (1988) stated, "Behavioral objectives are included as a basic ingredient of many commercially developed instructional programs available to speech clinicians" (p. 149). If you do not understand behavioral objectives, you will have difficulty conducting the programs and obtaining and recording responses in the intended manner. Mowrer (1988) also stated, "Most federal grant applications which pertain to any form of instruction require that objectives be clearly indicated and tied to performance measures" (p. 149). Although grant writing is not foremost at this point in your career, it may become important in the not too distant future. With the practice in writing behavioral objectives that is gained during the clinical practicum, you learn basic skills that can easily be applied to the grant-writing process. However, there are more immediate reasons for gaining expertise in writing behavioral objectives, such as for writing lesson plans, reports, and Individualized Education Programs (IEPs).

Lesson Plans

Behavioral objectives make up a major part of lesson plans (also referred to as pretherapy plans or clinical strategy outlines). Before entering each therapy session, the clinician must develop a lesson plan, which consists of realistic goals to be accomplished during that session. These goals are written in the form of behavioral objectives. Lesson plans can be developed for each session separately or for all sessions held within a week. The following factors need to be considered when determining the frequency with which lesson plans are written: the length of the sessions, the frequency of the sessions, and the client's progress. If progress is fast, a new plan should be devised for each session. If progress is slow, a weekly plan may be adequate.

Lesson plans are usually divided into two main parts. The first part consists of session objectives, which are called short-term objectives, short-range objectives, lesson objectives, subobjectives, or transitional objectives. Regardless of the terminology used, they are all expressed in behavioral objectives. The second part of a lesson plan consists of procedures used to meet each objective listed. Additional requirements for lesson plans vary from training program to training program. It is likely that you will be required to provide a written rationale for each objective.

Short-Range Objectives

According to Thompson (1977), "Short-term objectives are concerned with small units of behavior and should be attainable in a short time" (p. 54). Thompson (1977) also said, "The short-term objectives identify the appropriate activities through which the child will progress toward the expectancies stated in the long term plan" (p. 6). Silverman (1984) stated, "Short-term goals specify abilities that clients must acquire before they can achieve long-term goals" (p. 230).

A lesson plan for a child 10 years 3 months of age is in Figure 1.1. It includes short-term objectives and procedures for a mild articulation problem.

Long-Range Objectives

Behavioral objectives are also used when writing long-range objectives, also known as long-term objectives or long-term goals, and may or may not be the same as terminal objectives, which are the final objectives that need to be mastered prior to discharge. The length of time implied by "long term" varies. It could mean 3 months or 1 year; however, when one is functioning within a college or university setting, the term often is defined as the length of one semester, one quarter, or two quarters, depending on the administrative calendar. Thus, it seems reasonable that additional nomenclature could be semester or quarterly objectives.

Objectives that can realistically be accomplished within the designated time frame must be determined. This task is not always easy, and the initial long-range objectives may have to be revised at varying intervals. However, the number of revisions should decrease as the clinician gains experience. Silverman (1984) stated, "Long-term goals specify the outcome the clinician is attempting to achieve" (p. 224). Because long-range objectives are written in a behavioral objective style, you should now have the foundation necessary for their construction.

LESSON PLAN

Short-Term Objectives:

1. Steven will correctly produce the /s/ phoneme in all positions of words in 90% of his attempts.
2. Steven will correctly monitor (point to the appropriate light) his production of the /s/ phoneme in all positions of words in 90% of his attempts.
3. Steven will correctly imitate the /s/ phoneme in the initial position of words in sentences in 90% of his attempts.
4. Steven will correctly monitor (point to the appropriate light) his imitations of the /s/ phoneme in the initial position of words in sentences in 90% of his attempts.
5. Steven will correctly produce the /s/ phoneme in the initial position of words in sentences in 90% of his attempts.
6. Steven will correctly monitor (point to the appropriate light) his productions of the /s/ phoneme in the initial position of words in sentences in 90% of his attempts.

Procedures:

1. Steven will say words containing the /s/ phoneme in the initial, medial, and final positions. If /s/ is produced incorrectly, auditory stimulation or placement cues will be used to help him attain a correct response.
2. After saying each word, Steven will indicate the correctness of the /s/ production by pointing to a red light if incorrect and a green light if correct.
3. Sentences containing /s/ in the initial position of words will be presented for Steven to imitate. For each error made, Steven will produce the word by itself. If correct production is attained, he will again imitate the sentence, trying to incorporate this correct production. If production remains incorrect, the sentence will be broken into phrases and auditory stimulation will be used.
4. After imitating sentences containing /s/ in the initial position of words, Steven will indicate the correctness of each target production by pointing to a red light if incorrect and a green light if correct.
5. Steven will construct sentences containing /s/ in the initial position of words. For each error made, he will produce the word by itself. If correct production is attained, Steven will again produce the sentence, trying to incorporate this correct production.
6. After producing sentences containing the /s/ phoneme in the initial position of words, Steven will indicate the correctness of each target production by pointing to a red light if incorrect and a green light if correct.

Figure 1.1. Sample lesson plan.

Relationship Between Long-Range and Short-Range Objectives

Because short-range or short-term objectives are based on behavioral objectives, Thompson (1977) stated, "Short-term objectives must be consistent with the LTO [long-term objective] and should flow from it" (p. 49). He also stated that short-range objectives "are small segments of behavior and should be manageable units of instruction [and] ... should assist the instructional process, not interfere with it" (pp. 50, 52). Thus, it may be necessary for many short-range objectives to be accomplished before a long-range objective is achieved. For example, if a client cannot perform the short-range objectives listed below, it will be necessary to master them before being able to attain success on the long-term objective: correct production of the /s/ phoneme in spontaneous conversation in 90% of his attempts.

The client will

1. auditorily discriminate (indicate by raising his hand) the /s/ phoneme from dissimilar phonemes when presented in isolation in 90% of his attempts.
2. auditorily discriminate (indicate by raising his hand) the /s/ phoneme from similar phonemes presented in isolation in 90% of his attempts.
3. auditorily discriminate (indicate by raising his hand) the /s/ phoneme from similar phonemes in consonant–vowel combinations in 90% of his attempts.
4. auditorily discriminate (indicate by raising his hand) the /s/ phoneme in the initial position of words when presented in rhyming word pairs in 90% of his attempts.
5. correctly imitate /s/ in isolation in 90% of his attempts.
6. correctly produce the /s/ phoneme in isolation in 90% of his attempts.
7. correctly monitor (state if correct or not) production of the /s/ phoneme in isolation in 90% of his attempts.
8. correctly imitate /s/ in the initial position of words in 90% of his attempts.
9. correctly produce /s/ in the initial position of words in 90% of his attempts.
10. correctly monitor (state if correct or not) production of the /s/ phoneme in the initial position of words in 90% of his attempts.
11. correctly produce /s/ in the final position of words in 90% of his attempts.
12. correctly monitor (state if correct or not) production of the /s/ phoneme in the final position of words in 90% of his attempts.
13. correctly produce /s/ in the initial position of words in phrases in 90% of his attempts.
14. correctly monitor (state if correct or not) production of the /s/ phoneme in the initial position of words in phrases in 90% of his attempts.
15. correctly produce /s/ in the initial and final positions of words in phrases in 90% of his attempts.

16. correctly monitor (state if correct or not) /s/ in the initial and final positions of words in phrases in 90% of his attempts.
17. correctly produce /s/ in the initial and final positions of words in sentences in 90% of his attempts.
18. correctly monitor (state if correct or not) /s/ in the initial and final positions of words in sentences in 90% of his attempts.
19. correctly produce /s/ in structured conversation in 90% of his attempts.
20. correctly monitor (self-correct) 90% of the incorrect /s/ productions during structured conversation.

Depending on the client's progress, additional steps may have to be added, some may be combined, and some may be eliminated. For example, imitation of the target behavior may need to precede Objectives 11, 13, 15, 17, and 19 if the client has difficulty with production. The client's performance will provide guidance in making these decisions. The point is that, by accomplishing the previously listed short-range objectives, the client is working toward mastering the long-range objective. If the client masters each short-range objective, he should be able to master the long-range objective, which is to correctly produce the /s/ phoneme in spontaneous conversation in 90% of his attempts.

The following language example further clarifies the relationship between long-range and short-range objectives. Again, it will be necessary for the client to master the short-range objectives listed below before being able to attain success on the long-range objective (correct production of the singular present progressive tense in 90% of the obligatory contexts during all communication events).

The client will

1. correctly imitate Noun + is + Verb + ing immediately following a model in 90% of his attempts.
2. correctly imitate Noun + is + Verb + ing 2 seconds after the model is presented in 90% of his attempts.
3. correctly imitate Noun + is + Verb + ing when an intervening sentence is presented between the model and response in 90% of his attempts.
4. correctly produce Noun + is + Verb + ing in response to the question "What is the Noun doing?" in 90% of his attempts.
5. correctly produce Noun + is + Verb + ing in response to "What's happening in this picture?" in 90% of his attempts.
6. correctly produce Noun + is + Verb + ing in response to "Tell me about the Noun" in 90% of the obligatory contexts.
7. correctly produce Noun + is + Verb + ing when telling a story from pictures in 90% of the obligatory contexts.

8. correctly produce Noun + is + Verb + ing when looking out the window and discussing events of the people seen, in 90% of the obligatory contexts.
9. correctly produce Noun + is + Verb + ing during an oral presentation in the classroom in 90% of all obligatory contexts.

The client's performance determines when and if other steps should be added, combined, or eliminated. By accomplishing the short-range objectives listed, the client is working toward mastery of the long-range objective. If the client successfully passes through the various steps, he is well on his way toward correct production of the singular present progressive tense in obligatory contexts encountered during communication events.

Relationship Between Long-Range and Terminal Objectives

As previously mentioned, the long-range objectives may or may not be the same as the terminal objectives, which are also based on behavioral objectives. An explanation that focuses on the two long-range objectives discussed in the previous section is provided in this section. The articulation objective is "correct production of the /s/ phoneme in spontaneous conversation in 90% of his attempts." The language objective is "correct production of the singular present progressive tense in 90% of the obligatory contexts during all communication events."

If a client with an articulation problem misarticulates only the /s/ phoneme and has no other speech, language, or communication problem, the long-range objective stated in the previous paragraph is the same as the terminal objective, which Mowrer (1988) described as "one you wish to have accomplished when you are ready to dismiss a case" (p. 169). In other words, as soon as the client masters the long-range objective, he is discharged or terminated from therapy. If the client misarticulates other phonemes that he should have mastered, therapy would continue. In this latter example, the long-range objective and terminal objective are not synonymous. The client's terminal objective may be "correct production of the /s/, /l/, and /r/ phonemes in all contexts during spontaneous conversation in 90% of his attempts." The terminal objective may also be stated as "correct production of all phonemes in all contexts during spontaneous conversation in 90% of his attempts."

Likewise, the long-range *language* objective can be a terminal objective under certain circumstances. If the rest of the client's language, speech, and communication is appropriate for his age, he would be dismissed from therapy after mastering the present progressive tense. Thus, in this situation, this long-range objective is the same as the terminal objective. However, if the client has difficulty with other aspects of language, other long-range objectives would have to be mastered before discharge from therapy. In this latter case, a long-range objective and a terminal objective differ.

If the client will be dismissed from therapy upon attainment of an objective, the objective can be considered terminal. If the client will be returning for additional therapy, an objective is not terminal.

Reports

Behavioral objectives are written in both the initial evaluation and the progress report. Because progress reports are usually required at the end of the semester or quarter, they are sometimes called "end-of-semester progress reports" or "quarter progress reports." The objectives that will be emphasized in therapy are listed in the initial evaluation. These objectives are again included in the end-of-semester or quarter progress report, followed by an account of the progress made during the designated time frame. These reports are discussed in Chapter 4, but are mentioned here because it is important to understand the extent to which behavioral objectives are used in the speech–language pathology profession.

Individualized Education Program

The term *Individualized Education Program* (IEP), which had its origin in the Education for All Handicapped Children Act of 1975 (Public Law [P.L.] 94-142), is familiar to individuals working in the field of education. According to P.L. 94-142, an IEP is a written statement that describes the educational objectives for a child with disabilities and the special services to be provided. In the school setting, the term *IEP* is more widely used than *behavioral or instructional objectives.* The law requires that IEPs include annual goals and either short-term instructional objectives or benchmarks, which are "statements about reference points along the path toward learning a new skill or set of skills" (Lucas, 2000, p. 5). Thus, knowledge of behavioral objectives is incorporated into IEP writing. IEPs are explored in depth in Chapter 8.

A goal that you should accomplish as early as possible in the clinical practicum process is to understand the composition and construction of well-written behavioral objectives. Behavioral objectives have far-reaching effects because they form the basis for much of the paperwork required in speech–language pathology. Being able to skillfully write behavioral objectives and realize their importance during this part of the clinical experience will enhance future professional performance.

After reading this chapter, you should be able to

1. state three reasons why behavioral objectives are important.
2. state and explain the three components of a behavioral objective.
3. divide behavioral objectives into components in 90% of your attempts.
4. correctly write behavioral objectives in 90% of your attempts.

Appendix 1.A

Exercise: Identifying Components of Behavioral Objectives

Read the following sample objectives. Write the performance, condition, and criterion for each objective on the lines provided. Upon completion, check your responses with Appendix 1.B.

The lead-in "The client will ..." is used for all examples in this section.

Sample Objectives 1: Articulation

1. correctly produce the /r/ phoneme in all positions of words in 90% of his attempts.

   Performance: _____

   Condition: _____

   Criterion: _____

2. correctly imitate /s/ in isolation in 8 of 10 attempts.

   Performance: _____

   Condition: _____

   Criterion: _____

3. raise his tongue tip to the alveolar ridge with his mouth open at least 1½ inches on 8 of 10 trials.

   Performance: _____

   Condition: _____

   Criterion: _____

4. auditorily discriminate (by raising his hand) /s/ from /f/ in consonant–vowel combinations in 90% of his attempts.

   Performance: _____

   Condition: _____

   Criterion: _____

5. correctly monitor (state if correct or not) production of the /l/ phoneme during spontaneous conversation in 90% of his attempts.

Performance: _____

Condition: _____

Criterion: _____

6. correctly monitor (self-correct) 90% of the incorrect /s/ productions during reading.

Performance: _____

Condition: _____

Criterion: _____

Sample Objectives 2: Phonology

1. close syllables on spontaneously produced monosyllabic target words in 90% of his attempts. (*Note:* This objective addresses the process deletion of final consonants.)

Performance: _____

Condition: _____

Criterion: _____

2. correctly imitate the consonant clusters /sk/, /sp/, and /st/ without a pause between the two consonants in 90% of his attempts. (*Note:* This objective addresses the process cluster reduction.)

Performance: _____

Condition: _____

Criterion: _____

3. produce unstressed syllables in bisyllabic words in 90% of his attempts. (*Note:* This objective addresses the process deletion of unstressed syllables.)

Performance: _____

Condition: _____

Criterion: _____

4. produce voiceless consonants when preceding vowels in 90% of the appropriate contexts. (*Note:* This objective addresses the process prevocalic voicing of consonants.)

Performance: _____

Condition: _____

Criterion: _____

5. produce fricatives or affricates in 90% of the appropriate contexts. (*Note:* This objective addresses the process stopping.)

   Performance: _____

   Condition: _____

   Criterion: _____

6. produce liquids in 90% of the appropriate contexts. (*Note:* This objective addresses the process gliding.)

   Performance: _____

   Condition: _____

   Criterion: _____

Sample Objectives 3: Language

1. spontaneously name 20 of 25 pictures in a child's dictionary.

   Performance: _____

   Condition: _____

   Criterion: _____

2. expressively identify (name) pictures of common objects in 90% of his attempts.

   Performance: _____

   Condition: _____

   Criterion: _____

3. receptively identify (point to) pictures given in a field of three in 8 of 10 attempts.

   Performance: _____

   Condition: _____

   Criterion: _____

4. correctly use present progressive tense while describing 20 of 25 pictures that are not visible to the clinician.

   Performance: _____

Condition: _____

Criterion: _____

5. appropriately use the pronouns *he* and *she* during conversation in 90% of his attempts.

Performance: _____

Condition: _____

Criterion: _____

6. correctly use regular plurals in at least 90% of his attempts while telling a story.

Performance: _____

Condition: _____

Criterion: _____

Sample Objectives 4: Voice

1. identify (raise hand) at least 7 of his vocal abuses when all possible abuses are stated.

Performance: _____

Condition: _____

Criterion: _____

2. explain 3 steps in laryngeal functioning one session after the clinician's explanation.

Performance: _____

Condition: _____

Criterion: _____

3. use appropriate pitch while producing /ɑ/ in 8 of 10 trials.

Performance: _____

Condition: _____

Criterion: _____

4. produce easy onset of voice on the vowels /o/ and /i/ in 90% of his attempts.

Performance: _____

Condition: _____

Criterion: _____

5. produce appropriate oral resonance on vowel–consonant combinations in 90% of his attempts.

   Performance: _____

   Condition: _____

   Criterion: _____

Sample Objectives 5: Fluency

1. identify (say "there") 90% of his nonfluencies that consist of prolongations lasting longer than 2 seconds.

   Performance: _____

   Condition: _____

   Criterion: _____

2. read in front of his class with fewer than .5 stuttered words per minute.

   Performance: _____

   Condition: _____

   Criterion: _____

3. speak with fewer than .5 stuttered words per minute during 5 minutes of spontaneous conversation with the clinician.

   Performance: _____

   Condition: _____

   Criterion: _____

4. cancel 90% of the stuttering episodes that occur while talking on the telephone.

   Performance: _____

   Condition: _____

   Criterion: _____

5. identify (state) all factors in his stuttering equation one session after this discussion occurred.

   Performance: _____

   Condition: _____

   Criterion: _____

6. use pullouts during all episodes of blocking while speaking to the principal for 5 minutes.

   Performance: _____

   Condition: _____

   Criterion: _____

Sample Objectives 6: Pragmatics

1. request (by pointing or using eye gaze) an object that is out of reach twice during a 10-minute time segment.

   Performance: _____

   Condition: _____

   Criterion: _____

2. take 3 consecutive turns when a familiar joint action routine is initiated by a significant other.

   Performance: _____

   Condition: _____

   Criterion: _____

3. attend to (look at) the speaker during 2 of 3 communication episodes.

   Performance: _____

   Condition: _____

   Criterion: _____

4. initiate a greeting upon seeing the clinician on 4 of 5 appropriate occasions.

   Performance: _____

   Condition: _____

   Criterion: _____

5. specify a topic once during each therapy session.

   Performance: _____

   Condition: _____

   Criterion: _____

6. maintain a topic initiated by someone else for 3 conversational turns.

   Performance: _____

Condition: _____

Criterion: _____

Sample Objectives 7: Problem Behavior

1. walk into the therapy room without yanking the clinician's arm in 2 of the 3 weekly therapy sessions.

   Performance: _____

   Condition: _____

   Criterion: _____

2. sit without kicking for 5 minutes after the removal of restraints (your hands on the client's knees).

   Performance: _____

   Condition: _____

   Criterion: _____

3. attend to (look at) a picture for 2 minutes when a desirable toy is within reaching distance.

   Performance: _____

   Condition: _____

   Criterion: _____

4. perform a specified task for 25 minutes without throwing a temper tantrum.

   Performance: _____

   Condition: _____

   Criterion: _____

5. follow 8 of 10 directions within 2 seconds of the initial presentation.

   Performance: _____

   Condition: _____

   Criterion: _____

Sample Objectives 8: Phonological Awareness

1. provide a rhyming word when presented auditorily with a word in 90% of his attempts.

   Performance: _____

Condition: _____

Criterion: _____

2. clap once for each syllable in a word presented auditorily by the clinician in 90% of his attempts.

   Performance: _____

   Condition: _____

   Criterion: _____

3. clap once for each word in a sentence presented auditorily by the clinician in 90% of his attempts.

   Performance: _____

   Condition: _____

   Criterion: _____

4. correctly identify the beginning sound in a word presented auditorily by the clinician in 90% of his attempts.

   Performance: _____

   Condition: _____

   Criterion: _____

5. correctly blend the word when given its syllables auditorily in 90% of his attempts.

   Performance: _____

   Condition: _____

   Criterion: _____

6. correctly state the sounds that letters make when presented visually in 90% of his attempts.

   Performance: _____

   Condition: _____

   Criterion: _____

Sample Objectives 9: Dysphagia

1. masticate and transfer semisolids without pocketing in the buccal cavity during 90% of his swallows.

   Performance: _____

Condition: _____

Criterion: _____

2. protrude, elevate, and lateralize his tongue following auditory and visual cueing in 90% of his attempts.

   Performance: _____

   Condition: _____

   Criterion: _____

3. tuck his chin before each swallow and maintain this position during the swallow in 90% of his attempts.

   Performance: _____

   Condition: _____

   Criterion: _____

4. utilize a supraglottic swallow independently during 9 of 10 swallows.

   Performance: _____

   Condition: _____

   Criterion: _____

5. swallow single-teaspoon presentations of a puree diet using a double swallow without signs of choking, coughing, or wet, gurgly vocal quality.

   Performance: _____

   Condition: _____

   Criterion: _____

6. swallow a nectar-consistency liquid using single straw sips without signs of aspiration.

   Performance: _____

   Condition: _____

   Criterion: _____

Sample Objectives 10: Augmentative and Alternative Communication

1. use eye gaze to request an activity given a field of two icons in 90% of his attempts.

   Performance: _____

Condition: _____

Criterion: _____

2. request an object by pointing to an icon in his communication book in 9 of 10 attempts.

Performance: _____

Condition: _____

Criterion: _____

3. turn on his communication device in less than 30 seconds in 3 consecutive trials.

Performance: _____

Condition: _____

Criterion: _____

4. direct his older sister to dress a doll by pointing to 3 of 4 picture symbols in the correct order.

Performance: _____

Condition: _____

Criterion: _____

5. make the clown dance by activating the switch when requested in 9 of 10 attempts.

Performance: _____

Condition: _____

Criterion: _____

6. select appropriate greetings on his communication device using scanning in 90% of his attempts.

Performance: _____

Condition: _____

Criterion: _____

<u>**Appendix 1.B**</u>

Answers: Identifying Components
of Behavioral Objectives

Sample Objectives 1: Articulation

1. correctly produce the /r/ phoneme in all positions of words in 90% of his attempts.

   Performance: <u>correctly produce the /r/ phoneme</u>

   Condition: <u>in all positions of words</u>

   Criterion: <u>in 90% of his attempts</u>

2. correctly imitate /s/ in isolation in 8 of 10 attempts.

   Performance: <u>correctly imitate /s/</u>

   Condition: <u>in isolation</u>

   Criterion: <u>in 8 of 10 attempts</u>

3. raise his tongue tip to the alveolar ridge with his mouth open at least 1½ inches on 8 of 10 trials.

   Performance: <u>raise his tongue tip to the alveolar ridge</u>

   Condition: <u>with his mouth open at least 1½ inches</u>

   Criterion: <u>on 8 of 10 trials</u>

4. auditorily discriminate (by raising his hand) /s/ from /f/ in consonant–vowel combinations in 90% of his attempts.

   Performance: <u>auditorily discriminate (by raising his hand) /s/ from /f/</u>

   Condition: <u>in consonant–vowel combinations</u>

   Criterion: <u>in 90% of his attempts</u>

5. correctly monitor (state if correct or not) production of the /l/ phoneme during spontaneous conversation in 90% of his attempts.

   Performance: <u>correctly monitor (state if correct or not) production of the /l/ phoneme</u>

Condition: *during spontaneous conversation*

Criterion: *in 90% of his attempts*

6. correctly monitor (self-correct) 90% of the incorrect /s/ productions during reading.

Performance: *correctly monitor (self-correct) incorrect /s/ productions*

Condition: *during reading*

Criterion: *90%*

Sample Objectives 2: Phonology

1. close syllables on spontaneously produced monosyllabic target words in 90% of his attempts. (*Note:* This objective addresses the process deletion of final consonants.)

Performance: *close syllables*

Condition: *on spontaneously produced monosyllabic target words*

Criterion: *in 90% of his attempts*

2. correctly imitate the consonant clusters /sk/, /sp/, and /st/ without a pause between the two consonants in 90% of his attempts (*Note:* This objective addresses the process cluster reduction.)

Performance: *correctly imitate the consonant clusters /sk/, /sp/, and /st/*

Condition: *without a pause between the two consonants*

Criterion: *in 90% of his attempts*

3. produce unstressed syllables in bisyllabic words in 90% of his attempts. (*Note:* This objective addresses the process deletion of unstressed syllables.)

Performance: *produce unstressed syllables*

Condition: *in bisyllabic words*

Criterion: *in 90% of his attempts*

4. produce voiceless consonants when preceding vowels in 90% of the appropriate contexts. (*Note:* This objective addresses the process prevocalic voicing of consonants.)

Performance: *produce voiceless consonants*

Condition: *when preceding vowels*

Criterion: *in 90% of the appropriate contexts*

5. produce fricatives or affricates in 90% of the appropriate contexts. (*Note:* This objective addresses the process stopping.)

Performance: produce fricatives or affricates

Condition: the appropriate contexts

Criterion: 90%

6. produce liquids in 90% of the appropriate contexts. (*Note:* This objective addresses the process gliding.)

Performance: produce liquids

Condition: the appropriate contexts

Criterion: 90%

Sample Objectives 3: Language

1. spontaneously name 20 of 25 pictures in a child's dictionary.

Performance: spontaneously name pictures

Condition: in a child's dictionary

Criterion: 20 of 25

2. expressively identify (name) pictures of common objects in 90% of his attempts.

Performance: expressively identify (name) pictures

Condition: of common objects

Criterion: in 90% of his attempts

3. receptively identify (point to) pictures given in a field of three in 8 of 10 attempts.

Performance: receptively identify (point to) pictures

Condition: given in a field of three

Criterion: in 8 of 10 attempts

4. correctly use present progressive tense while describing 20 of 25 pictures that are not visible to the clinician.

Performance: correctly use present progressive tense

Condition: while describing pictures that are not visible to the clinician

Criterion: 20 of 25

5. appropriately use the pronouns *he* and *she* during conversation in 90% of his attempts.

   Performance: appropriately use the pronouns he and she

   Condition: during conversation

   Criterion: in 90% of his attempts

6. correctly use regular plurals in at least 90% of his attempts while telling a story.

   Performance: correctly use regular plurals

   Condition: while telling a story

   Criterion: in at least 90% of his attempts

Sample Objectives 4: Voice

1. identify (raise hand) at least 7 of his vocal abuses when all possible abuses are stated.

   Performance: identify (raise hand) vocal abuses

   Condition: when all possible abuses are stated

   Criterion: at least 7

2. explain 3 steps in laryngeal functioning one session after the clinician's explanation.

   Performance: explain steps in laryngeal functioning

   Condition: one session after the clinician's explanation

   Criterion: 3

3. use appropriate pitch while producing /ɑ/ in 8 of 10 trials.

   Performance: use appropriate pitch

   Condition: while producing /ɑ/

   Criterion: in 8 of 10 trials

4. produce easy onset of voice on the vowels /o/ and /i/ in 90% of his attempts.

   Performance: produce easy onset of voice

   Condition: on the vowels /o/ and /i/

   Criterion: in 90% of his attempts

5. produce appropriate oral resonance on vowel–consonant combinations in 90% of his attempts.

   Performance: produce appropriate oral resonance

   Condition: on vowel–consonant combinations

   Criterion: in 90% of his attempts

Sample Objectives 5: Fluency

1. identify (say "there") 90% of his nonfluencies that consist of prolongations lasting longer than 2 seconds.

   Performance: identify (say "there") his nonfluencies

   Condition: that consist of prolongations lasting longer than 2 seconds

   Criterion: 90% of his nonfluencies

2. read in front of his class with fewer than .5 stuttered words per minute.

   Performance: read

   Condition: in front of his class

   Criterion: with fewer than .5 stuttered words per minute

3. speak with fewer than .5 stuttered words per minute during 5 minutes of spontaneous conversation with the clinician.

   Performance: speak

   Condition: during 5 minutes of spontaneous conversation with the clinician

   Criterion: with fewer than .5 stuttered words per minute

4. cancel 90% of the stuttering episodes that occur while talking on the telephone.

   Performance: cancel stuttering episodes

   Condition: that occur while talking on the telephone

   Criterion: 90%

5. identify (state) all factors in his stuttering equation one session after this discussion occurred.

   Performance: identify (state) factors in his stuttering equation

   Condition: one session after this discussion occurred

   Criterion: all (implies 100%)

6. use pullouts during all episodes of blocking while speaking to the principal for 5 minutes.

   Performance: use pullouts during episodes of blocking

   Condition: while speaking to the principal for 5 minutes

   Criterion: all (implies 100%)

Sample Objectives 6: Pragmatics

1. request (by pointing or using eye gaze) an object that is out of reach twice during a 10-minute time segment.

   Performance: request (by pointing or using eye gaze) an object

   Condition: that is out of reach

   Criterion: twice during a 10-minute time segment

2. take 3 consecutive turns when a familiar joint action routine is initiated by a significant other.

   Performance: take turns

   Condition: when a familiar joint action routine is initiated by a significant other

   Criterion: 3 consecutive

3. attend to (look at) the speaker during 2 of 3 communication episodes.

   Performance: attend to (look at) the speaker

   Condition: during communication episodes

   Criterion: 2 of 3

4. initiate a greeting upon seeing the clinician on 4 of 5 appropriate occasions.

   Performance: initiate a greeting

   Condition: upon seeing the clinician

   Criterion: on 4 of 5 appropriate occasions

5. specify a topic once during each therapy session.

   Performance: specify a topic

   Condition: during each therapy session

   Criterion: once

6. maintain a topic initiated by someone else for 3 conversational turns.

   Performance: maintain a topic

Condition: initiated by someone else

Criterion: for 3 conversational turns

Sample Objectives 7: Problem Behavior

1. walk into the therapy room without yanking the clinician's arm in 2 of the 3 weekly therapy sessions.

   Performance: walk into the therapy room

   Condition: without yanking the clinician's arm

   Criterion: in 2 of the 3 weekly therapy sessions

2. sit without kicking for 5 minutes after the removal of restraints (your hands on the client's knees).

   Performance: sit without kicking

   Condition: after the removal of restraints

   Criterion: 5 minutes

3. attend to (look at) a picture for 2 minutes when a desirable toy is within reaching distance.

   Performance: attend to (look at) a picture

   Condition: when a desirable toy is within reaching distance

   Criterion: for 2 minutes

4. perform a specified task for 25 minutes without throwing a temper tantrum.

   Performance: perform a specified task

   Condition: without throwing a temper tantrum

   Criterion: for 25 minutes

5. follow 8 of 10 directions within 2 seconds of the initial presentation.

   Performance: follow directions

   Condition: within 2 seconds of the initial presentation

   Criterion: 8 of 10

Sample Objectives 8: Phonological Awareness

1. provide a rhyming word when presented auditorily with a word in 90% of his attempts.

   Performance: provide a rhyming word

Condition: when presented auditorily with a word

Criterion: in 90% of his attempts

2. clap once for each syllable in a word presented auditorily by the clinician in 90% of his attempts.

Performance: clap once for each syllable in a word

Condition: presented auditorily by the clinician

Criterion: in 90% of his attempts

3. clap once for each word in a sentence presented auditorily by the clinician in 90% of his attempts.

Performance: clap once for each word in a sentence

Condition: presented auditorily by the clinician

Criterion: in 90% of his attempts

4. correctly identify the beginning sound in a word presented auditorily by the clinician in 90% of his attempts.

Performance: correctly identify the beginning sound in a word

Condition: presented auditorily by the clinician

Criterion: in 90% of his attempts

5. correctly blend the word when given its syllables auditorily in 90% of his attempts.

Performance: correctly blend the word

Condition: when given its syllables auditorily

Criterion: in 90% of his attempts

6. correctly state the sounds that letters make when presented visually in 90% of his attempts.

Performance: correctly state the sounds that letters make

Condition: when presented visually

Criterion: in 90% of his attempts

Sample Objectives 9: Dysphagia

1. masticate and transfer semisolids without pocketing in the buccal cavity during 90% of his swallows.

Performance: masticate and transfer semisolids

Condition: without pocketing in the buccal cavity

Criterion: during 90% of his swallows

2. protrude, elevate, and lateralize his tongue following auditory and visual cueing in 90% of his attempts.

Performance: protrude, elevate, and lateralize his tongue

Condition: following auditory and visual cueing

Criterion: in 90% of his attempts

3. tuck his chin before each swallow and maintain this position during the swallow in 90% of his attempts.

Performance: tuck his chin

Condition: before each swallow and maintain this position during the swallow

Criterion: in 90% of his attempts

4. utilize a supraglottic swallow independently during 9 of 10 swallows.

Performance: utilize a supraglottic swallow

Condition: independently

Criterion: during 9 of 10 swallows

5. swallow single-teaspoon presentations of a puree diet using a double swallow without signs of choking, coughing, or wet, gurgly vocal quality.

Performance: swallow single-teaspoon presentations of a puree diet

Condition: using a double swallow

Criterion: without signs of choking, coughing, or wet, gurgly vocal quality

6. swallow a nectar–consistency liquid using single straw sips without signs of aspiration.

Performance: swallow a nectar-consistency liquid

Condition: using single straw sips

Criterion: without signs of aspiration

Sample Objectives 10: Augmentative and Alternative Communication

1. use eye gaze to request an activity given a field of two icons in 90% of his attempts.

Performance: use eye gaze to request an activity

Condition: given a field of two icons

Criterion: in 90% of his attempts

2. request an object by pointing to an icon in his communication book in 9 of 10 attempts.

Performance: request an object in his communication book

Condition: by pointing to an icon

Criterion: in 9 of 10 attempts

3. turn on his communication device in less than 30 seconds in 3 consecutive trials.

Performance: turn on his communication device

Condition: in less than 30 seconds

Criterion: in 3 consecutive trials

4. direct his older sister to dress a doll by pointing to 3 of 4 picture symbols in the correct order.

Performance: direct his older sister to dress a doll

Condition: by pointing to picture symbols in the correct order

Criterion: 3 of 4

5. make the clown dance by activating the switch when requested in 9 of 10 attempts.

Performance: make the clown dance

Condition: by activating the switch when requested

Criterion: in 9 of 10 attempts

6. select appropriate greetings on his communication device using scanning in 90% of his attempts.

Performance: select appropriate greetings on his communication device

Condition: using scanning

Criterion: in 90% of his attempts

If you correctly identified at least 90% of the components in this exercise and are satisfied with your performance, return to where you left off in Chapter 1. Begin reading the section titled "Application and Importance of Behavioral Objectives."

References

Education for All Handicapped Children Act of 1975, 20 U.S.C. § 1400 *et seq.*

Lucas, S. (2000). *The SLP's IDEA Companion.* East Moline, IL: LinguiSystems.

Mager, R. F. (1984). *Preparing instructional objectives* (rev. 2nd ed.). Belmont, CA: Fearon.

Mowrer, D. E. (1988). *Methods of modifying speech behaviors* (2nd ed.). Prospect Heights, IL: Waveland Press.

Silverman, F. H. (1984). *Speech–language pathology and audiology: An introduction.* Columbus, OH: Merrill.

Thompson, D. G. (1977). Writing long-term and short-term objectives. Champaign, IL: Research Press.

Wheeler, A. H., & Fox, W. L. (1977). *A guide to writing instructional objectives.* Lawrence, KS: H&H Enterprises.

Chapter 2

Behavioral Objectives: Common Writing Problems

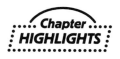

- Problems to avoid while writing behavioral objectives
- Writing problem-free behavioral objectives
- Critically analyzing behavioral objectives

Speech–language clinicians need to write behavioral objectives in a clear and acceptable fashion. As a beginning clinician, you might wonder why behavioral objectives cannot simply include performance, condition, and criterion components. You might question why behavioral objectives must be written in a particular manner. When your objectives are not approved, you do not always understand how to improve them. In this chapter, I discuss common problems in writing behavioral objectives to clarify how to prepare well-written objectives in speech–language pathology.

Problem 1: Incorrect Format Following the Lead-In

Problems occur frequently with the portion of the objective immediately following the lead-in, or introductory, statement. Typically, this problem is caused by lack of grammatical consistency between the lead-in and the actual objective. If the statement created by the lead-in *and* the objective creates a complete sentence, you should not add a colon after the lead-in, and you should begin each objective with a lowercase (not capital) letter. If the lead-in statement is a phrase that is correctly followed by a colon (e.g., "Lesson Objective:"), the objectives begin with a capital letter if they *are* complete sentences but with a lowercase letter if they *are not* complete sentences. To demonstrate, I give examples from beginning clinicians. These examples are coded with a "(U)" (for uncorrected) following the example number; the corrected versions of the examples are coded with a "(C)" (for corrected). The new or corrected information is underlined.

In this example, the lead-in and the objective together form a complete sentence, so the objective should not begin with a capital letter.

> **The client will**
> **1.1(U) Receptively identify (by pointing) 8 of 10 body**
> **parts.**
>
> **1.2(C) receptively identify (by pointing) 8 of 10 body**
> **parts.**

For the next and most other examples through the chapter, **"Lesson Objectives:"** is the assumed lead-in. Therefore, the objectives should begin with capital letters.

> **1.2(U) the client will receptively identify (by pointing) 8 of**
> **10 body parts.**

Because the portion following the colon is a complete sentence, "the" should begin with an uppercase letter:

> **1.2(C) The client will receptively identify (by pointing) 8**
> **of 10 body parts.**

QUICK CHECK

The lead-in is the introductory statement that precedes the list of behavioral objectives. If the lead-in and the objective form a complete sentence, the objective should begin with a lowercase letter. If the lead-in is followed by a colon and the portion following the colon is a complete sentence, the first word should be capitalized. If the portion following the colon is not a complete sentence, the first word should begin with a lowercase letter.

Problem 2: Consistency

A problem that frequently occurs when more than one objective is listed is a lack of consistency in how the objectives are written. An example follows:

> **2.1(U)** Scott will spontaneously produce two-word combinations twice during the session.
>
> to correctly imitate Noun + Verb + Object combinations presented while looking at a storybook in 90% of his attempts.

This example clearly shows a lack of consistency in the structure of the objectives. All objectives cited together should begin in the same manner. Either of the two formats can be used. Examples of each type follow:

> **Lesson Objectives:**
> **2.1(C.1)** <u>to</u> spontaneously produce two-word combinations twice during the session.
>
> <u>to</u> correctly imitate Noun + Verb + Object combinations presented while looking at a storybook in 90% of his attempts.
>
> **2.1(C.2)** <u>Scott</u> will spontaneously produce two-word combinations twice during the session.
>
> <u>Scott</u> will correctly imitate Noun + Verb + Object combinations presented while looking at a storybook in 90% of his attempts.

It is important to be consistent when writing objectives. Adopt one format and stick with it.

Problem 3: Performance Component

As discussed at length in Chapter 1, a common problem in the performance component is the use of verbs that are not specific. An example of an objective containing this error follows:

> **3.1(U.1) to discriminate among the /s/ phoneme and
> other phonemes in 7 of 10 attempts.**

Because the verb *discriminate* is not directly observable, an indicator behavior is needed so the clinician can know exactly what the client will be doing when demonstrating achievement of the objective. An example of this correction follows:

> **3.1(C.1) to discriminate <u>auditorily (by raising his hand)</u>
> among the /s/ phoneme and other phonemes in 7
> of 10 attempts.**

The indicator behavior, "by raising his hand," takes care of the initial problem. However, the writer must remember that anyone reading the objective should be able to picture the task to be performed. If "auditorily" is not included, one might expect a visual task in which the client raises his hand when shown the letter "S" and does not raise it when another letter is shown. Of course, if one knows the definition of a phoneme, this interpretation is excluded, but another exists: A deaf child may be discriminating the /s/ phoneme from other phonemes solely through the visual modality—that is, how each phoneme looks when produced. I include these possibilities to stress the importance of critically reading and evaluating objectives. The development of these skills should result in better written objectives.

To narrow the focus further, Objective 3.1 could still be more specific. From the original objective, it is unclear whether this beginning clinician really knew where she was headed in the remediation process. Additional information on the nature of "other phonemes" should be provided. Is the client being required to make gross or fine discriminations? This information can be provided in more than one way. Two suggestions follow:

> **3.1(C.2) to discriminate auditorily (raise his hand) the /s/
> phoneme <u>from all other fricatives</u> in 70% of his attempts.**

> **3.1(C.3) to discriminate auditorily (raise his hand) the /s/
> phoneme from /f/, /v/, /θ/, /ð/, /z/, /ʃ/, and /ʒ/
> presented in isolation in 70% of his attempts.**

This objective is now well written. Problems with the performance aspect have been rectified, and a condition has been added to eliminate ambiguity.

The problem occurring in the performance component of the next example may not be obvious on initial scrutiny, but should become apparent.

> **3.2(U) to discuss with Larry the visual and acoustic characteristics of the /s/ phoneme.**

Keep in mind that the performance component is being discussed. Problems with the other components will be corrected in the objective but not discussed in this section. The major problem with the performance part of the objective is that the focus is placed on the wrong person. The performance component is supposed to deal with how the client should demonstrate achievement of an objective and not what the clinician does. The following revision in the performance component places the emphasis on the client:

> **3.2(C) <u>to state</u> 2 visual and 2 acoustic characteristics of the /s/ phoneme.**

This objective clearly states what the client has to do to be successful.

Another objective is as follows:

> **3.3(U) to produce the /s/ phoneme in words with 90% accuracy.**

In this example, the problem in the performance component may not be initially obvious. The client may already be producing an /s/ phoneme, but it may be distorted. According to this objective, as written, distorted /s/ productions would be considered correct. The following revised objective does not consider distortions acceptable:

> **3.3(C) to produce the /s/ phoneme <u>correctly</u> in all positions of words in 90% of his attempts.**

The impact of simply adding *correctly* is important because a distorted /s/ will not be considered an acceptable production.

The next example states what the client will do, but the manner in which it is stated is not clear and precise.

> **3.4(U) to produce the /s/ phoneme in sentences by imitation with 90% accuracy.**

The word *imitation* is a key word in the objective because it states exactly what the client will be doing. Thus, it should receive more emphasis. A revised objective follows:

> **3.4(C) to <u>imitate</u> the /s/ phoneme correctly in sentences in 90% of his attempts.**

Because the word *imitate* is more strategically placed, it is less likely to be overlooked. The inaccurate impression from reading Objective 3.4(U) is that the client is spontaneously producing the phoneme in sentences. This conclusion is not reflected in revised Objective 3.4(C). Behavioral objectives must be written in a precise and specific manner to prevent misinterpretation.

In the following objective, try to determine what the client should be doing while demonstrating achievement:

> **3.5(U) to strengthen and stabilize the /s/ phoneme in 90% of his attempts.**

The words *strengthen* and *stabilize* are used in Van Riper and Erickson's (1996) articulation therapy program, but they are not used precisely enough in this statement to clarify exactly what the client should be doing. Many therapeutic techniques will lead to strengthening and stabilization of a particular phoneme if executed skillfully; therefore, the performance component must be more specific. Two possible corrections follow:

> **3.5(C.1) <u>to prolong correct production</u> of the /s/ phoneme in isolation for 15 seconds.**

> **3.5(C.2) to produce the /s/ phoneme correctly in isolation <u>15 times in 15 seconds.</u>**

Both of these objectives provide a clear idea of what the client must do to demonstrate achievement.

In summary, problems affecting the performance component of behavioral objectives have been identified and discussed in this section. Example 1 showed usage of a nonspecific verb and demonstrated that the entire objective had to be written in a more specific manner. Example 2 placed the focus on the clinician instead of the client. By not clearly stating the intention in the third example, distorted productions would have been acceptable. Example 4 conveyed the idea that the objective should be broken down into the smallest, most precise behavior and should clearly reflect what the client needs to do. Example 5 needed to state specifically what the client should do.

Two points are important to remember when constructing the performance portion of a behavioral objective: Be certain the objective reflects exactly what the client should do to demonstrate achievement of the objective, and be certain that the verbs used are specific.

Problem 4: Condition Component

Problems encountered in the condition component stem from either not stating or not clearly stating the circumstances under or in which the performance is done. Problems concerning components other than the condition will be corrected in these revisions but will not be discussed in this section. The first example follows:

> **4.1(U) to determine the location of the /t/ phoneme with 90% accuracy.**

Because the reader cannot readily determine the nature of this task, further description is necessary. An acceptable revision follows:

> **4.1(C) to determine (by pointing to train cars) the correct location of the /t/ phoneme <u>when 3 phonemes are presented in isolation</u> in 90% of his attempts.**

This revised objective enables the reader to predetermine the task that will be presented. Objective 4.1(U) did not specify whether the /t/ phoneme would be presented in isolation, syllables, words, or sentences. In the revised objective, there is no guesswork involved as the environment (isolation) is clearly specified in the condition component of the objective.

This next example further illustrates how the condition in an objective adds clarification.

> **4.2(U) to discriminate auditorily between the /p/ and /b/ phonemes in 90% of his attempts.**

To avoid misinterpretation, further clarification is necessary, which can be accomplished by including a condition in the objective. A revised objective follows:

> **4.2(C) to discriminate correctly and auditorily (by pointing to the corresponding picture) between the /p/ and /b/ phonemes <u>presented in isolation</u> in 90% of his**

> **attempts. (*Note:* A picture of a motor boat is associated with /p/ and a picture of a ball is associated with /b/ on this particular task.)**

The condition "presented in isolation" clarifies the task. The reader has been given enough information to develop a preconceived notion about the therapeutic task that the clinician and client will be performing to accomplish the objective. A well-defined objective is also likely to keep the clinician on task.

The next example gives an impression that the client is functioning on a higher level than he actually is.

> **4.3(U) to produce the /s/ phoneme correctly in sentences in 54 of 60 attempts.**

This objective seems to imply that the client can spontaneously produce sentences and maintain correct /s/ production. Because the client is not performing at this level, a condition needs to be stated in the objective.

> **4.3(C) to correctly produce the /s/ words <u>on his word list when incorporated into sentences</u> in 90% of his attempts.**

The fact that the client's production centered around incorporating a word containing the /s/ phoneme into a sentence indicates that a reminder is necessary for correct production to be achieved. When the objective is worded in this manner, one gets a more realistic idea of the level at which the client is functioning.

Notice how much more specific the next objective becomes when a condition is added.

> **4.4(U) to produce the /p/, /t/, /k/, and /v/ phonemes correctly in syllables in 4 of 5 attempts.**

As written, the objective indicates that the client will be producing all syllable types. If one thinks of all the different possibilities, it makes sense to add a clarifying statement or condition, as reflected in the revision.

> **4.4(C) to produce each of these phonemes /p/, /t/, /k/, and /v/ correctly <u>in consonant–vowel combinations</u> in 4 of 5 attempts.**

The condition "in consonant–vowel combinations" limits the type of syllable in which the phonemes will be produced.

In the next example, the condition also needs clarification.

4.5(U) to receptively identify 13 of 15 objects correctly.

The impression obtained from reading this objective is that 15 objects will be placed in front of the client, who will be responsible for selecting the object named from the entire field of 15. Because this is not the intent of the objective, the goal needs to be revised.

**4.5(C) to receptively identify (by <u>pointing</u> to) 13 of 15
objects <u>correctly given a field of 2</u>.**

This revised objective indicates that two objects will be presented to the client at a time. Selecting one object from a field of 15 is much more difficult than selecting an object from a field of 2. When the objective is worded in this manner, it is less likely to be misinterpreted.

In summary, objectives containing problems in the condition component have been discussed in this section. In all examples, the revisions consist of adding additional information to describe the circumstances under or in which the performance is to be done.

QUICK CHECK

> Be as specific as possible in writing the condition component. To prevent misinterpretation, include in the objective any pertinent and relevant situations and circumstances that are necessary for clarification.

Problem 5: Criterion Component

The criterion component specifies how well the client is expected to perform. Problems encountered with this component arise when the clinician does not state a criterion or does not state it accurately. The first example lacks a criterion.

5.1(U) to produce the /s/ phoneme correctly in isolation.

Because a criterion is not stated, it is not possible to know when the objective has been accomplished. A revision follows:

**5.1(C) to produce the /s/ phoneme correctly in isolation <u>in</u>
<u>90% of his attempts</u>.**

It is now possible to know when the objective is accomplished and to measure the client's progress.

Technically, there is nothing wrong with the manner in which the criterion is stated in the following objective. It is, however, needlessly binding.

5.2(U) to produce the /s/ phoneme correctly in sentences in 54 of 60 attempts.

Strictly speaking, there is no way the client can meet this criterion unless he is given 60 trials to produce /s/. Even if the child produces 40 sentences (each containing one /s/ phoneme) and correctly produces 36 of the /s/ phonemes, he cannot meet the criterion despite the high level of success (90%). Further, by stating the criterion in this manner, flexibility is stifled because it is not possible to move to another objective until the client has been given 60 opportunities to produce /s/. The following revision avoids the problem:

5.2(C) to produce the /s/ phoneme correctly in sentences in 90% of his attempts.

Stating the objective in this manner is conducive to flexibility. Moving to a higher level objective is contingent on the client's performance alone and not on an arbitrary number of trials. More specifically, if the client correctly produces 9 of 10 /s/ phonemes, he has met criterion and can move to a higher level objective. Additional time does not have to be spent on 50 more trials. The percentage of success is 90% for both objectives, but the second objective is clearly less restrictive and permits more effective use of time and allows more efficient and flexible therapy.

The next example is more abstract. The term *accuracy*, here defined as "correctness," leads to confusion in this objective.

5.3(U) to produce the /s/ phoneme in isolation with 90% accuracy in all attempts.

This objective can be paraphrased by saying that every time the client produces the /s/ phoneme, his production will be 90% accurate. This can be interpreted as meaning that the /s/ phoneme will not be totally correct because this would be indicated by "100% accuracy." Because 90% accuracy implies that the production is not quite right, would a distorted /s/ production be acceptable? The following revised objective is not as prone to multiple interpretations:

5.3(C) to produce the /s/ phoneme correctly in isolation in 90% of his attempts.

This criterion clearly indicates that the client must produce the /s/ phoneme correctly in at least 90% of the total number of attempts. If the total number of trials is 50, the client has to produce /s/ correctly in at least 45 of them to meet criterion.

The next objective is written in an imprecise manner so that the meaning is nearly beyond comprehension.

> **5.4(U) to produce the /s/ target phoneme in isolation 30 times in 100% of his attempts.**

The reader might interpret this objective as meaning that the client will produce the /s/ phoneme 30 times and that it has to be correct each time to meet criterion. To change this objective to a less confusing statement, the writer needs to determine what is important: the number 30, or 100% of the attempts, or both. If both are important, the objective can be revised in either of these ways:

> **5.4(C.1) to produce the /s/ phoneme correctly in isolation in 30 of 30 attempts.**

> **5.4(C.2) to produce the /s/ phoneme correctly in isolation in all 30 attempts.**

This objective has another problem, however. Requiring 100% correct productions is excessive. A criterion of 90% is adequate because a client typically continues to improve after training stops. It is not efficient to work on a behavior that will continue to show some spontaneous improvement. Thus, the objective should be revised from 100% to 90% of his attempts to allow for spontaneous growth. The revised objective follows:

> **5.4(C.3) to produce the /s/ phoneme correctly in isolation in 90% of his attempts.**

If the clinician decides that the number 30 is important, the objective can be written in a couple of ways, depending on whether the trials have to be consecutive:

> **5.4(C.4) to produce the /s/ phoneme correctly in isolation in 30 consecutive trials.**

> **5.4(C.5) to produce the /s/ phoneme correctly in isolation a total of 30 times.**

According to the wording in the latter objective, the number of trials is not important. The client can meet the criterion by producing /s/ in isolation correctly in 30 of 60 trials or in 30 of 70 trials. Stating the criterion in this manner is not suggested as the client can meet it without having adequate success and without actual mastery of the phoneme. In the former example, the client's percentage of correctness is 50%; in the latter example, it is 43%. Neither of these percentages warrants pro-gressing to a higher level objective.

This next objective does not state the criterion clearly:

> **5.5.(U) to produce the target /s/ phoneme in isolation in 90% of his attempts 25 times.**

After reading the discussions of the previous four objectives in this section, you probably can revise this objective immediately. Two suggested revisions follow:

> **5.5(C.1) to produce the /s/ phoneme correctly in isolation <u>in 90% of his attempts.</u>**

> **5.5(C.2) to produce the /s/ phoneme correctly in isolation <u>in 23 of 25 attempts.</u>**

The first revision is more acceptable than the second as it enables more flexibility (as discussed in relation to the second objective in this section).

In summary, problems specific to the criterion component have been discussed. The discussion about each objective should be instrumental in helping you to write criterion components that reflect how the client is expected to perform. Many of the revisions show how the criterion can be stated more clearly to avoid misinterpretation.

QUICK CHECK

Make certain the criterion portion of a behavioral objective is stated accurately so it is possible to determine when the client accomplishes the objective.

Problem 6: Lack of Support or Harmony

Many of the previously discussed problems can be identified simply by reading the behavioral objective. A more serious problem involves lack of support or harmony between the objective and the procedures initiated to meet that objective. This problem is less easily identified because the objectives are well written on the surface. A problem of this type does not appear until the behavioral objective is read immediately before or during the observation of the therapy session. Only then is it discovered that what is occurring in the therapy session does not support the objective. This problem frequently occurs if there is little or no direction in the client's therapy program or if no critical thought has gone into determining the objectives.

This lack of harmony between the objective and the procedure is usually observed first by your supervisor. When it is brought to your attention, you must decide if the objective is correct or if the procedure is correct. Based on this decision, appropriate changes must be made.

In the examples described in this section, assume that what was occurring in the session was appropriate. The problem in each case was that the goal was not written specifically enough, so it had to be revised. Although the revisions all required a more specific performance component, this problem warrants special discussion because it goes beyond merely rewriting the objective. For each of the following examples, (a) the behavioral objective is given as written by the beginning clinician, (b) behavior from the therapy session is described and discussed, and (c) the revised objective that supports the therapy session is provided.

The first objective follows:

> **6.1(U) to produce the /r/ phoneme correctly in sentences in 90% of his attempts.**

During the session, the child said "scarf" in the sentence "I have a scarf" and was reinforced for this production. According to the original goal, production of the word *scarf* should not be reinforced because the word does not contain the consonantal /r/ phoneme as found in the word *red*. Instead, the word *scarf* contains the centering diphthong /ɑr/.

After discussion with a supervisor, the beginning clinician determined that correct production of the centering diphthongs was the target behavior. The goal was then revised:

> **6.1(C) to produce <u>centering diphthongs</u> correctly in sentences in 90% of his attempts.**

By making the performance portion of the objective more specific, harmony was obtained between the objective and the procedure.

The second objective follows:

> **6.2(U) to produce the /s/ phoneme correctly during conversation in 90% of his attempts.**

During the session, the beginning clinician reinforced the client's production of the words *swim* and *state*. However, the *sw* and *st* combinations are blends or consonant clusters and are not included in the original objective. After reading the objective, the supervisor expected the client to be reinforced for the correct production of /s/ in words said during conversation such as *sun*, *ice*, and *bicycle*, but not *swim*. Based on observation of the session, the supervisor assumed that the objective should be revised as follows:

> **6.2(C.1) to produce /s/ blends correctly during conversation in 90% of his attempts.**

Continued observation of the session, however, revealed that the beginning clinician also reinforced production of the /s/ phoneme in the words *sit* and *nest*. Discussion with the beginning clinician revealed that she viewed the goal as being correct production of the /s/ phoneme in all possible contexts. Therefore, it was necessary to revise the goal:

> **6.2(C.2) to produce /s/ correctly in all contexts during conversation in 90% of his attempts.**

With the objective written in this manner, it is appropriate for the beginning clinician to reinforce correct productions of /s/ as singletons, blends, or sound combinations. Harmony between the objective and the procedure was accomplished by making the performance portion of the objective more specific.

The next objective to consider is as follows:

> **6.3(U) to produce the /s/ phoneme correctly during reading in 90% of his attempts.**

The client's production of the words *bees* and *was* was reinforced during the reading activity. However, because both of these words end in the /z/ phoneme, they are not included in the original objective.

Through discussion, the supervisor learned that the beginning clinician was looking for correct production of both members of the cognate pair. This information should have been reflected in the objective. Therefore, the objective was revised:

> **6.3(C) to produce the /s/ and /z/ phonemes correctly during reading in 90% of his attempts.**

The objective is now supported by the procedure. Once again, harmony was achieved by making the performance portion of the objective more specific.

In summary, the three examples cited in this section all involve what appear to be well-written behavioral objectives. The three components (performance, condition, and criterion) are intact—at least at first glance. When the therapy session is observed concurrent with reading the objectives, however, a lack of harmony between the objective and the procedure becomes evident. In the examples cited, harmony was achieved by making the performance aspect of the objective more specific.

Always make certain that there is harmony between your objectives and procedures. Make certain that all of your procedures support your objectives.

This chapter has shown various problems that arise in writing behavioral objectives. The first problem—incorrect format following the lead-in—deals with lack of consistency between the lead-in and the actual objective. The remaining problems deal with either the performance, condition, or criterion component of the behavioral objective. The final problem—lack of support or harmony—deals with the lack of agreement between the objective and the procedure. I have identified these common problems in hopes that you will give more analytic and critical thought to your behavioral objectives before submitting them to your clinical supervisor.

After reading this chapter, you should be able to

1. state at least three problems affecting the performance component of behavioral objectives.
2. explain the main problem affecting the condition component of behavioral objectives.
3. state at least three problems affecting the criterion component of behavioral objectives.
4. write at least four problem-free behavioral objectives reflecting four different communication disorders.
5. detect and fix all problems evident in your behavioral objectives.

Reference

Van Riper, C., & Erickson, R. (1996). *Speech correction: An introduction to speech pathology and audiology* (9th ed.). Boston: Allyn & Bacon.

Chapter 3

Evaluation and Progress Reports: Organization and Content

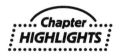

Chapter HIGHLIGHTS

- Critically analyzing evaluation reports
- Content to include in evaluation reports
- Organization of evaluation reports
- Problems to avoid while writing evaluation reports
- Developing a sense for writing evaluation reports
- Content to include in progress reports
- Organization of progress reports
- Developing a sense for writing progress reports

Writing evaluation and progress reports that are well organized and that have clear meaning to the various readers can be a challenge. However, learning to analyze and produce quality evaluation and progress reports is critical for beginning speech–language clinicians. Because all reports and evaluations remain in client files long after their preparation, they need to be understandable to a reader who may need to refer to them when the writer is no longer accessible or cannot decipher her writing from years ago. In this chapter, I analyze a poorly written evaluation report and describe guidelines for writing evaluation and progress reports.

Substandard Evaluation

Although the format and content of an evaluation report vary depending on (a) the professional setting in which the report is prepared and (b) the disorder exhibited, clinicians in all settings need to be able to write quality evaluation reports. A poorly written example of a professional evaluation report begins on the next page. This report, written by a clinician with a master's degree, came across my desk many years ago. Since then, it has been presented to many beginning clinicians as their first exposure to critically analyzing evaluation reports. As you read the introductory paragraph of the report, and before continuing to the next paragraph, you will see that it is a challenge to determine what is wrong and to suggest improvements.

After reading this evaluation report, some of you might wonder why it is unacceptable. If that is the case, do not worry. Reread the example and ask yourself these questions: Does this clearly and completely describe the client's condition and the proposed actions? Is it well organized and clearly written? Then read the analysis that follows. (*Note:* Names and addresses of people and agencies have been changed or omitted to preserve confidentiality.)

Analysis

Although the writing style might be acceptable for a social history evaluation, it is poorly organized for a speech–language evaluation. Information needs to be organized by topic with headings and subheadings to assist the reader in locating information. Also, some important information needs to be added (e.g., the telephone number for the foster parents). To help you understand the problems with this evaluation report, the following topics are discussed: background information, clinical assessment, and writing style and grammar. (No priority is implied by this order.) A later section of this chapter includes an organizational outline to use in your reports and instructions on how to use language to accurately convey your thoughts. Keep in mind that the problems discussed in this section were unique to the writer of this evaluation report. You may have other weaknesses, such as poor use of grammar or poor organizational skills. This chapter is intended to help you improve your evaluation and progress report writing immediately.

Background Information: Descriptive Data
Source. Certain data are basic to evaluation reports and are included because they aid the reader's comprehension. In the sample

EVALUATION REPORT: POOR EXAMPLE

Speech—Language Evaluation Report

Sally Smith
000 Main Street
Snowtown, PA 00000
D.O.B. May 17, [3 years ago]
Foster parents: Betty and Bill Brown

This is a 3-year, 2-month-old girl who is seen for a speech and language evaluation at the request of Snowtown's County Children's Services. Serena Phillips is the caseworker. It is felt that she is delayed in speech and language acquisition for her age. The history is quite involved. She was taken into a foster home at the age of 18 months. At that time, she was said to be deprived and almost in a catatonic state. She didn't talk at all and didn't smile. It took several weeks for the foster parents to get her to smile, and at 23 months of age she said "mommy."

Up until the age of 18 months, it was felt that Sally was on a very poor diet. She was taken care of at times by a half sister. Her mother died when she was 13 months old. Informally, it has been ascertained that the mother's health was quite poor during pregnancy. The cause of death was a stroke so we might get some hint of some of the problems that she had from this. Evidently the home situation was terrible.

She has been seen at Snowtown Medical Center and they have stated that she has delayed bone age. However, according to the foster mother, she has been progressing nicely as of late. The foster mother seems to be quite quick to explain Sally's slowness as functional and is quite adamant about the fact that she is not retarded. At present, she is beginning to put words together. Her intelligibility is quite poor. Therefore, I could not obtain much in the way of an articulation sample. I was able to obtain a raw score on Form A of the Peabody Picture Vocabulary test. This was 12, which converts to a mental age of 2–3, an intelligence quotient of 73 and a percentile score of 2. The reliability of these tests at the low end of the age spectrum is quite poor, and therefore the score is certainly no better than a ball park score. It is felt that Sally has not had any ear infections and that she can hear well. The hearing screening that we did was essentially normal.

Certainly, from the history that we obtained, it seems as though we are dealing with a case of delayed speech and language acquisition that may certainly be explained in part or in its entirety by the very poor situation in which this child found herself for the first 18 months of her life during which the linguistic foundation should have been built. She will be attending a nursery program at Snowtown College and it would seem as though it would be most convenient for the parent if her speech therapy session could be plugged in to this. Therefore, I will be contacting Mrs. White of Snowtown College Speech Dept. to see if she will be able to work this out. If this is not possible then we could consider seeing Sally down here for speech therapy, but in view of the

(continues)

EVALUATION REPORT (Continued)

convenience of the college to the parents I would suggest that they try to work it in up there.

　　I would like to see Sally back here in about six months for further speech evaluation.

Peggy Church

cc: Serena Phillips, SCCS [Snowtown's County Children's Services]
　　Mrs. White, Speech Dept. Snowtown College

Note: The *Peabody Picture Vocabulary Test* has been revised and Form A is no longer current. The newer editions of this test do not result in determining a mental age or intelligence quotient. The most current edition is the *Peabody Picture Vocabulary Test–Third Edition* (Dunn & Dunn, 1997).

evaluation report, the evaluator does not say where she obtained the information in the first two paragraphs and at the beginning of the third. Although Serena Phillips is cited as the caseworker, the report does not state that she provided any background information. The evaluator does not say if the caseworker accompanied the child to the evaluation. The sentence, "It is felt that she is delayed in speech and language acquisition for her age," does not clarify who initially felt that a delay was evident. The writer does not say who diagnosed delayed bone age at the Snowtown Medical Center. Although the evaluator mentioned in the report that the foster mother is adamant that Sally is not retarded, the source of that information is not stated. Was it related by the caseworker or the foster mother herself? Was the foster mother present? Was the information provided on a case history intake form, and if so, who completed it? Likewise, the source is not known for the following statement: "It is felt that Sally has not had any ear infections and that she can hear well."

　　Dates.　　The evaluator does not provide the date of this report, the date on which Sally was seen at the Snowtown Medical Center, or how old she was when delayed bone age was diagnosed. Likewise, the writer does not say when Sally's mother suffered the stroke or when she passed away. It is important to know how old Sally was at the time of these devastating events.

　　Social and Developmental History.　　The social and developmental history data must be presented in some logical order or sequence. Glancing at the ages stated in the first two paragraphs, for example, one sees 18 months, 23 months, 18 months, and 13 months. The information would be easier to follow if it were presented chronologically.

Unsupported Statements. All statements in the evaluation report should be supported by explanatory information. For example, after reading, "Up until the age of 18 months, it was felt that Sally was on a very poor diet," one wonders why. Nowhere in this report was information presented to support this statement. Other examples of unsupported statements include these: "Informally, it has been ascertained that the mother's health was quite poor during pregnancy" and "Evidently the home situation was terrible." The reader wonders whether these statements are based on fact because no information provided in the report backs up these statements. Evaluation reports should not include speculations that cannot be supported with data.

Clinical Assessment

Objectives. After performing an evaluation, the clinician should describe in the report exactly where the child is functioning in the area(s) of speech and/or language, where the child should be functioning given his or her chronological age or mental age, and what the best path is to help him or her get there. As described previously in this book, this path is a series of small steps called objectives. At the end of an evaluation report, the immediate objectives of therapy should be stated. However, they are absent in this report.

Diagnoses. The evaluator states that Sally has delayed speech, but this diagnosis is not supported in the body of the report. The only statements pertaining to her speech are these: "Her intelligibility is quite poor. Therefore, I could not obtain much in the way of an articulation sample." The writer does not provide any specific data about the child's speech. Important information needs to be included, such as phonemes the child can produce correctly, substituted phonemes and the nature of the substitutions, omitted phonemes, vowel production, stimulability, and phonological processes. If this information were provided, perhaps the diagnosis of delayed speech could be supported.

The evaluator also indicates that Sally has delayed language: "She is beginning to put words together" and she had "a percentile score of 2" on the *Peabody Picture Vocabulary Test.* Despite the provision of two statements about the child's language, the diagnosis is weakly supported and the child's present level of language functioning remains unknown. Much more relevant information needs to be included in the evaluation and all relevant aspects of language must be addressed in the report. For example, the following information would be helpful: How many different single words does the child use? How many two-word utterances does the child use and what type(s) (agent + action, action + object, agent + object, etc.)? Overall, how does the child communicate her wants and needs? In addition, the child's use of pragmatics and semantics was not addressed thoroughly.

Writing Style and Grammar

Precision and Clarity in Word Selection. The vocabulary used in an evaluation report should be precise, clear, and appropriate for professional writing. Otherwise, the evaluation will lose some or all of its validity. Substandard vocabulary from the sample evaluation report is underlined in the following examples:

> **The reliability of these tests at the low end of the age spectrum is quite poor, and therefore the score is certainly no better than a <u>ball park</u> score.... She will be attending a nursery program at Snowtown College and it would seem as though it would be most convenient for the parent if her speech therapy session could be <u>plugged</u> in to this.... If this is not possible, then we could consider seeing Sally <u>down here</u> for speech therapy, but in view of the convenience of the college to the parents, I would suggest that they try to work it in <u>up there</u>.... I would like to see Sally <u>back here</u> in about six months for further speech evaluation.**

The underlined words are not appropriate or meaningful in professional evaluation reports.

Use of Pronouns. Pronouns tend to confuse readers unless the referent for each pronoun is obvious. The reader should not have to search previous text to determine the referent for a pronoun. Referents that are not clear lead to ambiguity and inaccuracy. The first paragraph of the sample report is replete with examples of unclear pronoun use: "Mary Doe is the caseworker. It is felt that <u>she</u> is delayed in speech and language acquisition for her age." Although *she* clearly refers to Serena Phillips, the most recent person mentioned, Sally A. Smith is the person who has the speech and language delay. The next sentence, "<u>She</u> was taken into a foster home at the age of 18 months," also incorrectly refers to the caseworker and not the client. This referent problem continues throughout the first paragraph: "At that time, <u>she</u> was said to be deprived and almost in a catatonic state. <u>She</u> didn't talk at all and didn't smile." In the next example, the pronouns *she* and *her* both refer to the caseworker when they are supposed to pertain to the client: "It took several weeks for the foster parents to get <u>her</u> to smile and at 23 months of age <u>she</u> said 'mommy.'"

In the second paragraph, it is confusing as to whose mother died because in the sentence, "<u>Her</u> mother died when <u>she</u> was 13 months old," the most recent referent for both <u>her</u> and <u>she</u> is Sally's half sister. The following sentence is also problematic: "The cause of death was a stroke so we might get some hint of some of the problems that <u>she</u> had from this." Once again, the referent is inaccurate. Although the last mentioned noun was "mother," it appears that the evaluator's intent is to refer to Sally. The next example, the first sentence of the third paragraph, begins with a pronoun: "<u>She</u> has been seen at Snowtown Medical Center and <u>they</u> have stated that <u>she</u> has delayed bone age." The last referent mentioned was "mother" in the sentence, "Informally, it has been ascertained that the mother's health was quite poor during pregnancy." Another referent problem in the first sentence of the third paragraph concerns the pronoun *they*. The persons who diagnosed delayed bone age were never mentioned, and the "center" itself does not diagnose. Notice that *she* is used three times in the third paragraph before Sally is mentioned, and each use is ambiguous.

Contractions. Contractions are not generally acceptable in formal writing and are out of place except when used to cite specific examples of sentences used by the client. Two examples of contraction usage appear in the first paragraph of the report on Sally: "She <u>didn't</u> talk at all and <u>didn't</u> smile."

Abbreviations. As a general principle, abbreviations should not be used in formal writing. Only one example appears in this evaluation report: "Therefore, I will be contacting Mrs. White of Snowtown College Speech <u>Dept.</u>...."

Exceptions to the principle about abbreviation usage are allowed in technical writing where abbreviations of lengthy technical terminology are more easily recognized than the terms themselves. However, when a term is abbreviated, it must be spelled out completely the first time it appears and followed immediately by its abbreviation in parentheses. Thereafter, the abbreviation can be used in text without further explanation. An example not based on the preceding evaluation follows: "The *Peabody Picture Vocabulary Test–Third Edition* (PPVT–III) was administered to determine the client's functioning in receptive vocabulary."

First- or Third-Person Writing Style. Although active voice (i.e., use of first or third person) is typically preferred over passive voice in writing because the active voice is more forceful and direct, use of either first or third person in writing evaluation reports can cause problems. Use of first person—that is, referring to yourself as "I"—comes across as trying to increase your importance. Likewise, reference to yourself in the third person—that is, as "the evaluator"—is somewhat ambiguous and can give the impression of trying to deny your findings. Examples of first-person usage from the sample report follow:

> Therefore, I could not obtain much in the way of an articulation sample. I was able to obtain a raw score on Form A of the *Peabody Picture Vocabulary Test*.... Therefore, I will be contacting Mrs. White of Snowtown College Speech Dept. to see if she will be able to work this out. If this is not possible, then we could consider seeing Sally down here for speech therapy, but in view of the convenience of the college to the parents, I would suggest that they try to work it in up there. I would like to see Sally back here in about 6 months for further speech evaluation.

One way to avoid using first-person pronouns is to switch from active voice to passive voice. Suggestions for changing the previous excerpt to avoid using first person follow:

> Therefore, it was difficult to obtain an articulation sample. A raw score of 12 was obtained on the *Peabody Picture Vocabulary Test*.... Therefore, Mrs. White of Snowtown College Speech Department will be contacted to see if she can make suitable arrangements. If suitable arrangements cannot be made at Snowtown College, Sally will be scheduled to receive services at this facility. Because of the convenience for the parents if services were rendered at Snowtown College, it is strongly suggested that this avenue be pursued. Sally's speech and language should be reevaluated at this facility in 6 months.

The writer of the evaluation did not refer to herself in the third person. However, this problem can be rectified in the same manner as in the first-person example by using passive voice.

Another pronoun problem is that the writer used the third-person plural pronoun *we*, which should not have been used because the work was done by one person. One person performed the evaluation and that same person wrote the evaluation report. Therefore, the use of *we* is misleading:

> The hearing screening that <u>we</u> did was essentially normal. Certainly from the history that <u>we</u> obtained, it seems as though <u>we</u> are dealing with a case of delayed speech and

language acquisition…. If this is not possible then <u>we</u> could consider seeing Sally down here for speech therapy, but in view of the convenience of the college to the parents I would suggest that they try to work it in up there.

Now that you have experience critically analyzing evaluations, use this information to analyze your own evaluations. On what areas do you need to work?

General Guidelines for Speech–Language Evaluation Reports

Evaluation reports must be well written because they will be sent to other agencies or professionals. Although the following general guidelines will help you get a good start with the writing process, keep in mind that these are merely guidelines and you may have to modify your evaluation reports to meet the client's needs, a facility's format, or your supervisor's preferred format. The following content areas, which should be included in a report on the evaluation of a child's speech and language, are typically presented in the order listed: identifying information, background information, evaluation, impressions, and recommendations. Evaluations should use headings and subheadings to assist with organization and should contain the information specified later in this section. Headings and subheadings should be either underlined, boldfaced, or italicized for easy identification.

The heading for identifying information is merely implied and does not appear on written evaluations, although the actual information is presented. It is obvious what this information is, and thus a heading is not needed. However, I present this heading [in brackets] in the following text solely to emphasize organization through the use of headings.

No standard model exists for speech–language evaluation reports. However, two formats seem to be used more frequently than others. In one format, paragraphs are indented and an extra space exists between the paragraphs under the same heading; in a variation of this format, used in the examples of reports in Chapter 4, paragraphs are likewise indented but no extra space is added between paragraphs under the same heading. In the second format, which is block style, paragraphs are not indented and an extra space exists between paragraphs related to the same heading.

A question that most beginning clinicians ask is how long an evaluation report needs to be. Although there is no specific number of pages, evaluations must cover all of the basic information and then some. The amount of information depends on the nature of the client's problem(s), as well as the clinician's knowledge and ability to focus on important information.

[Identifying Information]

In the report samples in Chapter 4, I present the identifying information in the manner shown:

NAME:	FILE NUMBER:
ADDRESS:	EVALUATION DATE:
	BIRTH DATE:
PHONE:	AGE:
PARENTS (if applicable):	STUDENT CLINICIAN:
PROBLEM:	SEMESTER:

The format for this section, however, may vary across settings. Some settings require categories such as referral source, school/preschool, or family physician. A good rule of thumb is to familiarize yourself with the format used in your setting before writing your first evaluation.

The age category needs some explanation. If the client is a child, the exact age in years and months should be provided. After subtracting the child's birth date from the evaluation date, you have the child's age in years, months, and days. Generally, if the number of days is 16 or higher, you round up to the next month. For example, if a child's age is 3 years, 1 month, and 21 days, an age of 3 years 2 months should be stated. Once a child reaches adolescence, however, it usually is not necessary to state the age in years and months because typically there is no difference in speech, language, or communication functioning between, for example, age 14 years 0 months and age 14 years 11 months. The only exception is if a particular test administered differentiates between various months of a particular age, in which case it is necessary to provide the client's age in years and months.

Background Information

The background information to be obtained will vary depending on the client's age and condition. This section should include the reason the person is being evaluated as well as the source of referral. If the client is self-referred or parent referred, the reason for referral should be stated using the client's or parent's words as appropriate.

If the client was previously enrolled in therapy, state where therapy was obtained and name the clinician, if possible. Summarize the therapeutic objectives if the informant can provide this information. State when therapy began and when it ended. State the reason for termination.

If the client is a child, include speech and language milestones (e.g., age at which the first word was spoken, what the first word was, age at which two-word utterances were spoken). If the child is not yet producing two-word utterances, state how large the child's vocabulary is. If the child is not yet using words, state how he gets his wants and needs across.

Developmental milestones should be included for young children. Only include information pertaining to those milestones that should have been mastered previously. Specify at what age the child did the following: sit with support, move by creeping, sit easily unsupported, crawl, pull himself up to a standing position, take stepping movements, take the first independent step, walk when one hand was held, walk with feet slightly apart without falling, walk upstairs unassisted, walk up and down stairs alone without alternating feet, walk up stairs with alternating feet, become toilet trained during the day, and become toilet trained during the day and night.

Birth history should be reported, but again areas to emphasize will vary depending on each client. It might be important to obtain information about the following: length of pregnancy, child's birth weight, hazards present (e.g., whether labor was induced), mother's health during pregnancy, duration of labor, type of delivery (vaginal, breech, or cesarean section), instruments used during delivery, incubation at birth and length of incubation, child's color at birth, scars or bruises present at birth, length of time it took the child to regain birth weight, and whether the child had difficulty sucking.

Medical history should be included. Inquire about the client's general health and what diseases he has had. Find out if the child ever had a high fever, and if so, whether he ever had convulsions.

Additional information is needed if the client is an adult. It is important to include the client's educational and vocational history.

If much of this information appears in previous evaluations done at another or the current facility, state the significant information as well as any new information in your evaluation report. It is acceptable to refer the reader to another report by stating, "Additional background information may be found in the May [this year] evaluation report done at (complete name of the facility)," if performed at another facility, or "Additional background information may be found in the Spring [this year] evaluation report," if performed at the same facility.

In general, it will be up to you to determine the actual organization of the "Background Information" section. If you have a lot of information for particular topics (e.g., previous therapy, speech and language milestones, developmental milestones), the use of subheadings will be helpful for organizational purposes. If you do not have a lot of information, the use of new paragraphs for each topic will be adequate.

Evaluation

The "Evaluation" section should contain some brief introductory information before the discussion of specific evaluation information. Examples follow:

> **John performed all tasks willingly and interacted well with the examiner. He was quite verbal and appeared to be unaware of any communication difficulty.**

> **Ari was very cooperative at the beginning of the evaluation. After 20 minutes, his attention was lost and he could not be directed back to tasks.**

> **Zakia willingly separated from her mother and eagerly entered the evaluation room. She was extremely verbal and attempted all tasks enthusiastically.**

> **Sam performed all tasks willingly and interacted well with the examiner during the evaluation. However, he asked to have numerous items repeated on the various tests administered during the evaluation.**

> **Emily clung to her mother and tears welled in her eyes when the examiner extended a hand to lead her to the evaluation room. It was then decided that she should be accompanied by her mother, who remained present throughout the evaluation. With her mother present, Emily was cooperative and attempted all tasks.**

Speech

State the name of each speech test administered as well as what the test measures. Provide test scores and their interpretation. If the client exhibits an articulation problem, report findings in terms of omissions, substitutions, distortions, and additions. Include the position within words in which each type of error occurred. After analysis, state whether any entire phoneme class is in error. State which phonemes the child should already have mastered according to the norms accompanying the administered test or other published norms (e.g., Bowen, 1998; Lowe, 1986; Prather, Hedrick, Kern, 1975; Sander, 1972). Cite the norm used. If a client exhibits a phonological process problem, indicate the phonological processes present. Provide examples for all existing processes.

In addition to single-word production, evaluate the client's speech informally during conversation. Determine if the client's articulatory performance on single words is similar to his performance in conversation. Determine the client's percentage of intelligibility. Include a statement about the consistency of errors, the stimulability of the misarticulated sounds, and the highest level at which the client had success, if any, on errored phonemes (isolation, syllable, word, phrase, etc.). If the client has a problem, indicate whether he showed signs of awareness of the problem. If any errors are conspicuous, provide a description and explanation.

Fluency and Rate

If the client has obvious disfluencies and this is the reason that he or she is being evaluated, a different evaluation format should be followed. Analyze disfluencies in detail, and you probably do not need to look at speech and language in depth.

If the client has "normal nonfluencies," explain the nonfluencies in the report but indicate that they are to be expected for his age. If the client's fluency is within normal limits, so state.

If you are uncertain whether the client's rate is within the normal limits, tape-record a short sample of conversational speech and count the number of words produced in 1 minute. A normal speaking rate is approximately 175 words per minute.

Language

Receptive Ability. For each receptive language ability test administered, state the name and indicate what the test assessed (e.g., receptive vocabulary). Provide the results of each test and include the receptive language age if applicable. If the client has a delay, state the length of the delay. Be certain to include areas in which the client successfully performed, as well as areas in which the client experienced difficulty. In other words, thoroughly summarize the client's performance.

Go beyond formal tests, and provide evidence for all your findings. You may want to include some of the following information in your evaluation if pertinent. Does the client understand conversation, follow simple directions, understand basic concepts, identify common objects, identify body parts, identify common objects when their use is given, match colors, understand prepositions, and understand size (*big* and *little*) and quality (*more* and *less*)? Use your professional judgment to determine which aspects of receptive language should be pursued for each individual client. If these aspects were incorporated into a formal test that was administered, do not "test" them again.

Expressive Ability. The expressive language ability section should address syntax, morphology, semantics, and pragmatics. Provide the name of each test administered, and state what was assessed. State the results of each test and include the expressive language age. If the client has a delay, state the length of the delay. Include areas in which the client successfully performed, as well as areas of difficulty. Evaluate the client's language informally as well as formally. Overall, summarize the client's performance.

Oral-Peripheral Examination

The oral-peripheral examination should be performed toward the end of your evaluation. As the client is communicating and performing earlier tasks, you have the opportunity to observe the oral structure and function. Directly assess only those structures or functions that are suspect as a result of your observations.

In your report, discuss structure and function separately. It is not adequate to state that the structure and function are within normal limits; you also need to state the findings on which this conclusion of normalcy is based.

Structure. Examine the client's lips to determine if they are of normal size, shape, and symmetry. Examine the relationship of the mandible to the maxilla. Ascertain if the occlusion is normal. Examine the client's tongue to determine if it is of normal shape, size, and symmetry. Examine the hard and soft palates.

Function. Determine if the client can protrude and retract his lips at a normal speaking rate and in quick succession. Ascertain if the client can elevate, depress, protrude, retract, and lateralize his tongue. Determine if there is adequate velopharyngeal closure on the production of /ɑ/. Check the client's diadochokinesis.

Vocal Parameters

Even if the client's main complaint is not one dealing with voice, informally assess vocal parameters. Listen to the client during conversation. If his voice appears normal, state in the report that "Vocal parameters were informally assessed during conversation. Pitch, quality, and loudness were within normal limits for (name's) age, gender, and size."

However, if the client does have a voice problem, the parameters of pitch, quality, and loudness must be thoroughly evaluated.

Auditory Sensitivity

Conduct a pure-tone hearing screening test. State in your report that "A pure-tone hearing screening test was administered to assess (name's) hearing sensitivity." State the frequencies in hertz (Hz) tested and the decibel (dB) level used. Usually, the following frequencies are tested in each ear: 250, 500, 1000, 2000, and 4000 Hz. A 25-dB level is usually used. State the conditions in which the testing occurred (quiet, noisy, etc.). State if the client passed the screening in both ears, in the right ear, or in the left ear. State how the client indicated that he heard the tones.[1]

Impressions

The "Impressions" section follows from the rest of the written evaluation. In this section, you interpret the information presented in your report so the reader understands what the information means. Do not include information that is not supported by data or observations. The nature and severity of the client's speech–language problem is stated in this section and should be based on the analysis of formal and informal test results and the client's history, along with observations of the client and his parents (if applicable). Also include a statement summarizing areas of normal functioning, the prognosis for improvement and the basis for this prediction, and the type and severity of the client's problem.

---

[1]An important ethical issue regards the use of audiometry in clinical practice by speech-certified persons who are not certified in audiology. The American Speech-Language-Hearing Association (ASHA, 1994) has stated the following position:

> Individuals who hold only the Certificate of Clinical Competence in Speech–Language Pathology (CCC-SLP) may perform or supervise pure-tone air conduction hearing screening procedures for persons who can reliably participate in such procedures through conditioned play or conventional behavioral responses. The screening procedures used shall be developed in consultation with an individual holding the Certificate of Clinical Competence in Audiology and shall comply with current applicable ASHA policies. Individuals who hold only the CCC-SLP shall limit judgments and descriptive statements about the results of hearing screening procedures to a determination as to whether the person has passed or failed the screening. Persons who fail the hearing screening should be referred to a certified audiologist. (pp. 11–12)

The bottom line is that it is unethical for a speech–language pathologist to perform a hearing threshold test. Speech–language pathologists are only qualified to perform hearing screening tests and are only allowed to state if the person passed or failed. It is not ethical to interpret the findings in any other way.

Recommendations

Make certain that the report has previously provided an adequate basis for any recommendations you make. General and specific recommendations should be stated. An example follows:

> It is recommended that:
> 1. (Name) receive language therapy twice a week.
> 2. (Name) receive a thorough audiological examination to determine current hearing acuity.
> 3. Language therapy should emphasize production of two-word utterances.

Note: If you are not going to be providing the therapeutic services, it is best not to recommend particular tests or programs to be used with the client as the clinician who will provide the services may have individual preferences or limited access to materials.

[Signatures]

The heading "Signatures" is implied and does not overtly appear on evaluations. Because the signatures are obvious, they do not need to be identified with a heading. This heading appears here in brackets solely to emphasize the organizational structure of an evaluation. At the conclusion of an evaluation report, you and your supervisor need to sign it. You do not need to include your institutional affiliation if it is stated on the letterhead on which the report is prepared.

Jane Doe
Jane Doe
Undergraduate Student Clinician

Betty A. Brown
Betty A. Brown, MS, CCC/SLP
Clinical Supervisor

QUICK CHECK

> Upon completion of your evaluations, make certain you have adequately addressed all of the necessary content areas. Make certain that headings and subheadings are used appropriately.

Progress Reports: Organization and Content

As therapy progresses, you will need to write progress reports. Although these reports must also be written in a professional manner, writing progress reports is not as monumental a task as writing evaluations because many aspects of writing evaluations are incorporated into writing progress reports.

Progress reports are written on clients who have been receiving therapy to document any improvement that has been made. Progress reports are usually written at the end of each semester so the clinician who will be assigned to the client the following semester will have a good idea of what has been done and where to begin. Examples of progress reports are provided in Chapter 4.

Progress reports, like evaluations, must be of professional caliber because they will also be sent to other agencies or professionals. You may need to modify the guidelines presented in this section to meet the needs of each client. The following content areas should be included and can be presented in the order provided: identifying information, background information, additional testing, therapeutic objectives, progress and procedures, current status and impressions, and recommendations. To assist with organization, progress reports should use headings and subheadings, which should be underlined, boldfaced, or italicized for easy identification.

[Identifying Information]

In the progress report samples in Chapter 4, I present the identifying information in the manner shown:

NAME:	FILE NUMBER:
ADDRESS:	EVALUATION DATE:
	BIRTH DATE:
PHONE:	AGE:
PARENTS (if applicable):	STUDENT CLINICIAN:
	SEMESTER:

As for evaluation reports, some settings may require different formats for progress reports. Check with your supervisor before writing your first report.

Background Information

In sentence form, state the client's name and exact age in years (and months, if appropriate). State the exact name of the facility at which therapy was received. State the client's original diagnosis, the date of the diagnosis, and the severity at the time of the diagnosis. Provide the same information about diagnosis and severity for the most recent evaluation. Include the number of sessions the client attended out of the possible number he could have attended since the last evaluation. Specify the beginning and ending dates of these sessions. Any additional information that has not been included in one of the previous evaluation or progress reports should be noted in this section.

Additional Testing (Optional)

Include the "Additional Testing" section only if any additional testing was done after the initial evaluation report or most recent progress report. Frequently, tests that were administered as part of the initial evaluation are readministered later to measure progress; in this case, provide and compare the results of both test administrations.

Therapeutic Objectives

List the objectives for the current semester in the format shown:

The objectives for this semester were
1. _____
2. _____

Progress and Procedures

Address each objective individually. Summarize the actual procedure used to achieve each objective. Vary the lead-ins. An example follows: "Objective 1 (correct production of the /s/ phoneme in isolation) was accomplished by using a combination of phonetic placement and auditory stimulation." Briefly explain the techniques used. Do not state the materials used as they are not a part of the procedure. Another example is the following: "To accomplish Objective 2 (receptive identification of verbs) ...." Indicate progress, if made, by using percentages or some other objective measurement. Be certain to state the client's level of performance at the beginning of the semester as well as at the end of the semester. For example, "At the beginning of the semester, Hannah could not produce the /s/ phoneme correctly in isolation. She currently produces it correctly in 80% of her attempts." It would also be acceptable to include in this section activities that the client liked or specific techniques used to help control unwanted behaviors.

Current Status and Impressions

State the current diagnosis and compare it with the original diagnosis. Include the current severity of the problem(s). Include the prognosis for further improvement, if indicated, and support for this prognosis.

Recommendations

Indicate whether therapy should be continued or terminated. State whether the client should be reevaluated. State objectives for the next semester, if applicable, in this manner: "Pending a reevaluation in the (spring or fall) semester, possible therapeutic objectives are …" Be specific but it is not necessary to state criteria at this time.

[Signatures]

Both you and your supervisor need to sign the progress report, provide your degrees or credentials, and give your titles. An example follows:

Jane Doe
Jane Doe
Undergraduate Student Clinician

Betty A. Brown
Betty A. Brown, MS, CCC/SLP
Clinical Supervisor

QUICK CHECK

When writing progress reports, be certain to include the necessary content areas. Use appropriate headings and subheadings to assist with your organization.

After reading this chapter, you should be able to

1. state at least five problems found in the "substandard" sample evaluation provided at the beginning of the chapter.

2. state five content areas (headings) to include in a speech–language evaluation report.

3. state at least two general pieces of information to be included under each of the five content areas in a speech–language evaluation report.

4. state at least five problems to avoid while writing evaluation reports.

5. state seven content areas (headings) that might be included in a speech–language progress report.

6. state at least two general pieces of information to be included under each of the seven content areas (headings) in a speech–language progress report.

References

American Speech-Language-Hearing Association. (1994, March). Clinical practice by certificate holders in the profession in which they are certified. *Asha, 36*(Suppl. 13), 11–12.

Bowen, C. (1998). *Developmental phonological disorders: A practical guide for families and teachers.* Melbourne, Australia: ACER Press.

Dunn, L., & Dunn, L. (1997). *Peabody Picture Vocabulary Test–Third Edition.* Circle Pines, MN: American Guidance Service.

Lowe, R. (1986). *Assessment link between phonology and articulation (ALPHA).* East Moline, IL: LinguiSystems.

Prather, E., Hedrick, D., & Kern, C. (1975). Articulation development in children aged two to four years. *Journal of Speech and Hearing Disorders, 40*(2), 179–191.

Sander, E. (1972). When are speech sounds learned? *Journal of Speech and Hearing Disorders, 37*(1), 55–63.

Chapter 4

Evaluation, Reevaluation, and Progress Reports: Writing Reports That Shine

- Developing a deeper sense for writing evaluation reports
- Developing a sense for writing reevaluation reports
- Developing a deeper sense for writing progress reports

This chapter contains examples of evaluation, reevaluation, and progress reports. Although these reports are well written, some speech–language pathology supervisors may suggest revisions to reflect their preferred writing style or to meet the needs of a specific reporting agency. Because there is a zone of acceptance for professional reports, no single or best way to write reports can be offered. However, you should keep in mind a few basic guidelines when writing professional reports. According to Paul-Brown (1994, p. 41), writing should be clearly understood by the reader; therefore, content should be

1. accurate, concise, and informative
2. adapted for a potentially large readership
3. useful and relevant to other staff (i.e., so that anyone can pick up a record and continue treatment)
4. neat and legible

By following these guidelines, you can complete written material with a minimum number of rewrites and create a document that contains pertinent content and is easy to read.

One way to get a feel or sense for the flow and style of professional writing is to read and reread samples written by other professionals. The documents in this chapter provide you with a springboard into this process as you analyze the word choices and sentence structures used. Attend to the format: In these reports, paragraphs are indented with no space inserted between paragraphs. All identifying information has been changed to preserve the identity of persons involved. The actual years in which various events occurred are not provided so that information does not quickly become obsolete. (*Note:* Although reports typically do not include the authors and dates of tests, that information is added in brackets, and references are included for the purposes of this book.)

Evaluation Reports

Evaluation Report 1: Articulation

Evaluation Report 1 is an example of a report on a child referred for faulty articulation. Therefore, articulation was the area on which the clinician devoted the most time and attention. Formal assessment of the child's language ability was not necessary because no problems were evident in this area. (*Note:* "Identifying Information" appears in brackets throughout this chapter because this heading is typically only implied in these reports.)

Evaluation Report 2: Language

Evaluation Report 2 differs from the first in that background information must be obtained from the client's previous files. The major focus of the evaluation is on language. The findings are contradictory in that informal assessment revealed age-appropriate results whereas formal assessment did not. This contradiction is unusual.

Evaluation Report 3: Language and Articulation

Evaluation Report 3 is lengthy due to the clinician's thoroughness because of the extent of the child's problem. The clinician's thoroughness is evident in the background information section, which is quite comprehensive, and also in the way the language sample was analyzed and interpreted. The area of pragmatics is addressed. This child exhibits a problem in receptive language, expressive language, and articulation.

Evaluation Report 4: Fluency

When the focus of an evaluation is on fluency, as it is in Evaluation Report 4, speech and language do not necessarily have to be evaluated or included. The inclusion of speech and language varies according to the facility. Some facilities require that an informal statement be included for each speech or language area. However, if a problem is evident in any area of speech or language, it should be addressed. The structure and function of the oral-peripheral mechanism do not need to be written in detail as long as problems are not evident. Likewise, it is not necessary to discuss vocal parameters in any detail. However, if a problem is evident in any of these areas, it should be addressed thoroughly.

QUICK CHECK

Take the time to read and reread evaluations that you write upon completion. Make certain they shine! If they do not, rewrite any problematic section(s).

EVALUATION REPORT 1: ARTICULATION

Speech–Language Evaluation Report

[Identifying Information]

NAME: Rebecca Byers

ADDRESS: 00 Broad Street
Maintown, PA 00000

PHONE: 000-000-0000

PARENTS: Mary and Bill

PROBLEM: Articulation

FILE NUMBER:

EVALUATION DATE: February 4, [this year]

BIRTH DATE: December 9, [4 years ago]

AGE: 4 years 2 months

CLINICIAN: Celine Reynolds

SEMESTER: Fall [this year]

Background Information

Rebecca, age 4 years 2 months, was seen for a speech evaluation on February 4 of this year, after being referred by Alice Allan, a speech–language pathologist at the Maintown Hospital and Medical Center. Ms. Allan performed a speech and language screening. Rebecca failed the speech screening. According to Ms. Allan, Rebecca's errors consisted of /f, s, ʃ, p, t, k/. Rebecca's mother accompanied her to the screening and served as informant. When asked to describe the problem, Mrs. Byers stated, "Rebecca is difficult to understand at times."

According to Mrs. Byers, Rebecca started using sentences at 2½ years of age. Mrs. Byers was unable to provide other speech and language milestones. Developmental milestones include the following: sitting alone at 7 months, crawling at 7 months, standing at 11 months, walking at 1 year, feeding herself with a spoon at 16 months, toilet trained during the day at 2 years 8 months, and toilet trained at night at 3½ years.

Mrs. Byers stated that she had no problems with her pregnancy, but she could not provide specific information such as the length of labor or her daughter's birth weight. Regarding medical history, Rebecca has had no injuries, operations, or recent illnesses. She had the flu at 3 years of age and chicken pox at 3½ years of age.

Evaluation

Rebecca was very shy and hid behind her mother when it was time to separate from her and enter the testing room. She was able to be coaxed. Rebecca was very soft-spoken throughout the evaluation. She cooperated and performed all tasks.

Speech

The *Arizona Articulation Proficiency Scale: Third Revision* was administered to assess articulation on single words. The results were as follows:

(continues)

Omissions	Substitutions	Distortions
h (I)	b/f (I)	None
t (F)	g/k (I)	
ks (F)	d/j (I)	
ts (F)	b/p (I)	
	d/t (I)	
	w/v (I)	
	b/v (F)	
	w/r (I)	
	t/θ (I)	
	d/ð (I)	
	t/ʃ (F)	
	d/z (I,F)	
	d/s (I)	
	t/s (F)	
	b/pl (I)	
	t/tr (I)	
	t/st (I)	
	d/ld (F)	
	g/gr (I)	
	d/ʤ (I)	
	t/ʧ (I)	

Key: I = initial position; F = final position.

According to this test's norms, /h/ is mastered by 1½ years of age, /p/ by 2 years, /f/ and /k/ by 2½ years, and /j/ and /t/ by 3 years. The remaining errored phonemes are not expected to be mastered until 5 years or later. Therefore, according to the test norms, /f, k, j, p, t, h/ should have been mastered by Rebecca's age.

Rebecca's total score on this test was 71.5, which resulted in a standard score of 34 and a percentile of 6. This indicated a rating of "moderate" severity. Rebecca's intelligibility score was ranked level 4, which is interpreted as "speech is intelligible with careful listening."

Stimulability was performed to determine if Rebecca could imitate errored phonemes when given an auditory model. She was stimulable for /h/, /f/, and /j/ in the initial position of words. She was not stimulable for the remainder of the errored phonemes.

A sample of Rebecca's conversational speech was obtained to compare articulation on single words with articulation in connected speech, as well as to determine her intelligibility. The errors in connected speech were consistent with the errors on the formal test. Rebecca was unintelligible in 25% of her conversational speech.

(continues)

EVALUATION REPORT 1 (Continued)

Language Ability

Receptive

Rebecca's receptive language ability was not formally tested. Informal observation based on her ability to follow conversation and correctly answer questions indicated that her receptive language skills were within normal limits.

Expressive

Rebecca's expressive language ability was not formally assessed. Informal observation based on a sample of her conversation indicated that expressive language skills were within normal limits.

Oral-Peripheral Examination

Structure

Rebecca's lips and tongue were of normal size, shape, and symmetry. The relationship of the mandible to the maxilla was normal. Examination of the hard and soft palates revealed no abnormalities.

Function

Rebecca was able to protrude, retract, elevate, depress, and lateralize her tongue. She was able to protrude and retract both her lips and her tongue in quick succession. Adequate velopharyngeal closure was evident on production of /ɑ/. Diadochokinetic rate was judged as adequate on production of /pʌtəkə/ even though articulatory errors were present on /t/ and /k/.

Vocal Parameters

Rebecca's vocal parameters were informally assessed during conversation. Her pitch, quality, and loudness were within normal limits for her age, gender, and size.

Auditory Sensitivity

An attempt was made to screen Rebecca's hearing by administering a pure-tone screening test. However, she could not be conditioned to raise her hand upon hearing a tone. Therefore, Rebecca's hearing was informally assessed. Because she responded to questions and conversation presented at varying intensity levels, her hearing is probably within normal limits. In addition, Mrs. Byers indicated that Rebecca had passed an earlier hearing test. Further details could not be obtained as Mrs. Byers could not remember where Rebecca was tested, who tested her, or when the testing had occurred.

Impressions

Rebecca exhibits an articulation problem of moderate severity that is characterized by omissions and substitutions. A reduction in intelligibility is evident. Careful listening is necessary to understand single words. In conversation, 75% of Rebecca's output can be understood. Prognosis for improvement with therapy is good as Rebecca was stimulable to some of her errored phonemes.

(continues)

Recommendations

It is recommended that

1. Rebecca be enrolled in articulation therapy twice a week for individual half-hour sessions.
2. an attempt should be made to condition Rebecca so that reliable results can be obtained on a pure-tone hearing screening test.

Rebecca's initial therapeutic goals should be

1. to produce /p, t, f, k/ correctly in the initial and final positions of words in sentences in 90% of her attempts.
2. to produce /h/ correctly in the initial position of words in sentences in 90% of her attempts.

Celine Reynolds
Celine Reynolds
Undergraduate Student Clinician

Betty A. Brown
Betty A. Brown, MS, CCC/SLP
Clinical Supervisor

EVALUATION REPORT 2: LANGUAGE

Speech–Language Evaluation Report

[Identifying Information]

NAME: Carlos Ramirez   FILE NUMBER:
ADDRESS: 00 Mill Road   EVALUATION DATE: October 17, [this year]
          Maintown, PA 00000   BIRTH DATE: March 1, [3 years ago]
PHONE: 000-000-0000   AGE: 3 years 8 months
PARENTS: Ramon and Sue   CLINICIAN: Mary Miller
PROBLEM: Language   SEMESTER: Fall [this year]

Background Information

Carlos Ramirez, age 3 years 8 months, was initially screened for speech and language problems at the Middletown Head Start Center on September 26 of this year. The service was provided by a student from the Maintown University Speech and Hearing Center. At that time, the *Fluharty Preschool Speech and Language Screening Test–Second Edition* was administered. Carlos's chronological age at that time was 3 years 7 months. The results were as follows:

Identification Total = 5   Cutoff Score = 11
Articulation Total   = 26   Cutoff Score = 19
Comprehension Total = 6   Cutoff Score = 6
Repetition Total   = 2   Cutoff Score = 4

Carlos passed the Articulation and Comprehension portions of the test but failed the Identification and Repetition sections. Therefore, further evaluation was warranted. Thus, Carlos was seen for a language evaluation on October 17.

An informant was not present. Therefore, background information had to be obtained from Carlos's file at Middletown Head Start Center. According to the file, Carlos's medical history was not characterized by any illnesses or hospitalizations. It was also documented that Carlos had met his childhood milestones for motoric skills and normal speech and language development at the appropriate ages. However, specific ages were not provided for when each milestone was met.

Spanish is Carlos's native language and the primary language spoken in his home. However, Carlos's mother speaks English fluently. Mrs. Ramirez's description of Carlos, which appeared in his file, was "hyperactive." It was also noted in the file that Carlos's parents had been separated since he was 1 year 6 months old. Although Carlos lives with his mother and three brothers, his father visits regularly.

Additional information can be found in Carlos's file located at the Middletown Head Start Center.

(continues)

Evaluation

Carlos was cooperative during testing. He attempted all tasks.

Language Ability
Receptive

The *Peabody Picture Vocabulary Test–Revised* (Form M)[1] was administered to assess Carlos's performance on receptive vocabulary. His raw score of 8 resulted in a standard score equivalent of 61, a percentile rank of less than 1, a stanine score of 1, and an age equivalent of 2 years 2 months. His performance was 1 year 6 months below his chronological age.

Carlos correctly identified pictures of the following vocabulary words: *car, ball, money, bee, bottle, circle, plant,* and *ladder.* He did not correctly identify the following: *broom, candle, reading, full, mail, horn,* and *pulling.*

Carlos's receptive language was assessed informally. He responded appropriately to all questions asked and followed commands without difficulty. He was able to perform the following upon request: go to a shelf and select a specific toy, show how a toy worked, make a toy horse walk and jump, and put various toy animals in the barn.

Expressive

The *Expressive One-Word Picture Vocabulary Test–Revised*[2] was administered to assess Carlos's expressive semantic skills. His raw score of 27 resulted in a mental age of 2 years 9 months, a percentile rank of 3, and a stanine score of 2. His raw score was 1.3 standard deviations below the median. His performance was 11 months below his chronological age. He was able to name pictures of the following words: *boat, cat, apple, eyes, bus, tree, bear, truck, train, glasses, duck, knife, hammer, scissors, chicken,* and *tiger.* Carlos did not name the following: *pumpkin* (no response), *umbrella* (response was "rain"), *wagon* (response was "bus"), *kite* (response was "balloon"), *triangle* (response was "star"), *square* (response was "circle"), *ear* (response was "nose"), *wheel* (response was "boat"), *leaf* (response was "tree"), and *typewriter* (response was "Go like this" as typing movements were demonstrated).

The *Structured Photographic Expressive Language Test–Preschool* was administered to assess expressive language skills. Carlos's raw score of 2 placed him below the first percentile. He scored 5 standard deviations below the mean. Errors were noted on the following structures: prepositions; plural nouns /s/, /z/, and /ɨz/; plural present progressive tense verbs; possessive nouns; subject pronouns; singular present progressive tense verbs; regular past tense verbs; third-person singular copula *is;* third-person plural copula *are;* third-person singular marker on present tense of the verb; simple negation;

(*continues*)

---

[1] The *Peabody Picture Vocabulary Test–Revised* (Form M) [Dunn & Dunn, 1981] has been revised and Form M is no longer current. The most recent edition is the *Peabody Picture Vocabulary Test–Third Edition* [Dunn & Dunn, 1997].

[2] The *Expressive One-Word Picture Vocabulary Test–Revised* [Gardner, 1990] has been updated. The current edition is the *Expressive One-Word Picture Vocabulary Test–2000* [Gardner, 2000].

EVALUATION REPORT 2 (Continued)

and irregular past tense verbs. Better than 80% of the children in Carlos's age group (3-6 to 3-11) had success on the above-mentioned structures except third-person singular, regular past tense, simple negation, and irregular past tense. Therefore, Carlos did not demonstrate age-appropriate syntactic skills.

An informal language sample was obtained to assess Carlos's expressive language skills in spontaneous conversation. The mean length of utterance (MLU) computed from the sample was 4.14, with an upper bound of 11. According to Brown's stages, Carlos is functioning in Stage V. The following are some examples of his utterances: "I wanna check one more time," "Right here there are two turtles," "What do you got there?" "What is that?" "Is it like that?" "I wanna put that back," "It could fall down on the book," "But this will take it off," "This don't fit right there," "The Ninja Turtle can't fit," "I have those at home," "I'm gonna put the cow right here," "It came out," "It broke the window," "It's running," "But this will take it off," and "I will get it."

Oral-Peripheral Examination
Structure

Carlos's lips and tongue were found to be of normal size, shape, and symmetry. The relationship of the mandible to the maxilla was within normal limits. The soft palate appeared to be within normal limits. However, the hard palate was extremely high and narrow.
Function

Carlos was able to protrude and retract his lips. He could also perform these movements in quick succession. Carlos could elevate, depress, protrude, retract, and lateralize his tongue. Velopharyngeal closure was assessed on production of /ɑ/ and found to be within normal limits. Diadochokinetic rate was not within normal limits as productions were slow and arythmic.

Vocal Parameters

Pitch and loudness were within normal limits for Carlos's age, gender, and size. Vocal quality was slightly hyponasal. However, Carlos appeared to have a cold as there were several episodes of sneezing and coughing during the evaluation.

Auditory Sensitivity

A pure-tone hearing screening test was administered to assess Carlos's hearing sensitivity. The frequencies 500, 1000, 2000, and 4000 were tested at 25 dB. Carlos responded correctly to all frequencies in both ears.

Impressions

Formal test results indicate that Carlos's receptive and expressive language skills are not commensurate with his chronological age. However, informal assessment of his receptive and expressive language reveals different results in that Carlos's language func-

(continues)

tioning is appropriate for his chronological age. In Carlos's case, it is felt that formal test results are not a true indication of his language functioning.

Recommendations

Language therapy is not warranted at this time as informal assessment indicated functioning within normal limits. However, due to the disparity found between formal and informal results, Carlos's language should be reevaluated during the spring semester.

Mary Miller
Mary Miller
Undergraduate Student Clinician

Betty A. Brown
Betty A. Brown, MS, CCC/SLP
Clinical Supervisor

EVALUATION REPORT 3: LANGUAGE AND ARTICULATION

Speech–Language Evaluation Report

[Identifying Information]

NAME:	Patrick Agee	FILE NUMBER:	
ADDRESS:	00 Main Street	EVALUATION DATE:	June 30, [this year]
	Maintown, PA 00000	BIRTH DATE:	June 20, [5 years ago]
PHONE:	000-000-0000	AGE:	5 years 0 months
PARENTS:	Debra and David	CLINICIAN:	Jane Smith
PROBLEM:	Language and	SEMESTER:	Fall [this year]
	Articulation		

Background Information

Patrick Agee, a Caucasian male age 5 years 0 months, was seen at the Maintown University Speech and Hearing Center on June 30 of this year. He was referred by Mary Jones, a speech–language pathologist at Maintown Hospital's Speech and Hearing Center. Patrick's father, Mr. Agee, accompanied him to the evaluation and served as the informant during the case history interview.

Regarding prenatal history, it was reported that Mrs. Agee was under a physician's care throughout her pregnancy. Mr. Agee reported that the pregnancy was "normal" with no illness, emotional upset, or special diet. Concerning natal history, Mrs. Agee's labor lasted approximately 7 hours and Patrick was born by cesarean section. According to the informant, Patrick's birth weight was 7 pounds 3 ounces. Postnatal history revealed that Patrick has had all immunizations to date and has not had any childhood diseases. It was also reported that when Patrick was approximately 2½ to 3 years of age, he was hospitalized for 2 weeks due to urinal retention. When asked to describe Patrick's general health, Mr. Agee reported that it was "good."

According to the informant, there were no speech or language problems in the family. It was reported by Mr. Agee that he himself has a slight hearing loss. When asked to compare Patrick's development to that of other children, Mr. Agee stated, "His physical development is normal. He is below others in social–emotional development and language or communication skills."

Mr. Agee described Patrick's motor development as "normal." However, Mr. Agee stated that Patrick is still in the process of toilet training. It was reported that Patrick is able to dress himself but still has difficulty with snaps and buttons. He is able to use crayons and pencils to draw and color.

With regard to social development, Mr. Agee reported that Patrick's eye contact is not good, but is presently improving. He also stated that Patrick enjoys playing with cars and looking at books when indoors. Outdoors he enjoys playing on his swing set,

(continues)

riding his bike, and playing in his swimming pool. Mr. Agee described Patrick's personality as "pleasant, but if he is frustrated, he can be nasty."

Concerning speech and language development, Mr. Agee reported that Patrick babbled and his first word, "dada," appeared around 15 months. It was also reported that Patrick started putting words together at 2½ to 3 years of age. Mr. Agee reported that at the present time, Patrick speaks in short phrases or is echolalic. His vocabulary was reported to consist of several hundred words. Mr. Agee also stated that Patrick occasionally uses gestures alone or with short phrases. Patrick's speech–language problem was first noticed when he was around 18 months to 2 years of age.

Information regarding education was obtained. Patrick is presently attending the Middletown Head Start Center. Mr. Agee stated that Patrick gets along well with his teachers and peers. Reportedly Patrick receives speech and language therapy once a week for 30 minutes.

In addition, Mr. Agee reported that "a few months ago," Patrick went through a period of "speaking with a rough voice." He also reported that the "roughness" has since disappeared.

Evaluation

Patrick initially was unwilling to separate from his father. He sat on his father's lap for a few minutes while refusing to cooperate. However, he showed interest in the testing materials and was easily enticed into cooperating. Once Patrick became involved in the testing procedure, Mr. Agee was able to leave the room. It was sometimes difficult to keep Patrick on task during testing. Token reinforcement was necessary during part of the evaluation to maintain Patrick's attention. Periodically during the evaluation, Patrick turned away and started whining when he did not want to continue. This behavior appeared to increase as the test items became more difficult.

General Language

The *Verbal Language Development Scale, Revised,*[3] a parent report inventory that assesses a child's general language ability, was administered to Mr. Agee. A language age equivalent of 4 years 6½ months was obtained.

Receptive Language

The *Peabody Picture Vocabulary Test–Third Edition* was administered to assess single-word receptive vocabulary skill through picture identification. However, because a basal set could not be obtained, an estimate of Patrick's receptive vocabulary could not be made.

The *Preschool Language Scale–3* (PLS–3) was administered to assess Patrick's ability to receive auditory information involving concrete and abstract concepts, parts of speech, and grammatical language features. Patrick's raw score of 34 corresponds to an Auditory Comprehension Age of 3 years 5 months. Weaknesses noted include recognizing actions,

(continues)

---

[3]Mecham's *Verbal Language Development Scale* was published in 1971 and is used infrequently in current assessments.

EVALUATION REPORT 3 (Continued)

distinguishing parts, grouping objects, distinguishing prepositions, and understanding the concept of "three." Strengths were not evident.

Expressive Language

The expressive communication portion of the PLS–3 was administered to measure vocabulary, verbalized memory span, concrete and abstract thought, concept acquisition, articulation, and the ability to use grammatical features of language. A raw score of 26 was obtained, which corresponds to an Expressive Communication Age of 2 years 10 months. Weaknesses noted include using pronouns, naming objects, using plurals, conversing in sentences, answering questions logically, repeating sentences, stating opposites, and telling about remote events. Areas of strength were not evident.

During the evaluation, Patrick often imitated the clinician's utterances and intonation patterns. The function of these echoic responses was to maintain communication.

A 10-minute sample of Patrick's communication with the clinician during play was recorded. Interactions, intents, and consequences of the communication sample were analyzed to obtain pragmatic information. Patrick's interactions were classified as initiating, responding, or maintaining behaviors through three modes: paralinguistic, vocal, and verbal. His role in the interaction can be classified as follows:

	Paralinguistic	**Vocal**	**Verbal**	**Total**
initiating	0/86 = 0%	5/86 = 6%	6/86 = 7%	11/86 = 13%
responding	2/86 = 2%	14/86 = 16%	29/86 = 34%	45/86 = 52%
maintaining	0/86 = 0%	10/86 = 12%	19/86 = 22%	29/86 = 34%

Included in the vocal category were nine quick, short ventricular phonations that Patrick produced spontaneously. These included two instances of initiating, three of maintaining, and four responding behaviors during the 10-minute sample. These voiced gasps were often produced in conjunction with other communication behaviors (e.g., pointing) during the entire evaluation.

In addition, 42 spontaneous, intelligible verbal communicative behaviors were analyzed according to communicative intent by categorizing them as instrumentals (22/42 = 52%), statements (20/42 = 48%), or negations (0/42 = 0%). The instrumentals and statements were categorized as follows:

Instrumentals		**Statements**	
joint attention	3/42 = 7%	informative	20/42 = 47%
objects	3/42 = 7%	emotive	0/42 = 0%
actions	11/42 = 26%	social	0/42 = 0%
regulation of behavior	5/42 = 12%	experimental	0/42 = 0%
assistance	0/42 = 0%		
information	0/42 = 0%		

(*continues*)

Negative behaviors indicating rejection, nonexistence, or denial were not evident in the sample.

A semantic case analysis was performed on the 42 intelligible, non-echoic responses. Little semantic diversity was evident; however, the following semantic relations were observed (only semantic relations used two or more times are listed):

Action + Locative (e.g., "Put in the box")	14/42 = 33%
Action + Object (e.g., "Open the door")	4/42 = 9%
Experiencer + State + Entity (e.g., "I want baby")	2/42 = 5%
Action + Object + Locative (e.g., "Put dog on chair")	2/42 = 5%

A Type Token Ratio was computed on Patrick's 42 intelligible, non-echoic utterances to explore his use of referential meaning. The total number of different words Patrick produced was divided by the total number of words produced. A Type Token Ratio of .29 (32/110) was obtained, which indicates that very little lexical diversity was evident in the sample.

The mean length of utterance (MLU) was determined from the utterances in the 10-minute language sample. The MLU was calculated to be 3.17 morphemes when echoic utterances were excluded. The mean length of all verbal utterances was calculated to be 3.02 morphemes, which corresponds to a predicted chronological age of 34.8 months, with a standard deviation of 6.8 months. Patrick's chronological age of 58 months places him 3 standard deviations below the mean. This MLU corresponds to Brown's Stage IV. Structures normally evident at this stage that were not observed in Patrick's sample include correct use of auxiliary verbs; copulas; prepositions *on, with, of, for,* and *to;* demonstrative pronouns *this* and *that;* personal pronouns *you, me,* and *my;* and plural noun inflections /s/, /z/, and /ɨz/.

Speech

The *Goldman–Fristoe Test of Articulation 2* was administered to assess single-word articulation skills. When spontaneous productions could not be elicited, productions were obtained imitatively. Forty-nine errors were recorded out of a total of 73 phonemes tested, for an error rate of 67%. The following errors were noted:

	Initial	**Medial**	**Final**	**Blends**	
p	*	—	*	bl	b/bl
m		X*	—	br	b/br
n	X			dr	w/dr
b		*	*	fl	f/fl
g	k/g		ʔ/g	kl	kw/kl*
k		ʔ/k	—	kr	b/kr
f	*			pl	ʔ/pl
d	*			skw	θkw/skw*

(continues)

EVALUATION REPORT 3 (Continued)

	Initial	Medial	Final	Blends	
ŋ		ʔ/ŋ		sl	θ/sl
j	l/j			st	θ/st
ʃ	s/ʃ*	X*	X*	tr	tw/tr
ʧ	t/ʧ*	t/ʧ*	θ/ʧ*	hw	w/hw*
r	w/r	w/r	—		
ʤ	d/ʤ*	d/ʤ*			
θ	f/θ	f/θ			
v	b/v	f/v			
s	d/s*	X*	X*		
z	d/z				
ð	d/ð*	d/ð			

Key: ʔ = glottal stop; X = distortion; — = omission; * = interdental or labiodental.

Although some sounds were judged as correct perceptually, they were produced with incorrect placement. Many phonemes were produced with either interdental or labiodental placement. Informal analysis revealed that the following phonological processes were evident: final consonant deletion (/dʌ/ for /drʌm/ and /dʌ/ for /dʌk/), devoicing (/kʌn/ for /gʌn/), and stopping (d/s, d/z, and d/ð). Patrick was stimulable for /p, m, n, k/ at the syllable, word, and two-word phrase level. He was also able to imitate /d/ at all levels, although it was made labiodentally. Patrick was stimulable for /j/ at the syllable and word levels. Imitatively, Patrick's intelligibility is good, although the intelligibility of his spontaneous speech is poor.

Voice
Patrick's vocal parameters were informally assessed during conversation. Pitch and loudness were within normal limits for Patrick's age, gender, and size. However, his quality varied from breathy to normal to strained. Ventricular phonations were also produced in the manner of voiced gasps.

Auditory Sensitivity
An attempt was made to administer a pure-tone hearing screening test. Results could not be obtained as Patrick would not wear the headset. However, he did not have any difficulty hearing speech at varying levels of loudness throughout the evaluation.

Oral-Peripheral Examination
Structure
Patrick's lips and tongue were of normal size, shape, and symmetry. The relationship of the mandible to the maxilla was within normal limits. Examination of the hard and soft palates revealed no abnormalities.

(continues)

Function

Patrick rounded his lips, placed his upper teeth on his lower lip, and elevated, depressed, and lateralized his tongue tip upon imitation. Velopharyngeal closure was adequate on production of /ɑ/. Patrick's diadochokinetic rate was within normal limits on production of /pʌtəkə/.

Impressions

Patrick exhibits a moderate delay in receptive language, a moderate to severe delay in expressive language, and a moderate delay in articulation. Prognosis for improvement is favorable. Positive prognostic indicators include stimulability for errored phonemes as well as his young age. A negative prognostic sign is that an impairment exists in all areas tested—receptive language, expressive language, and articulation.

Recommendations

It is recommended that Patrick continue to receive speech and language therapy. If possible, he should be seen three times a week. A low-structured setting centering around Patrick's interests and daily routines may be beneficial. Relevant linguistic codes provided by the speech–language pathologist within this setting may stimulate similar relevant verbalizations from Patrick. Modification of Patrick's environment by creating various contextual situations may enhance his ability to induce content–form–use interactions. By providing appropriate contexts and functions, Patrick's attempts to use content–form interactions will be promptly rewarded by his successful communication. Modeling successful communication by another child may also be beneficial. In this manner, Patrick can first observe another child's effective use of appropriate content–form behaviors. Interpersonal functions of language (commenting about ongoing events, pretend or fantasy, and expression of emotion) can also be incorporated into the intervention procedures.

The following receptive language goals are recommended:

1. to increase recognition of actions
2. to improve ability to distinguish parts
3. to improve ability to categorize objects
4. to increase receptive vocabulary
5. to improve ability to distinguish prepositions

The following expressive language goals are recommended:

1. to increase the number of utterances that serve interpersonal functions (e.g., to obtain objects—"I want baby;" to regulate behavior of others—"Sit down"; and to call attention to self or objects and events in the environment—"Look")
2. to produce utterances in order to obtain information or assistance ("Help me")
3. to increase the number of utterances that are initiated by Patrick through joint attention activities (identify objects or events that Patrick takes an interest in—"Baby." Promptly reinforce all of Patrick's attempts at initiation.)
4. to eliminate inappropriate echoic responses

(continues)

EVALUATION REPORT 3 (Continued)

5. to eliminate inappropriate vocal behaviors
6. to increase semantic diversity by coding Agent + Action, Agent + Object, Agent + Action + Object, and Agent + Action + Object + Place relations
7. to produce Pronoun + Noun combinations in coding possession
8. to increase correct use of auxiliary verbs, copulas, prepositions, and plural nouns

The following articulation goal is recommended:

1. to produce /p, m, k, g, ŋ, ʃ, ʧ/ correctly in spontaneous speech

Jane Smith
Jane Smith
Undergraduate Student Clinician

Betty A. Brown
Betty A. Brown, MS, CCC/SLP
Clinical Supervisor

EVALUATION REPORT 4: FLUENCY

Fluency Evaluation Report

[Identifying Information]

NAME:	William Samuels	FILE NUMBER:	
ADDRESS:	00 Maintown Lane	EVALUATION DATE:	September 9, [this year]
	Maintown, PA 00000	BIRTH DATE:	March 14, [20 years ago]
PHONE:	000-000-0000	AGE:	20 years
PROBLEM:	Fluency	CLINICIAN:	Janis Foster
		SEMESTER:	Fall [this year]

Background Information

William Samuels, age 20, presently attends Maintown University. His major is undeclared at this time. His speech was evaluated at Maintown University's Speech and Hearing Center on September 9 of this year.

William's speech problem was diagnosed as stuttering in fourth grade. He received fluency therapy for 8 years while in public school. He also received therapy from Easter Seals. William indicated that these two therapy programs, which he received simultaneously, were not coordinated and contradicted each other. However, he was not able to provide details about the therapy received while enrolled in either program. William stated that his fluency problem has worsened over the years. He is very aware of his problem and would like to remediate it.

On the case history form, William indicated that his stuttering becomes more severe when he is in a new situation. He also indicated that his stuttering worsens when he is under stress. When around familiar people, William does not have as much difficulty. He indicated that he has no history of hearing problems, respiratory problems, or any illnesses or accidents that could have caused his speech problem.

Evaluation

William was very attentive during this evaluation. He was extremely cooperative. He performed all tasks completely and willingly.

(continues)

EVALUATION REPORT 4 (Continued)

Fluency

Parts of the *Stuttering Standard Interview Procedure* were administered to assess the number of stuttered words William had in various contexts. The results are as follows:

Task	Part-Word	Struggle	Prolongation	Time
		Type of Stuttering		
Automatic		1		44 sec.
Echoic		2	3	14 sec.
Reading	6	4		54 sec.
Pictures		1		3 sec.
Monologue	2	1		47 sec.
Questions	1	2	1	20 sec.
Conversation	1	2	1	39 sec.
Observation in another setting	11	2		42 sec.

Overall total = 4 minutes 23 seconds or 4.38 minutes

Part-word repetitions = 21
Struggles = 15
Prolongations = 5

Total Stuttered Words Per Minute = 9.36

According to the *Stuttering Standard Interview Procedure* norms, a normal speaker should not exceed a rate of 0.5 stuttered words per minute. William's rate of 9.36 stuttered words per minute exceeds this limit by 8.86 stuttered words per minute.

The *Stuttering Severity Instrument for Children and Adults–Third Edition* (SSI–3) was administered to assess William's fluency during reading and conversation. The results were as follows:

Frequency Task Score = 12
Duration Score = 4
Total Physical Concomitant Score = 9
Total Overall Score = 25
Severity = Moderate

According to the SSI–3 test norms, William is exhibiting stuttering of moderate severity. The estimated length of his three longest blocks was approximately 3 seconds. He exhibited all four of the physical concomitants: distracting sounds (score 2), facial grimaces (score 3), head movements (score 3), and movement of extremities (score 1).

(continues)

Auditory Sensitivity

A pure-tone hearing screening test was administered to ascertain whether William's hearing was within normal limits. William responded to 25dB tones in his right and left ears at all frequencies presented (250, 500, 1000, 2000, and 4000 Hz).

Oral-Peripheral Examination

Structure

The structure of William's oral mechanism is adequate for normal speech production.

Function

The function of William's oral mechanism is adequate for normal speech production.

Vocal Parameters

Pitch, quality, and loudness are within normal limits for William's age, gender, and size.

Impressions

William has a stuttering problem of moderate severity. Due to his awareness of his problem and strong desire to change it, prognosis for improvement is good.

Recommendations

It is recommended that William be enrolled immediately to receive fluency therapy. He should be seen individually for two ½-hour sessions per week. The following goals should be emphasized:

1. to stutter less than .5 stuttered words per minute during reading
2. to stutter less than .5 stuttered words per minute during monologue
3. to stutter less than .5 stuttered words per minute during conversation

Janis Foster
Janis Foster
Undergraduate Student Clinician

Betty A. Brown
Betty A. Brown, MS, CCC/SLP
Clinical Supervisor

Reevaluation Reports

The most noticeable difference between an evaluation report and a reevaluation report is that the background information section of the reevaluation does not include all the information contained in the initial evaluation. It does, however, refer the reader to the previous evaluation by date or possibly to the client's entire file. Previous therapy may be cited in this section. Another obvious difference is if the client's oral-peripheral examination and hearing sensitivity were within normal limits when previously evaluated, they will not be evaluated again.

Reevaluation Report 1: Articulation and Language

Reevaluation Report 1 focuses on articulation as well as receptive and expressive language. This child's native language is Spanish.

Reevaluation Report 2: Voice

Because the focus of Reevaluation Report 2 is voice, aspects pertinent to voice are emphasized. Some important information that is not described in the report is available in the client's file: Prior to receiving therapy, this client was referred to an otolaryngologist to obtain the status of the vocal cords. The results of this evaluation revealed a "normal" larynx.

QUICK CHECK

After you complete writing your reevaluations, reread them. Make certain they are reports you are proud of.

REEVALUATION REPORT 1: ARTICULATION AND LANGUAGE

Speech–Language Evaluation Report

[Identifying Information]

NAME:	Vicente Munoz	FILE NUMBER:	
ADDRESS:	00 Main Lane	EVALUATION DATE:	March 10, [this year]
	Maintown, PA 00000	BIRTH DATE:	October 4, [4 years ago]
PHONE:	000-000-0000	AGE:	4 years 5 months
PARENT:	Jesus and Elena	CLINICIAN:	Theresa Ramos
PROBLEM:	Articulation and	SEMESTER:	Spring [this year]
	Language		

Background Information

Vicente Munoz is 4 years 5 months old. He attends the afternoon class at the Maintown Preschool. He has been receiving services from Maintown University's Speech and Hearing Center since the fall of last year. These services have been provided by a student clinician. After Vicente was evaluated last November, he was placed in group language stimulation, where the emphasis is on naming body parts in English. Vicente's native language is Spanish, which is the language spoken in his home. His English vocabulary is quite limited. Please refer to his initial evaluation dated November 10 of last year for further information.

Evaluation

Vicente was very quiet. It was difficult for him to attend to a task for more than 10 minutes.

Speech

The *Goldman–Fristoe Test of Articulation 2* was administered to assess Vicente's articulation on single words. The results follow:

Substitutions		Omissions	
Consonants	**Blends**	**Consonants**	**Blends**
v/b (M)	kw/kl	/m/ (M)	/r/ in /dr/
s/f (F)	pw/pl	/n/ (F)	/l/ in /fl/
t/d (F)	sk/skw	/b/ (F)	
t/ʃ (F)	tw/tr	/g/ (F)	
t/ʧ (I)		/ŋ/ (F)	
ʃ/ʧ (M,F)		/v/ (F)	
w/l (F)		/z/ (F)	
w/r (M,F)			

(continues)

REEVALUATION REPORT 1 (Continued)

Substitutions		**Omissions**	
Consonants	**Blends**	**Consonants**	**Blends**
j/ʤ (F)			
ʃ/ʤ (F)			
f/θ (I)			
d/θ (M,F)			
b/v (I,M)			
d/z (M)			
d/ð (I,M)			

Key: M = medial position; F = final position; I = initial position.

According to Sander's norms, the phonemes /m/, /n/, and /b/ should be mastered before age 2 and /g/, /ŋ/, and /d/ should be mastered at age 2. The phonemes /f/, /r/, and /l/ should be mastered at 3 years of age and /ʧ/, /ʃ/, /ʤ/, /z/, and /v/ at age 4. Because Vicente is 4 years 5 months old, the phonemes stated above should all be mastered. Vicente's other errored phonemes are not expected to be mastered at his age. However, many of his misarticulations may be the result of his Spanish-speaking background. Vicente had 34 errors, which resulted in a percentile rank of 4.

Vicente's stimulability was assessed to determine which errored phonemes could be imitated in the initial, medial, and final positions of syllables, words, and sentences. Vicente was stimulable on /v/ in the initial, medial, and final positions of words in sentences; /n/ in the initial and medial positions of words in sentences; /ʃ/, /l/, and /d/ in the initial, medial, and final positions of words; /f/ in the initial and final positions of words; and /b/ in the initial and medial positions of words. Vicente was not stimulable for other errored phonemes at any position.

A conversational speech sample was taken to determine Vicente's intelligibility, to assess his ability to articulate in connected speech, and to compare his misarticulations in conversation to those on the *Goldman–Fristoe Test of Articulation 2*. The results indicated that Vicente is unintelligible in connected speech when the context is not known. When context is known, only a few key words are intelligible. Errors noted in conversation were consistent with errors noted on the formal articulation test.

Language

Receptive

The *Preschool Language Scale–3* (PLS–3) was administered to formally assess Vicente's receptive language. His raw score of 28 resulted in a standard score of 70, a percentile rank of 2, and an age equivalent of 2 years 10 months. Performance is 17 months below his chronological age. Vicente passed all items between the ages of 2-6 and 2-11, which included descriptive concepts, part–whole relationships, and under-

(continues)

standing pronouns. However, he did not perform successfully on items between the ages of 3-0 and 3-11, which included understanding negatives, comparing objects, and indicating body parts on himself.

Expressive

The PLS–3 was administered to formally assess expressive language. Vicente's raw score of 20 is equivalent to a standard score of 61, a percentile rank of 0, and an age equivalent of 2 years 2 months. His performance is 2 years 3 months below his chronological age. Vicente passed all items between the ages of 1-6 and 1-11, which included having a vocabulary of at least 10 words, naming objects, producing a succession of single-word utterances, and using one pronoun. Vicente was not successful on items at the next age level (2-0 to 2-11), as he was unable to combine three or four words in spontaneous speech, answer wh– questions, produce basic sentences, or use possessives.

A language sample was obtained to further assess expressive language. The majority of Vicente's responses consisted of single words used for labeling. Expanded utterances could not be elicited. However, Vicente asked one question, "What's that?" Twenty-five utterances, containing 32 morphemes, were obtained, which resulted in a mean length of utterance of 1.3. This placed Vicente in Brown's Stage I of early language development. These results were consistent with formal testing.

Overall Language

Vicente's standard score total of his receptive and expressive performance was 131, which resulted in a total language standard score of 62, a percentile rank of 1, and an age equivalent of 2 years 7 months. He is functioning 1 year 10 months below his chronological age.

Oral-Peripheral Examination

Structure

Vicente's lips and tongue are of normal size, shape, and symmetry. The relationship of the mandible to the maxilla is within normal limits. Examination of the hard and soft palates revealed no abnormalities.

Function

Vicente rounded his lips; placed his upper teeth on his lower lip; and elevated, depressed, and lateralized his tongue tip. Velopharyngeal closure was adequate on production of /ɑ/. Diadochokinetic rate was within normal limits as assessed on production of /pʌtəkə/.

Auditory Sensitivity

A pure-tone hearing screening test was not administered as hearing sensitivity was within normal limits when previously assessed on November 10 last year. Informal assessment during this reevaluation further indicated that hearing was not a problem at this time.

Impressions

Vicente has a severe receptive and severe expressive language impairment in English, which is probably the result of Spanish being his native language as well as Spanish being

(continues)

the only language spoken in his home. Vicente also has a severe articulation problem in English. However, a number of his misarticulations are the result of his Spanish-speaking background. It is thought that with continual language stimulation in English, Vicente's ability to imitate words and, if Vicente's attention can be maintained, prognosis for improvement of the English language are favorable.

Recommendations

It is recommended that Vicente receive language therapy on an individual basis three times a week for half-hour sessions. It is further recommended that Vicente's receptive and expressive Spanish be evaluated to make certain that an impairment exists only in English. Goals should consist of the following:

1. correct receptive identification of pictures in 90% of his attempts
2. correct expressive identification of pictures in 90% of his attempts
3. correct categorization of pictures in 90% of his attempts

Theresa Ramos
Theresa Ramos
Undergraduate Student Clinician

Betty A. Brown
Betty A. Brown, MS, CCC/SLP
Clinical Supervisor

REEVALUATION REPORT 2: VOICE

Speech–Language Evaluation Report

[Identifying Information]

NAME: Alice Kerr

ADDRESS: 00 Market Street

           Maintown, PA 00000

PHONE: 000-000-0000

PROBLEM: Voice

FILE NUMBER:

EVALUATION DATE: October 8, [this year]

BIRTH DATE: May 2, [21 years ago]

AGE: 21 years

CLINICIAN: Betsy Maher

SEMESTER: Fall [this year]

Background Information

Alice Kerr is 21 years old. She received voice therapy during the spring semester last year at Maintown University's Speech and Hearing Center. Therapy focused on the use of relaxation techniques to improve vocal quality. Progress was made throughout the semester, although occasional regression was noted. Alice's long-term goal of using good vocal quality during conversation in 90% of her attempts was not met. A reevaluation took place on September 22 of this year.

Alice described definite vocal abuse situations. She also stated that her voice tires after using it for an extended amount of time. Please refer to her file for additional information.

Evaluation

Vocal Parameters

The *Voice Assessment Protocol for Children and Adults* was administered to assess Alice's pitch, loudness, and quality. Breathing and rate of speech were also assessed.

Pitch

Alice's habitual pitch was 196 Hz, which corresponds with the musical note G3. This was found by having her count to 5 and prolong the vowels. Her optimal pitch was 293 Hz, which corresponds with the musical note D4. This was determined by using both the loud-sigh technique and the natural speech method. Alice's pitch ranges from 169 Hz to 659 Hz. In musical terms, Alice's range goes from C3 to E5. Alice did not use her optimal pitch while speaking; instead she used a lower pitch. This lower pitched voice seemed to be a habit. Pitch breaks were not demonstrated and normal inflections were used.

Loudness

Alice demonstrated a typical level of loudness that was comfortably maintained. Her range of loudness was normal and was evenly emphasized. She has specific situations in her life, such as band and teaching twirling, that cause her to use increased loudness levels.

(continues)

REEVALUATION REPORT 2 (Continued)

Quality

The quality of Alice's voice was assessed. Her voice was moderately breathy and hoarse. There was a definite harsh strain heard in her voice. Her speech was also characterized by slight hypernasality.

Breath Features

Speech breathing was assessed. Alice used the clavicular region. A slight audible inhalation was evident during speech breathing. Alice stated that she uses an excessive amount of words per breath. She also commented that she sometimes runs out of breath when trying to finish sentences. Alice was able to prolong the /ɑ/ sound for the normal amount of time, but her voice fatigued toward the end. The s/z ratio was 1.07, which suggested a normal larynx, but her voice tired at the end.

Rate

Alice's rate of speech was assessed. Her rate of 180 words per minute was within normal limits.

Connected Speech

A sample of conversation was obtained to assess Alice's voice in connected speech, compare findings to those obtained during formal testing, and evaluate intelligibility. Alice's voice was found to be breathy and harsh with slight hypernasality. Her breathing was clavicular instead of diaphragmatic. Alice's speech is intelligible. The problems found in connected speech were consistent with those found during formal testing.

Oral-Peripheral Examination

An oral-peripheral examination was performed to assess the structure and functioning of the oral mechanism.

Structure

Alice's oral structures are adequate for speech production.

Function

Alice had some difficulty performing diadochokinetic movements. While repeating /p/, /t/, and /k/ individually in rapid succession and while repeating /pʌtəkə/, her voice demonstrated fatigue.

Auditory Sensitivity

No formal hearing test was administered at this time. Alice's hearing was found to be within normal limits when tested last semester. Based on informal assessment, there was no reason to question whether her hearing status changed.

Impressions

According to the test results, Alice has a voice problem of moderate severity. Her vocal quality is characterized as being breathy and hoarse with periodic episodes of a harsh

(continues)

strain. Both hypernasality and clavicular breathing are evident. Alice's habitual pitch is lower than her optimal pitch by 97 Hz. An improvement in quality would probably result in usage of optimal pitch. Alice frequently finds herself involved in vocal abuse situations; she is aware of these situations. Prognosis for improvement is good if Alice attends therapy and actively participates on a regular basis, applies facilitating techniques in all speaking situations, uses diaphragmatic breathing, and eliminates all episodes of vocal abuse.

Recommendations

It is recommended that Alice receive half-hour sessions of voice therapy twice a week on an individual basis. Goals should include the following:

1. using diaphragmatic breathing during conversation in 90% of her attempts
2. using good vocal quality during conversation in 90% of her attempts
3. decreasing the number of vocal abuse episodes to less than two per week

Betsy Maher
Betsy Maher
Undergraduate Student Clinician

Betty A. Brown
Betty A. Brown, MS, CCC/SLP
Clinical Supervisor

Progress Reports

A progress report is a statement of a client's performance during therapy. The frequency with which progress reports are written varies depending the type of client as well as the setting. In a university setting, the academic calendar determines when such reports are written. Progress reports are usually written at the end of each semester; however, exceptions may be made if the same clinician services a client for both the fall and spring semesters.

Progress Report 1: Articulation

Progress Report 1 indicates improvement in the area of articulation, but not enough to change the diagnosis. This client had difficulty self-monitoring; therefore, this aspect was not emphasized. Additional testing was not warranted.

Progress Report 2: Articulation

Progress Report 2 also shows improvement in the area of articulation. Self-monitoring was emphasized. A comparison of formal test results is also included.

Progress Report 3: Language and Attending Behavior

Language and attending behavior are the areas of focus in Progress Report 3. A comparison of formal test results is made.

QUICK CHECK

Check and recheck your progress reports. When a client demonstrates progress, make certain it is clearly stated. Make certain the procedures used to accomplish the various objectives are clear to the reader.

PROGRESS REPORT 1: ARTICULATION

Progress Report

[Identifying Information]

NAME: Maria Little   FILE NUMBER:
ADDRESS: 00 Pine Street   EVALUATION DATE: April 30, [this year]
               Maintown, PA   BIRTH DATE: December 9, [4 years ago]
PHONE: 000-000-0000   AGE: 4 years 5 months
PARENTS: Louisa and Jacob   CLINICIAN: Chris Pratt
PROBLEM: Articulation   SEMESTER: Spring [this year]

Background Information

Maria Little, age 4 years 5 months, was seen for articulation therapy at the Speech and Hearing Center at Maintown University. She attended 20 sessions out of the 23 held from February 6 to April 30 this year. Tests indicated that Maria's articulation errors consisted of the following substitutions: b/f, b/p, and g/k. Omissions of /h/ and /t/ were also evident. These errors resulted in unintelligibility at times. Please refer to previous reports for further information.

Therapeutic Objective

The long-range goal for this semester was for Maria to

1. produce /p, t, f, k/ correctly in the initial, medial, and final positions of words in sentences and /h/ in the initial position of words in sentences during 90% of her attempts.

Progress and Procedures

The objective—production of /p/, /t/, /f/, and /k/ in all positions of words in sentences and /h/ in the initial position of words in sentences—was accomplished by first explaining how the articulators were used to produce speech sounds. Maria then imitated /p/, /t/, /f/, /k/, and /h/ in isolation when given a model and a visual cue. Placement cues were given if necessary. When successful on imitation, Maria produced each phoneme after being shown a visual cue. She then progressed to imitating phonemes in consonant–vowel (CV) syllables, although branch steps were needed. The branch step for /p/ and /h/ consisted of production of the target sound, followed by a pause and then the vowel sound. The branch step for /f/ consisted of prolonging /f/ and then producing the vowel sound. Maria imitated /p/, /t/, and /k/ in CV syllables and then progressed to production in vowel–consonant (VC) syllables. Imitation of /t/, /k/, and /p/ in VC syllables was attempted next. A branch step of saying the vowel followed by a

(continues)

PROGRESS REPORT 1 (Continued)

pause and then saying /t/ was necessary. This step was accomplished by showing Maria the phoneme symbol card and modeling the syllable. Maria then advanced to a branch step, which led her to the original objective of imitating the syllable without a branch step. She then progressed to the production of /p/, /t/, and /k/ in VC syllables. Maria then advanced to production of /k/ in words. She was shown pictures containing the target in the initial position and had to imitate a model.

Although the semester's goal was not met, progress is evident. Maria is now able to correctly imitate /p/ and /t/ in the initial position of syllables in 70% and 75% of her attempts, respectively. She is now able to correctly produce /p/ and /t/ in the final position of syllables in 100% and 90% of her attempts, respectively. She correctly imitates the phonemes /f/ and /h/ in the initial position of syllables in 90% and 85% of her attempts, respectively, and the /k/ phoneme in the initial position of words in 90% of her attempts.

Current Status and Impressions

Maria continues to exhibit an articulation problem of moderate severity that is characterized by omissions, substitutions, and a reduction in intelligibility. However, Maria is now able to correctly produce /p/ and /t/ in the final position of syllables, imitate /f/ and /h/ in the initial position of syllables, and imitate /k/ in the initial position of words. Based on Maria's good attendance, her active participation in therapy, Mrs. Little's follow-through with all therapy assignments, and Maria's gains made thus far, prognosis for further improvement is favorable.

Recommendations

It is recommended that Maria be reevaluated at the beginning of the next fall semester and continue to receive therapy if warranted. Possible goals for future therapy for Maria are

1. to correctly produce /h/, /p/, /t/, and /f/ in all positions of words in 90% of her attempts.
2. to correctly produce /k/ in all positions of sentences in 90% of her attempts.

Chris Pratt
Chris Pratt
Undergraduate Student Clinician

Betty A. Brown
Betty A. Brown, MS, CCC/SLP
Clinical Supervisor

PROGRESS REPORT 2: ARTICULATION

Progress Report

[Identifying Information]

NAME: Kerry Payne
ADDRESS: 00 University Road
                 Maintown, PA 00000
PHONE: 000-000-0000
PROBLEM: Articulation

FILE NUMBER:
EVALUATION DATE: May 14, [this year]
BIRTH DATE: April 1, [19 years ago]
AGE: 19
CLINICIAN: Sandy Storm
SEMESTER: Spring [this year]

Background Information

Kerry Payne, age 19, received therapy for a mild articulation problem from September 10 to December 12 during the fall semester last year. She was then reevaluated at the Maintown University's Speech and Hearing Clinic on February 4 of this year. She continued to be diagnosed as having a mild articulation problem characterized by distortions of the /tʃ/ and /ʃ/ phonemes. Therefore, Kerry was again enrolled in therapy. This semester the therapeutic emphasis was placed on correct production of the /ʃ/ phoneme in conversation. Kerry attended 26 of 28 sessions from February 4 to May 14. For further information, please refer to the client's file.

Therapeutic Objectives

The objectives for therapy were to enable Kerry

1. to produce the /ʃ/ phoneme correctly as a releasor and arrestor in syllables in 90% of her attempts.
2. to monitor her productions of the /ʃ/ phoneme correctly as both releasor and arrestor in syllables in 90% of her attempts.
3. to produce the /ʃ/ phoneme correctly as a releasor and arrestor in words in 90% of her attempts.
4. to monitor her productions of the /ʃ/ phoneme correctly as both releasor and arrestor in words in 90% of her attempts.
5. to produce the /ʃ/ phoneme correctly as a releasor and arrestor in phrases in 90% of her attempts.
6. to monitor her productions of the /ʃ/ phoneme correctly as both releasor and arrestor in phrases in 90% of her attempts.
7. to produce the /ʃ/ phoneme correctly in conversation in 70% of her attempts.
8. to monitor her productions of the /ʃ/ phoneme correctly in conversation in 90% of her attempts.

(continues)

PROGRESS REPORT 2 (Continued)

Progress and Procedures

Objective 1 (correct production of /ʃ/ in syllables) was accomplished by having Kerry correctly produce the /ʃ/ phoneme in isolation without a model. These productions were then incorporated into syllables as releasors and arrestors. Kerry was not able to correctly produce /ʃ/ in syllables at the beginning of the semester, but now produces it in 95% of her attempts.

Objective 2 (correct monitoring of /ʃ/ in syllables) was met by using ear training and tape recordings. Kerry was required to listen to recordings of her syllable lists and identify and self-correct each error. Her monitoring ability in syllables has increased from 10% at the beginning of the semester to 98% currently.

Objective 3 (production of /ʃ/ in words) was fulfilled by having Kerry incorporate her correct productions of the /ʃ/ phoneme in syllables into words. At the beginning of the semester, she was unable to correctly produce /ʃ/ in words. Currently, Kerry correctly produces /ʃ/ in words in 90% of her attempts.

The procedure used to meet Objective 4 (correct monitoring of /ʃ/ in words) was Kerry's use of ear training to locate her errors. She was required to stop immediately after each error in a word and self-correct it. Her monitoring ability in words has increased from 10% previously to 95% presently.

Objective 5 (production of /ʃ/ in phrases) was accomplished by having Kerry maintain her correct productions of /ʃ/ in words and integrate these words into phrases. Initially, Kerry was not able to produce the /ʃ/ phoneme correctly in phrases. Currently, she produces it correctly in 96% of her attempts.

Objective 6 (correct monitoring of /ʃ/ in phrases) was fulfilled by using ear training and self-correction. Kerry was asked to state whether each of her productions was correct. She was required to self-correct errors. Initially, Kerry was not able to monitor her productions in phrases. She now correctly monitors 90% of her productions.

Objective 7 (correct production of the /ʃ/ phoneme in conversation) was obtained by having Kerry engage in spontaneous conversation while concentrating on the proper production of the /ʃ/ phoneme. Her ability to produce /ʃ/ correctly in conversation has increased from 0% at the beginning of the semester to 96% currently.

To accomplish Objective 8 (correct monitoring of the /ʃ/ phoneme in conversation), ear training and self-correction were used. Kerry was asked to correct any mistakes she made on /ʃ/ in conversation immediately after they occurred. She was also told to anticipate any problems with producing /ʃ/ spontaneously and to prevent any distortions from occurring. Her monitoring ability at the beginning of therapy was 10%. She is now able to correctly monitor 98% of her productions.

(continues)

Results of Standardized Testing

The *Screening Deep Test of Articulation* was administered on February 4 and readministered on May 7. The results of both tests were as follows:

Consonant Correctly Articulated	In Percentage of 10 Contexts	
	February	May
/s/	100	100
/l/	100	100
/r/	100	100
/ʧ/	10	10
/ʃ/	0	90
/θ/	100	100
/k/	100	100
/f/	100	100
/t/	100	100

Correct productions of the /ʃ/ phoneme increased from 0% in February to 90% in May. Emphasis has not yet been placed on production of the /ʧ/ phoneme; therefore, the percentage of correct production remained the same.

The *Deep Test of Articulation* (sentence form) was also administered during February and May to reassess production of the /ʃ/ and /ʧ/ phonemes. The results follow:

Phoneme	February		May	
	Number of Contexts	Percentage of Attempts	Number of Contexts	Percentage of Attempts
Releasor				
/ʧ/	5 of 22	23	18 of 22	82
/ʃ/	0 of 22	0	20 of 22	91
Arrestor				
/ʧ/	2 of 24	8	16 of 24	67
/ʃ/	0 of 24	0	23 of 24	96

Improvement was noted from February to May on production of the /ʃ/ phoneme as both a releasor and arrestor. Improvement was also noted on production of /ʧ/ in both releasing and arresting positions.

Current Status and Impressions

Although progress was evident this semester, Kerry's initial diagnosis of a mild articulation problem characterized by distortions of the /ʃ/ and /ʧ/ phonemes remains correct.

(continues)

PROGRESS REPORT 2 (Continued)

Prognosis for further improvement is good based on her performance this semester (good attendance, active participation in therapy, and follow-through on all assignments).

Recommendations

Kerry should receive further remediation at the Maintown University's Speech and Hearing Center next fall. She should be seen individually twice a week for half-hour sessions. Therapeutic goals, pending reevaluation after summer vacation, may consist of the following:

1. to maintain correct production of /ʃ/ in conversation in 90% of her attempts
2. to maintain correct monitoring of /ʃ/ in conversation in 90% of her attempts
3. to produce /tʃ/ correctly in all positions of words in 90% of her attempts
4. to monitor /tʃ/ correctly in words in 90% of her attempts
5. to produce /tʃ/ correctly in words within phrases in 90% of her attempts
6. to monitor productions of /tʃ/ correctly in phrases in 90% of her attempts
7. to produce /tʃ/ correctly in conversation in 90% of her attempts
8. to monitor productions of /tʃ/ correctly in conversation in 90% of her attempts

Sandy Storm
Sandy Storm
Undergraduate Student Clinician

Betty A. Brown
Betty A. Brown, MS, CCC/SLP
Clinical Supervisor

PROGRESS REPORT 3: LANGUAGE AND ATTENDING BEHAVIOR

Progress Report

[Identifying Information]

NAME: Joshua Fox

ADDRESS: 00 Center Street
                  Maintown, PA 00000

PHONE: 000-000-0000

PARENTS: Jamie and Bill

PROBLEM: Language and
                  Attending Behavior

FILE NUMBER:

EVALUATION DATE: December 15, [this year]

BIRTH DATE: January 19, [5 years ago]

AGE: 5 years 11 months

CLINICIAN: Jalisa Davis

SEMESTER: Fall [this year]

Background Information

Joshua Fox, age 5 years 11 months, received language therapy at the Maintown Medical Center from September 20 to December 15 this year. Services were provided by a student majoring in speech–language pathology at Maintown University. Joshua attended 19 of 22 sessions. He also receives physical and occupational therapy at Allville Speech Clinic in Allville, Pennsylvania, to remediate his developmental delays. Joshua received speech and language therapy last fall and spring semesters to remediate a moderate articulatory and language delay. For further information, please see the evaluation dated September 20.

Therapeutic Objectives

Joshua's therapeutic objectives for this semester were

1. to attend for 25 minutes in a structured therapy session.
2. to increase expressive vocabulary by 10 words.
3. to comprehend 5 prepositions of location and time in 90% of his attempts.

Progress and Procedures

Objective 1—to attend for 25 minutes—was accomplished by using a variety of techniques. Sessions were held in an environment that was as quiet and clutter-free as possible. When extraneous noises distracted Joshua and he looked away, his head was turned in the direction of the therapy materials and he was immediately reinforced verbally. The activities and materials used in a session were changed to maintain Joshua's attention. Visual memory activities were used to increase Joshua's attention and concentration. He was presented with two pictures that were then placed face down. The clinician pointed to a picture, and Joshua named the picture, which remained face down. This

(continues)

PROGRESS REPORT 3 (Continued)

activity enabled Joshua to increase his visual memory such that he could name concealed pictures on three cards. Joshua is now able to attend for a 25-minute structured therapy session with only an occasional reminder to sit up and look at the therapeutic materials.

To accomplish Objective 2—increase expressive vocabulary by 10 words—the *World Book Dictionary* was consulted to obtain a list of age-appropriate words. The objective was accomplished using materials such as pictures, blocks, and puzzles. "Happy" and "sad" were explained using pictures and actual facial expressions. The clinician discussed with Joshua items and occurrences that made Joshua happy. The shapes of blocks (*square, round, triangle, rectangle*) were explained using visual, auditory, and tactile senses. Joshua felt each shape in both hands to learn the concept of shapes. He first grouped and sorted blocks of similar shape, and he also receptively identified the shapes. Expressive identification of the shapes of the blocks is sporadic, but when Joshua is motivated, he is able to name the different shapes appropriately. Words expressing qualities (*hot, cold, empty, full*) were emphasized during play situations. When Joshua washed his hands, the difference between hot and cold water was discussed. Joshua is able to receptively identify hot and cold water, but he expressively identifies all water as "hot." "Empty" and "full" were explained using boxes of blocks and puzzles that have individual pieces. Joshua learned that the spaces without a puzzle piece were "empty," and when the puzzle was completed, it was "full." He also removed all the blocks from a box to make it "empty" and replaced them to make it "full." The concept of "another" was explained while Joshua built with blocks and drew happy face cards. Whenever he wanted another card, he had to ask for it using the word "another." Joshua now uses these words correctly and spontaneously in the therapy session.

Objective 3—comprehension of locative and time prepositions—was accomplished using play therapy including blocks, trucks, and farm animals. The words *before, behind, after, in,* and *under* were emphasized. Joshua was exposed to the locative prepositions in play activities where he was told to "put the block behind the cow," "put the block in the dump truck," and "make the truck go behind the dump truck." *Under* was illustrated using a sheet and various toys, placing everything under the sheet. Joshua put blocks *in* the box, *under* chairs, and *behind* chairs. The word *before* was explained using sequencing puzzles such as building a snowman. Joshua also looked at pairs of pictures and pointed to the one that came *before*. Joshua comprehends these prepositions in 90% of his attempts.

Results of Testing

Receptive Language
The *Utah Test of Language Development–Third Edition* was administered in September and again in December to formally assess Joshua's receptive language ability. Joshua

(*continues*)

achieved a language age equivalent of 2 years 10 months in September and an age equivalent of 3 years 3 months in December. In September, Joshua was able to identify pictures of objects and actions and was able to follow two-step directions such as "point to your ears and touch your nose." By December, Joshua is able to follow simple three-step directions. He receptively identified the colors red, blue, and yellow. Joshua also recognized body parts on the doll, the clinician, and himself. (Joshua did not have success on these latter items during the September testing.)

Expressive Language

The *Utah Test of Language Development–Third Edition* also was administered in September and again in December to formally assess Joshua's expressive language ability. Joshua achieved language age equivalents of 2 years 10 months in the initial testing and 3 years 3 months in the final testing. During the final testing, Joshua did not name colors, but he was able to name pictures of common objects. Joshua repeated three digits and four words in a complex sentence. The length of the utterances Joshua uses to communicate his needs has increased from "Go play now" to "We're going to play." Although progress was evident, Joshua is functioning at a level 2 years 8 months below his chronological age.

Informal assessment of Joshua's language ability reveals an increase in original spontaneous language such as greetings and questions. Joshua immediately says "hi" to those people he recognizes and says "bye" when they leave. He also asks many wh–questions about things in the environment that distract him (e.g., "Where you going?" "What's he doing?"). Joshua occasionally initiated conversation about himself (e.g., "I have my pictures at home," "My mom's coming"). He has been observed interacting with his classmates during free play as well as structured activity.

Current Status and Impressions

Joshua's language ability in September was 2 years 11 months below his chronological age and is now only 2 years 8 months below his chronological age. Joshua's attention span has improved so that he is able to concentrate on structured therapeutic activities for the duration of the session. Joshua continues to exhibit moderate receptive and expressive language delays. Progress is evident, although it is slow. Prognosis for further improvement is good due to Joshua's good attendance, his improved attending behaviors, and his family's motivation, cooperation, and follow-through.

(continues)

PROGRESS REPORT 3 (Continued)

Recommendations

Joshua should continue to receive language therapy on an individual basis twice a week for half-hour sessions. Objectives for next semester are the following:

1. increasing the length of utterances
2. increasing spontaneous language
3. increasing expressive vocabulary

Jalisa Davis
Jalisa Davis
Undergraduate Student Clinician

Betty A. Brown
Betty A. Brown, MS, CCC/SLP
Clinical Supervisor

KNOW IT, USE IT!

After reading this chapter, you should be able to

1. write an evaluation with less than five corrections as determined by your supervisor.
2. write a reevaluation with less than five corrections as determined by your supervisor.
3. write a progress report with less than five corrections as determined by your supervisor.

References

Dunn, L. M., & Dunn, L. M. (1981). *Peabody Picture Vocabulary Test–Revised.* Circle Pines, MN: American Guidance Service.

Dunn, L. M., & Dunn, L. M. (1997). *Peabody Picture Vocabulary Test–Third Edition.* Circle Pines, MN: American Guidance Service.

Fluharty, N. (2000). *Fluharty Preschool Speech and Language Screening Test–Second Edition.* San Antonio, TX: Psychological Corp.

Fudala, J. (2000). *Arizona Articulation Proficiency Scale: Third Revision.* Los Angeles, CA: Western Psychological Services.

Gardner, M. F. (2000). *Expressive One-Word Picture Vocabulary Test–2000.* Novato, CA: Academic Therapy Publications.

Gardner, M. F. (1990). *Expressive One-Word Picture Vocabulary Test–Revised.* Novato, CA: Academic Therapy Publications.

Goldman, R., & Fristoe, M. (2000). *Goldman-Fristoe Test of Articulation 2.* Circle Pines, MN: American Guidance Service.

McDonald, E. T. (1964). *A Deep Test of Articulation: Sentence Form.* Pittsburgh, PA: Stanwix House.

McDonald, E. T. (1976). *A Screening Deep Test of Articulation with Longitudinal Norms.* Pittsburgh, PA: Stanwix House.

Mecham, M. (1971). *Verbal Language Development Scale, Revised.* Circle Pines, MN: American Guidance Service.

Mecham, M. (1989). *Utah Test of Language Development–Third Edition.* Austin, TX: PRO-ED.

Paul-Brown, D. (1994). Clinical record keeping in audiology and speech–language pathology. *Asha, 36,* 40–42.

Pindzola, R. H. (1987). *Voice Assessment Protocol for Children and Adults.* Austin, TX: PRO-ED.

Riley, G. D. (1994). *Stuttering Severity Instrument for Children and Adults–Third Edition.* Austin, TX: PRO-ED.

Ryan, B. P., & VanKirk, B. (1971). *Monterey Fluency Program.* Monterey, CA: Monterey Learning Systems.

Sander, E. (1972). When are speech sounds learned? *Journal of Speech and Hearing Disorders, 37*(1), 55–63.

Werner, E., & Kresheck, J. (1983). *Structured Photographic Expressive Language Test–Preschool.* San Antonio, TX: Psychological Corp.

World book dictionary. (1990). Chicago: World Book.

Zimmerman, I., Steiner, V., & Pond, R. (1992). *Preschool Language Scale–3.* San Antonio, TX: Psychological Corp.

Chapter 5

Progress Notes

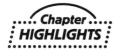 • Background information on progress notes
• Writing progress notes
• Analyzing progress notes
• Problems to avoid while writing progress notes

This chapter provides information and examples to help you write progress notes, which are also called daily logs. These notes become part of the client's permanent file. Following a discussion of the functions of progress notes, examples of cumulative progress notes are presented and analyzed. Samples of problematic progress note entries and suggestions for improvement are then provided.

Background

Accurate records are needed to record therapy and ensure the integrity and accountability of the clinicians. Paul-Brown (1994) stated, "clear and comprehensive records are necessary to justify the need for treatment, to document the effectiveness of that treatment, and to have a legal record of events" (p. 40). Cornett and Chabon (1988) further noted that "progress notes provide a complete and continuous record of all contacts (e.g., phone calls, letters, observations, therapy services, cancellations, clients' expressions of satisfaction or complaints about therapy, clinicians' suggestions or referrals) with or on behalf of the client" (p. 106). The American Speech-Language-Hearing Association (ASHA, 1992) requires that "accurate and complete records are maintained for each client and are protected with respect to confidentiality" (p. 64).

Knepflar and May (1992, p. 23) advised that

good progress notes will usually include the following:

1. Brief notes concerning specific clinical management techniques and materials used.
2. Interpretation of how the patient responded and statements regarding the patient's progress.
3. Suggestions or assignments given to the patient and, when appropriate, recommendations for the next session.

Not all authorities agree on the necessity to include all of Knepflar and May's suggestions in every progress note entry, but each entry must at the minimum include the client's performance on each objective. There is no standard length for a progress note entry. It has to be accurate and complete, and it does not have to be long. The number of objectives worked on during a particular therapy session is a good predictor of the length of the entry. A progress note entry addressing a client's performance on two objectives should not be as long as one including performance on five objectives.

Progress notes must be objective rather than subjective. That is, they must be based on observable and verifiable behaviors rather than on personal reflections, feelings, prejudices, or perceptions. Paul-Brown (1994) stated that, with regard to clinical records, one should enter "only what has taken place, not anticipated activities or observations" (p. 42).

Each progress note entry should be dated for the day the therapy session was conducted, *not* the date the entry was written (it is recommended that entries should always be written on the day of the session). In addition, each entry should be signed *except* when more than one entry appears on a page. In this case, the first entry should be signed and all other entries on that page can be initialed. For organizational purposes, each page should be numbered. If you are making entries on both sides of the paper, it is less confusing if the front and back of each page has either a different number (1, 2, ...) or a different letter (1A, 1B, ...).

Each progress note entry should be self-contained. It should be understood without reading the progress note preceding or following it. The note should not refer the reader to other entries.

Writing progress notes is not an end in and of itself. Progress notes should be scrutinized to determine the flow and direction of the therapeutic program. It should be possible to understand the therapeutic regimen simply by looking at and comparing the client's performance on each objective across sessions. Questions such as these should be answered: Is the client having success? If so, is it appropriate to increase the complexity of the task? Is the client not performing successfully? If not, is it appropriate to continue to work on that objective? Should a different procedure be used? Is a branch step necessary? Is the objective not appropriate at this time?

If the client is performing successfully on an objective, the complexity should be increased. Success is measured by whether or not the client has met the criterion, which is usually, but not always, set at correct performance in 90% of the attempts. Sometimes this 90% criterion must be achieved in two or three consecutive sessions. Likewise, if the client is not performing successfully, the complexity should be decreased. If the client does not perform successfully on a particular objective, it is necessary to determine why. Perhaps the complexity is still too difficult, or perhaps the objective is not appropriate for the client at this time. In any case, it is necessary to make changes in the therapeutic program. At times it is appropriate for progress notes to include the types of errors made when a client is not successful. It is often possible to gain insight by analyzing the client's errors or error patterns. Progress note entries can also be used to examine the response rate and determine whether it is adequate or needs to be increased.

Progress notes can follow different formats. Although the objectives and the client's performance must be provided, performance can be stated either in sentence form or by simply stating the results. If using the latter format, do not use any more words than necessary. Sometimes a charting format is used. The actual format used is up to the discretion of the supervisor.

Cumulative Progress Note Entries

Sample

The client about whom the following progress notes were written was 6 years 1 month old at the time the initial entry was made. A phonological problem of moderate severity was diagnosed. The focus of therapy was on the processes of deletion of final consonants and cluster reduction. This client was expected to meet a criterion of 90% correct on 2 consecutive days prior to advancing in therapy. These entries do not reflect the beginning of the client's therapy program. The numbers of the objectives do not remain constant, and objectives are numbered according to the order of focus within each session. These progress note entries, covering 12 consecutive sessions, are written in narrative form. It is not necessary to number the sessions when writing progress notes; however, it was done here for the sole purpose of providing ease of reference for the analysis that appears later in this chapter. Stating the nature of the errors made in this particular case is unnecessary because they are either the use of open syllables or cluster reduction, depending on which objective is emphasized. This information was clearly stated in the initial entries. (In the entries that follow, the objective appears first and then the client's performance.)

Session 1

3/20/[year]

Objective 1: Tom will close syllables in spontaneously produced monosyllabic target words in 90% of his attempts.

> He closed syllables in 16 of 20 monosyllabic target words (80%). When a cloze procedure was used, he closed syllables in 14 of 20 attempts (70%).

Objective 2: Tom will correctly imitate the consonant clusters /st/, /sk/, and /sp/ when a pause is evident between the two consonants in 90% of his attempts.

> He correctly imitated /s/ + /t/ in 6 of 8 attempts (75%); /s/ + /k/ in 5 of 8 attempts (63%); and /s/ + /p/ in 7 of 8 attempts (88%).

3/22/[year]–4/3/[year]

> Spring Break. Client did not receive services.

Session 2

4/4/[year]

Objective 1: Tom will close syllables in spontaneously produced monosyllabic target words in 90% of his attempts.

> He closed syllables in 24 of 25 target words (96%). When a cloze procedure was used, he closed syllables in 18 of 20 attempts (90%).

Objective 2: Tom will correctly imitate the consonant clusters /st/, /sk/, and /sp/ when a pause is evident between the two consonants in 90% of his attempts.

> He correctly imitated /s/ + /t/ in 7 of 8 attempts (88%); /s/ + /k/ in 6 of 9 attempts (75%); and /s/ + /p/ in 8 of 8 attempts (100%).

Session 3

4/7/[year]

Objective 1: Tom will close syllables in spontaneously produced monosyllabic target words in 90% of his attempts.

> He closed syllables in all 25 target words (100%). When a cloze procedure was used, he closed syllables in 19 of 20 attempts (95%).

Objective 2: Tom will close syllables in spontaneously produced monosyllabic target words in a carrier phrase in 90% of his attempts.

He closed syllables in 35 of 45 monosyllabic target words in a carrier phrase (78%).

Objective 3: Tom will correctly imitate the consonant clusters /st/, /sk/, and /sp/ when a pause is evident between the two consonants in 90% of his attempts.

He correctly imitated /s/ + /t/ in 9 of 10 attempts (90%); /s/ + /k/ in 8 of 10 attempts (80%); and /s/ + /p/ in 9 of 10 attempts (90%).

Session 4

4/9/[year]

Objective 1: Tom will close syllables in spontaneously produced monosyllabic target words in a carrier phrase in 90% of his attempts.

He closed syllables in 50 of 55 attempts (91%).

Objective 2: Tom will correctly imitate the consonant clusters /st/ and /sk/ when a pause is evident between the two consonants in 90% of his attempts.

He correctly imitated /s/ + /t/ in 18 of 20 attempts (90%) and /s/ + /k/ in 23 of 24 attempts (96%).

Objective 3: Tom will correctly imitate the consonant clusters /st/ and /sp/ in isolation without a pause in 90% of his attempts.

He correctly imitated /st/ in 16 of 20 attempts (80%) and /sp/ in 17 of 20 attempts (85%).

Session 5

4/10/[year]

Objective 1: Tom will close syllables in spontaneously produced monosyllabic target words in a carrier phrase in 90% of his attempts.

He closed syllables in 40 of 42 attempts (95%).

Objective 2: Tom will close syllables in monosyllabic target words in spontaneously produced phrases in 90% of attempts.

He closed syllables in 13 of 20 monosyllabic target words (65%) in spontaneously produced phrases.

Objective 3: Tom will correctly imitate the consonant cluster /sk/ when a pause is evident between the two consonants in 90% of his attempts.

He correctly imitated /s/ + /k/ in 19 of 20 attempts (95%).

Session 6

4/11/[year]

Objective 1: Tom will close syllables in monosyllabic target words in spontaneously produced phrases in 90% of his attempts.

He closed syllables in 27 of 36 monosyllabic target words (75%) in spontaneously produced phrases.

Objective 2: Tom will correctly imitate the consonant clusters /st/, /sk/, and /sp/ in isolation without a pause in 90% of his attempts.

He correctly imitated /st/ in 9 of 10 attempts (90%); /sk/ in 14 of 15 attempts (93%); and /sp/ in 18 of 20 attempts (90%).

Session 7

4/14/[year]

Objective 1: Tom will close syllables in monosyllabic target words in spontaneously produced phrases in 90% of his attempts.
Tom closed syllables in 20 of 25 monosyllabic target words in spontaneously produced phrases (80%).

Objective 2: Tom will correctly imitate the consonant clusters /st/, /sk/, and /sp/ without a pause in 90% of his attempts.
He correctly imitated /st/ in 18 of 20 attempts (90%); /sk/ in 9 of 10 attempts (90%); and /sp/ in 24 of 25 attempts (96%).

Objective 3: Tom will correctly imitate the consonant clusters /st/, /sk/, and /sp/ in the initial position of words in 90% of his attempts.
He correctly imitated /st/ in 7 of 10 words (70%); /sk/ in 6 of 10 words (60%); and /sp/ in 8 of 10 words (80%).

Session 8

4/17/[year]

Objective 1: Tom will close syllables in monosyllabic target words in spontaneously produced phrases in 90% of his attempts.
Tom closed syllables in 18 of 22 monosyllabic target words in spontaneously produced phrases (82%).

Objective 2: Tom will correctly imitate the consonant clusters /st/, /sk/, and /sp/ in the initial position of words in 90% of his attempts.
He correctly imitated /st/ in all 10 attempts (100%); /sk/ in 7 of 10 attempts (70%); and /sp/ in 9 of 10 attempts (90%).

Session 9

4/19/[year]

Objective 1: Tom will close syllables in monosyllabic target words in spontaneously produced phrases in 90% of his attempts.
Tom closed syllables in 18 of 20 monosyllabic target words in spontaneously produced phrases (90%).

Objective 2: Tom will correctly imitate the consonant clusters /st/, /sk/, and /sp/ in the initial position of words in 90% of his attempts.
He correctly imitated /st/ in all 12 attempts (100%); /sk/ in 16 of 20 attempts (80%); and /sp/ in 14 of 15 attempts (93%).

Objective 3: Tom will correctly spontaneously produce the consonant clusters /st/ and /sp/ in the initial position of words in 90% of his attempts.
He correctly produced /st/ in the initial position of 6 of 10 words (60%) and /sp/ in 7 of 10 words (70%).

Session 10

4/22/[year]

Objective 1: Tom will close syllables in monosyllabic target words in spontaneously produced phrases in 90% of his attempts.

Tom closed syllables in 25 of 26 monosyllabic target words in spontaneously produced phrases (96%).

Objective 2: Tom will close syllables in all words in spontaneously produced phrases in 90% of his attempts.

He closed syllables in 8 of 10 words (80%) in spontaneously produced phrases.

Objective 3: Tom will correctly imitate the consonant cluster /sk/ in the initial position of words in 90% of his attempts.

He correctly imitated /sk/ in the initial position in 18 of 20 attempts (90%).

Objective 4: Tom will correctly spontaneously produce the consonant clusters /st/ and /sp/ in the initial position of words in 90% of his attempts.

He correctly produced /st/ in the initial position of 9 of 10 words (90%) and /sp/ in 18 of 20 words (90%).

Session 11

4/25/[year]

Objective 1: Tom will close syllables in all words in spontaneously produced phrases in 90% of his attempts.

He closed syllables in 18 of 20 words (90%) in spontaneously produced phrases.

Objective 2: Tom will correctly imitate the consonant cluster /sk/ in the initial position of words in 90% of his attempts.

He correctly imitated the consonant cluster /sk/ in the initial position of all 10 words (100%).

Objective 3: Tom will correctly spontaneously produce the consonant clusters /st/, /sk/, and /sp/ in the initial position of words in 90% of his attempts.

He correctly produced /st/ in 19 of 20 words (95%); /sk/ in 6 of 10 words (60%); and /sp/ in 9 of 10 words (90%).

Session 12

4/27/[year]

Objective 1: Tom will close syllables in all words in spontaneously produced phrases in 90% of his attempts.

Tom closed syllables in 45 of 48 words (94%) in spontaneously produced phrases.

Objective 2: Tom will correctly spontaneously produce the consonant cluster /sk/ in the initial position of words in 90% of his attempts.

He correctly produced /sk/ in 14 of 40 words (70%).

Objective 3: Tom will correctly spontaneously produce the consonant clusters /st/ and /sp/ in the initial position of words in sentences in 90% of his attempts.

He correctly produced /st/ in the initial position of 8 of 10 words in sentences (80%) and /sp/ in 12 of 16 words in sentences (75%).

4/29/[year]
Cancelled due to client illness

Analysis of Progress Note Entries

Objective: Addition of Final Consonants

In this section, the previous progress note entries are analyzed and discussed to determine if the flow and direction of the therapeutic program are sound. It is important to again note that the criterion is correct usage in 90% of the client's attempts and that this criterion must be achieved on 2 consecutive days. The first objective, "Tom will close syllables in spontaneously produced monosyllabic target words ..." was worked on in Session 1, but criterion was not met. Criterion was met in Session 2. Because criterion had to be met on 2 consecutive days, this objective remained a focus during Session 3. Criterion was again met. Therefore, later in Session 3, a new objective, related but more complex, was introduced: "Tom will close syllables in spontaneously produced monosyllabic target words in a carrier phrase...." Criterion was not met in this session, but it was met in Sessions 4 and 5. The complexity of this task was then increased in Session 5 by changing the focus from carrier phrases to spontaneously produced phrases: "Tom will close syllables in monosyllabic target words in spontaneously produced phrases...." Criterion was not met in Sessions 5, 6, 7, or 8; however, improvement in performance can be seen (65%, 75%, 80%, and 82%, respectively). Criterion was met in Sessions 9 and 10. Therefore, the task was again increased in complexity during the latter portion of Session 10: "Tom will close syllables in all words in spontaneously produced phrases...." Criterion was not met during Session 10, but was met during Sessions 11 and 12. A further increase in complexity is now warranted. Although additional sessions were not provided in the progress note entries, realistic future objectives might be as follows: "Tom will close syllables in all words in spontaneously produced sentences," "Tom will close syllables in all words spoken during 30 seconds of conversation," and "Tom will close syllables in all words spoken during 1 minute of conversation." If believed necessary, reading could be incorporated between the focus on sentences and conversation.

Objective: Cluster Production

The objective, "Tom will correctly imitate the consonant clusters /st/, /sk/, and /sp/ when a pause is evident between the two consonants ...," was introduced in Session 1. Criterion was not met on any of the clusters during this session (75%, 63%, and 88%, respectively). Criterion was met for the first time on /s/ + /p/ (100%) in Session 2, but not on /s/ + /t/ (88%) or /s/ + /k/ (75%). Criterion was met for the second time on /s/ + /p/ and for the first time on /s/ + /t/ (90%) in Session 3. Criterion was met for the second time on /s/ + /t/ in Session 4. Therefore, it was appropriate to again increase the complexity on /sp/ and /st/ during the latter part of Session 4. However, /s/ + /k/ was worked on first and criterion was met (96%) for the first time. Therefore, the next objective, "Tom will correctly imitate the consonant clusters /st/ and /sp/ in isolation without a pause …," was introduced. Criterion was not met on either cluster during this session. The cluster /sk/ was still being worked on with a pause between the consonants, and criterion was met for the second time (95%) in Session 5. Therefore, all three clusters imitated without a pause could be emphasized in Session 6. Criterion was met for the first time on all three clusters during this session and for the second time during Session 7. Therefore, the complexity was again increased as can be seen in the objective, "Tom will correctly imitate the consonant clusters /st/, /sk/, and /sp/ in the initial position of words…." Criterion was not met on any of the clusters during this session, but was met on /st/ (100%) and /sp/ (90%) for the first time during Session 8 and for the second time during Session 9 (100% and 93%, respectively). During the latter half of Session 9, the objective, "Tom will correctly spontaneously produce the consonant clusters /st/ and /sp/ in the initial position of words …," was introduced. Criterion was not met in this session, but was met in both Sessions 10 and 11. Because the objective, "to imitate the consonant cluster /sk/ in the initial position of words …," met criterion in Sessions 10 and 11, /sk/ was also included with /sp/ and /st/ in the objective, "spontaneous production in the initial position of words …," during the latter part of Session 11. The clusters /st/ and /sp/ had already met criterion in Session 10 and did so again in Session 11. Criterion was not met on /sk/ during Session 11. Because criterion was met on /st/ and /sp/, complexity on these two clusters was again increased. The new objective, "Tom will correctly spontaneously produce the consonant clusters /st/ and /sp/ in the initial position of words in sentences …," was introduced in Session 12. Criterion was not met during this session.

Summary of Progress Note Entries

In analyzing Tom's performance, it is apparent that the objectives were appropriate. They were not so easy that he was immediately successful. They were not so difficult that success could not be attained. The objectives were appropriately graded in complexity in that each was slightly more difficult than the preceding one. Success on a preceding objective was necessary for all following objectives. Analysis of the progress note entries enables one to conclude that the flow and direction of the therapeutic program was appropriate for this client. All of these points are reflected in these progress notes, as they should be. Progress notes that are not well written are neither clear nor useful, as discussed in the next section.

QUICK CHECK

> After writing a progress note entry, make certain it follows from the previous entry. Compare entries to make certain progress is evident on a particular objective. Use the information recorded in your progress notes to help guide you in further planning the client's therapy program.

Problematic Entries

Several examples of problematic progress note entries are presented and discussed in this section, followed by revisions. Entries are not based on the same client; therefore, there is no continuity between or among entries.

Problem 1: No Objective Stated

11/13/[year]
Mary did not meet the objective.

$$/b/ \; 17/20 = 85\%$$
$$/d/ \; 17/20 = 85\%$$
$$/g/ \; 15/20 = 75\%$$

Mary was tired today. However, she watched me carefully as I produced the sounds in consonant–vowel (CV) combinations in the mirror.

Discussion and Revision. The objective was never stated. Based on the commentary, the objective can be hypothesized but might be misconstrued. Many readers would get the impression that the client is spontaneously producing the phonemes when in fact the client is imitating. The statement, "Mary was tired today," is subjective. An acceptable revision follows:

11/13/[year]
The objective is to imitate the /b/, /d/, and /g/ phonemes correctly in CV combinations.

Results:
/b/ 17/20 = 85%
/d/ 17/20 = 85%
/g/ 15/20 = 75%

Mary yawned 10 times and put her head on the table twice during this session.

QUICK CHECK

Always make certain that the objective is clearly stated in each progress note entry.

Problem 2: No Objective—Client's Performance Ignored

11/20/[year]
> **Four objectives were attempted. The results fol-**
> **low: review of imitation on two-syllable words**
> **5/10 (50%); production of two-syllable words 4/10**
> **(40%); imitation of three-syllable words 2/10**
> **(20%); and production of three-syllable words 1/10**
> **(10%). Criterion was not met on any objective.**

Discussion and Revision.   Again, the objective is not stated, but can be inferred and possibly misconstrued. The biggest problem inherent in this entry involves ignoring the client's performance. The client did not meet criterion on the review, which was imitation of two-syllable words, the least complex objective attempted during this session. Because the client did not have success imitating two-syllable words, the clinician should not have progressed to producing two-syllable words, let alone imitation and production of three-syllable words, which are all not only more complex but naturally build on the less complex objective. This clearly is an example of not letting the client's performance guide clinical decisions. In this case, decreasing the complexity of the task, not increasing it, would have been appropriate. An acceptable revision follows:

11/20/[year]
> **The first objective is to correctly imitate two-sylla-**
> **ble words. David did so on 5 of 10 words (50%).**
> **This task was then modified. As each word was**
> **presented, the clinician tapped each syllable on the**
> **table. David correctly imitated both the word and**
> **the tapping in 9 of 10 attempts (90%). The next**

task consisted of the clinician saying the words, but not tapping. David correctly imitated the production and tapped the syllables on his own in 8 of 10 attempts (80%) on his first trial and 10 of 10 attempts (100%) on his second trial. David then imitated 18 of 20 two-syllable words (90%) without tapping.

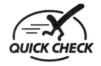

QUICK CHECK

Use the client's performance to determine whether the therapeutic focus is on target or whether it needs to be changed or modified.

Problem 3: Data Incomplete

2/15/[year]
> **Jon will correctly produce /n/, /p/, /f/, /k/, /d/, /b/, and /g/ in the initial position of words in 90% of his attempts.**

> **Result: 36/40**

Discussion and Revision. On the surface, the entry looks well written. Both the objective and the result are clearly stated. The percentage was omitted, but 36 of 40 is 90%, so criterion was met. It is best, however, to keep separate data and record results on each phoneme so problematic areas are not masked. In actuality, the results were /n/, 5 of 5 (100%); /p/, 5 of 5 (100%); /f/, 6 of 6 (100%); /k/, 6 of 6 (100%); /d/, 4 of 8 (50%); /b/, 5 of 5 (100%); and /g/, 5 of 5 (100%). Note that Jon did not have success on the phoneme /d/. However, when cumulative results were provided (36 of 40), it appeared that criterion was met. Therefore, the specific results on each phoneme were masked. It would be unfair to expect the client to function at a higher level on the /d/ phoneme, which would be the next step in his therapeutic program. An acceptable revision follows:

2/15/[year]
> **Jon will correctly produce /n/, /p/, /f/, /k/, /d/, /b/, and /g/ in the initial position of words in 90% of his attempts.**

> **Results:**
> **/n/ 5 of 5 (100%) /d/ 4 of 8 (50%)**
> **/p/ 5 of 5 (100%) /b/ 5 of 5 (100%)**

/f/ 6 of 6 (100%) /g/ 5 of 5 (100%)
/k/ 6 of 6 (100%)

Provide data for each objective, as well as for each part of each objective in your progress notes.

Problem 4: Ambiguity

10/25/[year]

> **Mercedes will auditorily and tactually discriminate between voiced and voiceless phonemes during 90% of her attempts.**

> **Results: 35 trials; 63%**

> **Mercedes was bored at times. She had difficulty sitting properly on her chair. Her attention span was extremely short.**

Discussion and Revision. Either the voiced and voiceless phonemes should have been listed, or the objective should have read, "between *all* voiced and voiceless phonemes." Otherwise, the phonemes included are ambiguous. The client attempted 35 trials, but the number correct was not stated. Because the client was only successful on 63% of her attempts, the errors should have been listed. More information is necessary. The clinician should have included the client's performance on each phoneme, as this is most beneficial for designing the therapeutic program. The last three statements in the entry are subjective. An acceptable revision follows:

10/25/[year]

> **Mercedes will auditorily and tactually discriminate between the voiced and voiceless phonemes /p/, /b/, /t/, /d/, /k/, /g/, /f/, and /v/ during 90% of her attempts.**

> **Results:**
> **/p/ 8 of 10 (80%) /b/ 6 of 10 (60%)**
> **/t/ 9 of 10 (90%) /d/ 7 of 10 (70%)**
> **/k/ 8 of 10 (80%) /g/ 6 of 10 (60%)**
> **/f/ 7 of 10 (70%) /v/ 6 of 10 (60%)**

Overall results:
voiced 32 of 40 (80%)
voiceless 25 of 40 (63%)

Errors: Mercedes stated that 8 voiced phonemes were voiceless and 15 voiceless phonemes were voiced.

Mercedes frequently looked out the window—eight times during the session. She got up out of her chair four times during this session. The longest she attended to a task today was 3 minutes.

QUICK CHECK

Upon completion of your progress note entries, reread them. Make certain to provide as much information as possible about the client's performance. Everyone reading your entries should be able to interpret them in the manner in which you intended.

Problem 5: Wrong Emphasis

2/16/[year]

Today's session consisted of elicitation of the /s/ and /z/ phonemes in monologue. The client was required to describe visual stimuli provided by the clinician in the form of action pictures while correctly producing the target phonemes in continuous speech. Marco correctly produced the target phoneme with the following results:

/s/ 34 of 36 attempts (94%)
/z/ 33 of 36 attempts (92%)

The clinician provided a verbal prompt upon presentation of each stimulus picture, such as "What is the girl doing?" or "What is the boy wearing?" Marco is constantly able to monitor his speech during monologue, as evidenced by his frequency of self-corrections without the presence of a model. The client must continue to be reminded to monitor his speech during informal conversation with the clinician.

Discussion and Revision. One problem intrinsic to this entry is that the focus appears to be on the clinician more than on the client. In the opening sentence, "Today's session consisted of elicitation of the /s/ and /z/ phonemes in monologue," the word *elicitation* is incorrect; it is the clinician who elicits and the client who produces. Therefore, the emphasis should be placed on the client and the client's production to meet the criterion, not the clinician's elicitation. There are three additional unnecessary references to the clinician in this entry. Furthermore, stating the stimulus materials used, action pictures, is not necessary as it does not serve any purpose in this particular entry. It is not a particular program being followed. Upon further analysis, the implied objective—production of stated phonemes in monologue—was not even attempted. Asking questions such as "What is the girl doing?" or "What is the boy wearing?" does not engage the client in monologue, but instead prompts the client to produce responses to specific questions within a structured situation. The phrase "while correctly producing the target phonemes in continuous speech" is misleading for the reasons given above. Lack of accountability is evident regarding Marco's ability to "monitor his speech during monologue, as evidenced by his frequency of self-corrections without the presence of a model." How accurate is his monitoring? How many self-corrections were made? To be accountable, the clinician must address and answer these questions.

It is difficult to revise this entry because the objective is not clearly stated and, upon analysis, is ambiguous. Is the objective "Marco will correctly produce the /s/ and /z/ phonemes while answering specific questions in 90% of his attempts" or "Marco will correctly produce the /s/ and /z/ phonemes during monologue in 90% of his attempts"? Because of the ambiguity, the entry will be revised reflecting both of these possible objectives. An acceptable revision for the first interpretation follows:

2/16/[year]

> **The objective was correct production of /s/ and /z/ while answering specific questions (e.g., "What is the girl doing?" "What is the boy wearing?").**
>
> > **Results:**
> > **/s/ 34 of 36 (94%)**
> > **/z/ 33 of 36 (92%)**
>
> **Marco monitored all 72 productions correctly (100%) and self-corrected 4 of his 5 erred productions (80%).**

An acceptable revision for the second interpretation follows:

2/16/[year]
> **The objective—Marco will correctly produce the /s/ and /z/ phonemes in monologue—was accomplished by having Marco select three topics to discuss. While talking, he correctly produced the /s/ phoneme in 34 of 36 attempts (94%) and /z/ in 33 of 36 attempts (92%). He correctly monitored all 72 productions (100%) and self-corrected 4 of his 5 errors (80%).**

QUICK CHECK

> Remember that the client is the recipient of your therapy. State all objectives in your progress note entries in terms of what the client will do, not what you will do.

Subjective-Objective-Assessment-Plan Format

Another format for problem-oriented progress notes is the subjective-objective-assessment-plan (SOAP) format (Hegde & Davis, 1995, p. 129). Often used in medical and other settings, the SOAP note format is used to record and analyze data pertinent to a client's performance in therapy. The frequency with which SOAP notes are written varies. Some settings require one SOAP note to be written for the week regardless of the number of therapy sessions rendered, whereas other settings require one SOAP note to be written per therapy session. SOAP notes should be written as concisely and neatly as possible. It is not necessary to use complete sentences. Abbreviations may be used as long as they are meaningful to those persons reading the notes. Each part of the SOAP note is addressed separately here.

Subjective

The first part of the SOAP note includes subjective observations. The information included in this section varies depending on the patient, his problem(s), and his situation. Subjective notes might include the following:

- A description of how the patient feels (e.g., "Mr. Gadani was in good spirits today.")
- The client's, the clinician's, or the family's impressions of the client's behavior (e.g., the clinician's observation that "Mr. Lee's attention span was very limited," or a report on a spouse's observation: "Mrs. Jones reported that her husband was communicating better today.")
- A description of physical characteristics (e.g., "Mr. Herring seemed to have greater use of his right hand today.")
- A report on sensory characteristics (e.g., "The patient's wife reported that her husband's hearing aid is not working right.")
- Comments about conditions of the testing situation (e.g., "Johnny was distracted by the sound of the lawn mower cutting grass outside," or "Mr. and Mrs. Smith were both in the room when Johnny was being tested.")

Use direct quotes, such as the following, to support statements when possible.

Stephanie appeared upset today. She stated, "My best friend isn't talking to me."

Matt's mother is pleased. She said, "Matt is talking so much better!"

Holly looked better today. Her nurse stated, "She's very alert today."

Other subjective statements include "Johnny is very motivated" and "Jeffrey's behavior interfered with the session." Although it is important to use facts to support statements when possible, this becomes problematic because facts are not a part of the subjective portion but instead belong in the objective portion. Therefore, the use of facts to support statements is demonstrated in the next section, on the objective part of the SOAP format.

Objective

The facts belong in the objective part of the SOAP note. For example, facts are needed to support the last two statements made in the previous section on the subjective part. A fact supporting the subjective statement, "Johnny is very motivated," is "Instead of finding ten objects beginning with /s/, he found twenty." A fact supporting the subjective statement, "Jeffrey's behavior interfered with the session," is "He refused to respond 18 times during the session." It is up to the person writing the SOAP note to choose whether to use numerals or to write the words for the numerals. Most clinicians prefer to use numerals because they are shorter and take less time.

Measurable information is included in the objective section. If any testing was done, list the test(s) as well as the client's performance. An example follows:

The following tests were administered:

Peabody Picture Vocabulary
    Test–III   **Age: 8 years 8 months**

Expressive Vocabulary Test   **Age: 5 years 3 months**

Test of Language Development–Primary:3
    Picture Vocabulary   **Age: 6 years 0 months**
    Relational Vocabulary   **Age: 5 years 8 months**
    Oral Vocabulary   **Age: 4 years 8 months**
    Grammatic Understanding   **Age: 4 years 6 months**
    Sentence Imitation   **Age: 4 years 7 months**
    Grammatic Completion   **Age: 4 years 5 months**

If therapy was the session's focus, state the goal(s) in a behavioral objective format and then indicate the client's performance. If applicable, compare the client's performance with that of his previous session, as in the following examples:

Vijay will correctly produce /s/ in the initial position of words in 90% of his attempts. He correctly produced /s/ in the initial position of words in 30 of 40 attempts (75%), as compared to 25 of 40 (63%) in the last session. A 12% improvement is evident.

Derrick will spontaneously use noun + verb combinations 8 times during the session. Today he spontaneously produced 6 noun + verb combinations compared to 3 during the last session.

Assessment

In the assessment portion of the SOAP note, interpret the subjective observations and objective data; summarize the data; and if possible, make a statement regarding the severity of the problem. An example follows:

The client presents with a severe phonological process problem. It is characterized by consistent deletion of final consonants, fronting, and stopping.

This section also includes comments on the client's performance, including both strengths and weaknesses. Hypotheses for why change did or did not occur may also be included.

Plan

Recommendations for future action and the course of treatment are outlined in the plan section. The initial SOAP note addresses whether or not therapy is recommended. If therapy is recommended, the location (unless implied) and frequency of therapy should be stated. The plan part of the first SOAP note is the place to recommend therapy on a trial basis or suggest a reevaluation in 3 or 6 months. The plan section is also the appropriate place to suggest referrals to other specialists. If a therapy program is already in progress, specifically state the therapy goals for the next session and future diagnostic goals, if applicable. All goals must be written in a behavioral objective format:

> **Connor will correctly imitate /s/ in the final position of words in 70% of his attempts.**

> **Rachel will spontaneously use noun + verb combinations in 90% of the obligatory contexts.**

It is important to remember that all new goals should be derived from the client's performance on the previous therapy goals. Examples of behavioral objectives dealing with recommended action follow:

> **It is recommended that Ryan receive an audiological reevaluation due to his fluctuating hearing.**

> **It is recommended that Kaitlin have a neurological evaluation.**

Writing Notes in SOAP Format

SOAP notes can be written in various ways. Two ways are demonstrated in this section. One way shows a clear delineation between the subjective, objective, assessment, and plan portions:

> **7/19/[year]**
>
> **S: Joe appeared happy today. He smiled frequently throughout the session.**
>
> **O: He correctly imitated 20 of 25 (80%) monosyllabic words beginning with /s/. He correctly**

produced 45 of 50 (90%) words beginning with /l/ in phrases. Joe demonstrated progress on both phonemes today. The production of /s/ increased from 65% to 80% and /l/ from 75% to 90%.

A: Joe continues to present with an articulation problem of moderate severity.

P: Continue current treatment goals and activities next session.

Another example of this format follows:

1/22/[year]

S: Mrs. Gibbs appeared tired today. Her eyes closed several times during the session. The nurse reported that she was awake most of the night.

O: When overexaggerating her articulatory movements, Mrs. Gibbs was intelligible on 10 of 15 (66%) monosyllabic words. She was intelligible on 4 of 5 (80%) carrier phrases. Her performance increased from 60% on monosyllabic words and 72% on carrier phrases.

A: Mrs. Gibbs continues to present with severe dysarthria.

P: Overexaggeration of articulatory movements to improve intelligibility will be continued next session.

A third example follows:

2/15/[year]

S: Mr. Robertson seemed uncomfortable today. He frequently moaned as he tried to change position.

O: Mr. Robertson correctly pointed to 6 of 10 common objects given a field of 2 and 4 of 10 pictures of common objects also given a field of 2. He named 2 of 10 common objects. Mr. Robertson pointed to the correct printed word in 5 of 10 attempts given a choice of 2.

Automatic speech: Mr. Robertson said his name, counted to 20, and said the days of the week.

A: Mr. Robertson presents with severe receptive and expressive aphasia.

P: Current treatment goals and activities will continue next session.

The second way to write SOAP notes uses a narrative format. Although the parts are not clearly delineated, the information is presented in the established order of subjective, objective, assessment, and plan. The examples previously presented in the delineated form are rewritten below using this second format:

7/19/[year]

Joe appeared happy today. He smiled frequently throughout the session. He correctly imitated 20 of 25 (80%) monosyllabic words beginning with /s/. He correctly produced 45 of 50 (90%) words beginning with /l/ in phrases. Joe demonstrated progress on both phonemes today. The production of /s/ increased from 65% to 80% and /l/ from 75% to 90%. Joe continues to present with an articulation problem of moderate severity. Continue with current treatment goals and activities next session.

1/22/[year]

Mrs. Gibbs appeared tired today. Her eyes closed several times during the session. The nurse reported that she was awake most of the night. When overexaggerating her articulatory movements, Mrs. Gibbs was intelligible on 10 of 15 (66%) monosyllabic words. She was intelligible on 4 of 5 (80%) carrier phrases. This performance increased from 60% on monosyllabic words and 72% on carrier phrases. Mrs. Gibbs continues to present with severe dysarthria. Overexaggeration of articulatory movements to improve intelligibility will be continued next session.

2/15/[year]

Mr. Robertson seemed uncomfortable today. He frequently moaned as he tried to change position. He correctly pointed to 6 of 10 common objects given

a field of 2 and 4 of 10 pictures of common objects also given a field of 2. He named 2 of 10 common objects. Mr. Robertson pointed to the correct printed word in 5 of 10 attempts given a choice of 2. Automatic speech: Mr. Robertson said his name, counted to 20, and said the days of the week. He presents with severe receptive and expressive aphasia. Current treatment goals and activities will continue next session.

Note that the same information is included in all of the entries. Only the format varies.

QUICK CHECK

If you are using the SOAP format, make certain that information supportive of the subjective, objective, assessment, and plan parts is included in each progress note entry.

SUMMARY

The information presented in this chapter was intended to advance your understanding of the importance and usefulness of well-written progress notes and to help you write acceptable progress notes from the start. The value of well-written progress notes can best be learned and truly understood in a situation when a client, previously seen by a fellow beginning clinician, is switched to your caseload and progress notes are either lacking or sketchy at best. Hopefully, neither you nor your peers will be guilty of writing unacceptable entries.

KNOW IT, USE IT!

After reading this chapter, you should be able to

1. state how you can use your progress notes to help determine the flow and direction of the client's therapeutic program to the satisfaction of your supervisor.
2. correctly write progress notes in 90% of your attempts as determined by your supervisor.
3. state and explain in detail at least four problems that can occur when writing progress notes.
4. correctly determine if your progress notes are well written or problematic in 90% of your attempts.
5. explain two variations of the SOAP format in detail to your supervisor.

References

American Speech-Language-Hearing Association. (1992). Standards for professional service programs in speech–language pathology and audiology. *Asha, 34,* 63–70.

Cornett, B., & Chabon, S. (1988). *The clinical practice of speech–language pathology.* Columbus, OH: Merrill.

Hegde, M. N., & Davis, D. (1995). *Clinical methods and practicum in speech–language pathology* (2nd ed.). San Diego: Singular.

Knepflar, K., & May, A. (1992). *Report writing in the field of communication disorders: A handbook for students and clinicians* (2nd ed.). Rockville, MD: National Student Speech-Language-Hearing Association.

Paul-Brown, D. (1994). Clinical record keeping in audiology and speech–language pathology. *Asha, 36,* 40–42.

Chapter 6

Taming the Paper Giant: Assuring Accuracy and Accountability

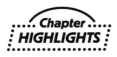

- Importance of accountability
- Efficient system for handling paperwork
- Record-keeping systems
- Record keeping during individual therapy sessions
- Record keeping during group therapy sessions
- Tracking clinical hours
- ASHA's certification requirements
- Continuing education requirements

One of the most valuable pieces of advice when you start clinical practicum is to stay on top of the paperwork from the very beginning. If you fall behind, you will soon find that it is difficult to catch up, and you might find yourself playing catch-up for the rest of the semester. If you follow the advice presented here, you will likely have a more positive clinical experience. Ignoring this tip might lead to a negative clinical experience, undesirable grades, or even the need to retake the clinical experience. Learning to stay in control of the paperwork from the beginning will prevent the feeling of being overwhelmed (see Figure 6.1).

To avoid this stumbling block, you may be tempted to use one of the many computer programs designed to assist with the administration of clinical functions. Although you may feel that use of software will help you be a better clinician, this is not necessarily true. I hope that this chapter will give you a better understanding of the "how" and

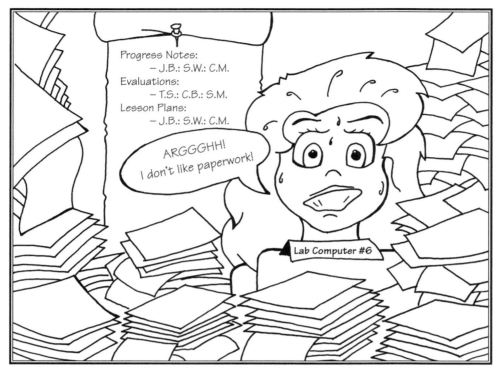

Figure 6.1. Death by paperwork.

"why" of the paperwork process. Later, when you understand the conceptual elements, you will be able to make an informed decision on the use of software.

This chapter also raises the sometimes sensitive topic of accountability and its link to the paperwork process. Leahy (1995) interprets accountability "as having readily accessible complete records of clients served, along with a justifiable rationale to document need for service" (p. 88). Records are evidence of what will happen or what has happened from initial contact through discharge from therapy. Swigert (2002) stated, "In the 'real' situations in which we work, documenting what we do is as important as providing the service" (p. 1). At some point during your professional career, it is highly probable that you will be involved with Medicare. When this happens, Swigert (2002) says you will "realize that the only way a claims reviewer can make judgment about compliance is to read our documentation" (p. 1). Therefore, it is important for speech–language pathologists to be accountable, and the only way this can be accomplished is through thorough documentation. Accurate records are also essential to guide and shape the therapeutic regimen and to document client performance. The more accurate these records are, the fewer misinterpretations can occur over what was the intent and outcome of the clinician's work. Swigert (2002) adequately sums it up by saying,

> Though we all get frustrated at the amount of paperwork that has to be done, it is crucial that we clearly document what we did, why we did it, and what the results were. It is only through clear documentation that we can demonstrate that patients are receiving appropriate services. (p. 17)

Paperwork Process and a System for Streamlining

Although the types of paperwork required of service providers will vary across programs, there is some consistency within collegiate programs. Most programs require the writing of behavioral objectives, evaluation reports, reevaluations, treatment plans, lesson plans, session evaluations, progress notes, and progress reports (all of which are addressed in this book). Although other documents are used in speech–language pathology, this section focuses on those that are linked directly to the therapy session: lesson plans, progress notes, session evaluations, and response sheets. An efficient and effective, or streamlined, system is described for handling these paperwork elements.

The first step toward the implementation of therapy is the *evaluation*. After a client is evaluated and therapy is recommended, the second step is to construct a *semester plan of treatment*. This plan comprises both long-range goals and short-term objectives. The ideas and content for constructing this plan are based on formal and informal testing and observations made during the initial evaluation. The next step is to create a *lesson plan* for each session or to cover all sessions held during an entire week. Lesson plans contain objectives for the session (short-term objectives), as well as the procedures (specific techniques, tasks, materials, and method of reinforcement) used to meet these objectives. In addition, many supervisors request a written rationale for each procedure. Following each session, *progress notes* need to be written. It is best to write them immediately following the session while your memory is fresh and the records containing data on the client's performance are at your fingertips. Immediately following the session, you need to write a detailed and insightful *evaluation* of the therapy session. This evaluation is usually written on the back of the lesson plan. You need to consider the following questions when you write your evaluation: Were the objectives met or not? What were the results?

Likewise, you need to consider the procedures: Which procedures were helpful and which were not? Why? Was progress made? Why or why not? If something did not go well, what could have been done differently? What were the strengths of the session? Why? What were the weaknesses? Why? What will be done differently during the next session?

Although you may think that the paperwork is complete, it starts all over again for the next session. At this point, you can streamline your paperwork by completing at the same time the progress notes and session evaluation for the session just completed, and a lesson plan and response sheet for the next session. Often beginning clinicians consider progress notes, session evaluations, lesson plans, and response sheets as being separate entities and work on them at separate times. This is not the best approach, however, because these records constitute an ongoing "reporting system," as shown in Table 6.1.

The most efficient way to tackle the paperwork is to do it immediately after conducting the therapy session. The session evaluation, progress notes, lesson plan for the next session, and response sheet (discussed later in this chapter) for the next session can be completed in approximately 20 minutes. This paperwork is easier if you are organized and if you actively think about and evaluate session performance (both yours and the client's) *during* each session.

If the progress notes and session evaluation for the current session, and the lesson plan and response sheet for the next session are done at four different times, efficiency decreases and time is wasted. It is necessary to rethink and review the previous therapy session four separate times: before writing the session evaluation, before writing the progress notes, before writing the lesson plan for the next session, and yet again, before designing the response sheet for the next session. Inefficiency results because you need to re-create the therapy set each time, which takes more time than the actual writing. Keep in mind that the writing cannot be done unless your mind and thoughts are focused on the therapy session. If these four parts are completed immediately following the session, your mind and thoughts are already on that session and what the focus should be for the next session.

QUICK CHECK

Make certain you are streamlining the paperwork process. Focus on one client at a time. Write your progress notes immediately following the session. Then continue with your written evaluation of that same session. Next, get your lesson plan and response sheet written for your next session with this same client. By completing all the necessary paperwork on one client immediately after a session, efficiency is increased and time is used wisely.

TABLE 6.1

Steps in the Therapeutic Process and Paperwork Requirements

Therapy Stage and Recording Requirement	Frequency of Preparation	Documentary Requirement(s) (*Partial List*)
Pretherapy Procedures		
Evaluation	Initially (and as ordered)	Testing (formal and informal)
		Observations
Plan of Treatment	1 per semester (may be modified)	Long-range goals
		Short-term objectives
Lesson Plan	1 per session (or week)	Short-term objectives
		Procedures
		Rationale (optional)
Response Sheet(s)	1 (or more) per session	Performance on objectives
Therapy Session		
Posttherapy Procedures		
Progress Notes	1 per session	Client's summarized performance
Session Evaluation (becomes part of lesson plan)	1 per session	Were objectives met?
		Were procedures appropriate?
		Was session productive?
Lesson Plan	1 for next session or week	Short-term objectives
		Procedures
		Rationale (optional)
Response Sheet(s)	1 (or more) for next session	Performance on objectives
Discharge from Therapy		

Note. Steps are repeated or modified as required.

Record Keeping During Individual Sessions

Excellent record keeping does not guarantee good care, but poor record keeping is an obstacle to clinical excellence (Kibbee & Lilly, 1989). Therefore, it is necessary to keep accurate records. Two methods are useful for keeping records when seeing clients for individual therapy sessions.

One method consists of keeping continuous records during the entire therapy session. All responses that are relevant to the objectives are recorded while the session is in progress. These records are then used to write the progress notes. If records are not kept, it is not possible to write accurate, objective progress notes.

When the recording of every response interferes with the naturalistic setting or has a negative impact on the flow of the session, another method of record keeping must be implemented. This second method involves recording samplings of behaviors during the therapy session rather than continuously recording responses. Each objective should be targeted for record keeping for a set time limit, which you will determine. For example, if there are three objectives, you may decide to keep records on Objective 1 for 2 minutes, Objective 2 for 2 minutes, and so on. Depending on the nature of the objective, the 2-minute time frame should be limited to responses by the client.

Regardless of the record-keeping method used, beginning clinicians frequently neglect to record some responses, which results in inaccurate data. Reasons for failing to record responses include getting too involved in the task at hand and simply forgetting, not realizing that a target response was attempted, not realizing that a target response was produced, or concentrating too much on what to do next rather than on what is being done at the moment. To increase the likelihood of recording all responses (continuous record keeping) or all responses during the set time (sampling), you should set up a response sheet (record sheet, tally sheet, data sheet) prior to the session. Position this response sheet so that responses or their outcomes can easily be recorded, and place your pen or pencil point on the paper at the place where the next response should be written. If this sheet is within easy reach and if your writing instrument remains in position, it will serve as a constant reminder to record the client's responses. This sheet should have each objective stated in abbreviated form with enough space available to keep a tally of responses. An example is shown in Figure 6.2.

Note that because Objectives 1 and 2 in Figure 6.2 were clearly defined at a previous time, the actual stimulus items are known prior to beginning the session. Therefore, it is possible to list the actual stimulus items on the response or tally sheet prior to the session, saving time by eliminating the need to write them while the client's responses are occurring. However, the stimulus items in Objective 3 cannot be formulated prior to the session because the client will be selecting a book and discussing actions of various people or animals. In such cases, the specific stimulus items cannot be predetermined. In this instance, it is best to simply write down the portion of the client's response that resembles the target structure (is + Verb + ing) as it is being produced. In this manner, it will be possible to further analyze the client's responses.

Objective 1 (receptive identification)	**Objective 2** (expressive identification)	**Objective 3** (production of is + Verb + ing)
1. eye	1. eye	
2. ear	2. ear	
3. knee	3. knee	
4. hand	4. hand	
5. foot	5. foot	
6. mouth	6. mouth	
7. elbow	7. elbow	
8. chin	8. chin	
9. face	9. face	
10. finger	10. finger	

Figure 6.2. Sample response sheet.

Make certain you are keeping records on the client's responses. Decide whether you will use continuous record keeping or sampling prior to the start of the session.

Record Keeping During Group Sessions

During a group therapy session, it is unlikely that a clinician can record all responses produced by each client on every objective. This is especially true if three or more clients are in attendance or if the session is actually one of *group therapy* as opposed to *therapy in groups* (as discussed in Chapter 9). Nevertheless, it is still necessary to keep records because accountability is required. Because continuous record keeping of all responses for all clients is not possible, the sampling method previously discussed is a feasible alternative.

To keep records in a group setting, record each client's responses for only one or two objectives targeted for that particular session. If the size of the group is large (five or six clients), it will not be possible to record responses for each client during each session. If this is the

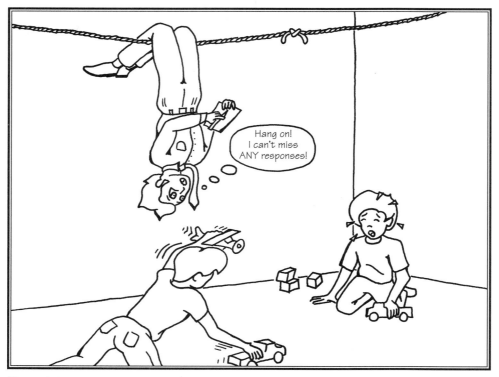

Figure 6.3. At *all* costs.

case, target objectives for half of the clients during one session and then target the rest of the clients during the next session.

If a client is working on more than two objectives, target different ones for each session to compensate for the limits imposed by the group setting. Ideally, each objective should be targeted at least every week and a half. The frequency will vary depending on the number of sessions each client receives per week, the number of clients present during a session, and the length of the session. This sampling approach is acceptable when recording all responses produced by each client during each session is simply not possible (see Figure 6.3).

Make certain you have adequate records for all clients in the group and all objectives worked on over a realistic time period.

Record Keeping with Young or Very Active Children

Oftentimes, student clinicians have difficulty keeping records during sessions when they are manipulating lots of materials in an attempt to keep a child's interest or when they are following a child's lead. Moving around the room with a child makes it difficult to keep records in the conventional manner, by marking on a sheet of paper that is on a table or that you are carrying as you move around. A better way is to stick a self-adhesive paper or masking tape on your nondominant arm for writing records. As long as you have a pen, pencil, or marker handy, record keeping in these situations should not be problematic.

QUICK CHECK Make certain your record-keeping system is working for you. If not, experiment.

Ways To Record

There are many ways to record responses. When a clear-cut response is required (as in Objectives 1 and 2 in Figure 6.2), a choice of the following notations would be appropriate: 1 (correct) or 0 (incorrect), + (correct) or − (incorrect), check mark (correct) or X (incorrect), check mark (correct) or − (incorrect), and Y(es) (correct) or N(o) (incorrect). If the notation may be confusing to your supervisor, provide a key on your record sheet to avoid misunderstanding. Be consistent, however, with your choice. Use the same notation across clients and over time.

An important consideration is whether to use horizontal or vertical record-keeping systems. Horizontal record keeping entails keeping track of responses in a left-to-right sequence across the page. Vertical record keeping involves recording responses from top to bottom. Vertical record keeping is considered a "deep" system in that more information is obtained. It is conducive to recording all attempts made at a stimulus item. However, a horizontal system is considered "shallow" because less information is obtained. This system usually looks at first attempts only and ignores second, third, or additional attempts at a stimulus item. However, there are adaptations that can be made so that horizontal record keeping can be slightly more effective.

Horizontal Example
In this example, Y (for Yes) is used to denote a correct response and N (for No) is used to indicate an incorrect response:

NNYYYNYYYNYY

Based on the recorded data, the client responded correctly on 8 of 12 stimulus items, or on 67% of the attempts, and it appears that the client was not given further opportunities to achieve success on the 4 incorrect stimulus items. This horizontal record may represent poor practice, as appropriate techniques should be used to elicit correct responses when the client experiences difficulty. However, if other opportunities to succeed *were* given, this horizontal system tends to inhibit recording the responses.

The horizontal system can be modified so that every response made on a stimulus item is recorded. A response sheet might then contain the following record:

NNNYNNYYYNNYYYYYNYYYY

Most people would interpret these data in the following manner: The client correctly responded on 12 of 20 stimulus items, or on 60% of the attempts. This interpretation is not accurate because there were only 12 stimulus items. The client's performance is misrepresented. Each attempt on a particular stimulus item cannot be weighted equally. That is, a second attempt cannot be counted the same as a first attempt, and a third attempt cannot be counted the same as a second attempt, and so forth. The faux pas that occurred in this example is that all the responses were weighted equally. It is not possible, however, to determine where one stimulus item ends and the next begins.

In Example A, a minor modification is made to rectify this problem.

Example A: NNNY, NNY, Y, Y, NNY, Y, Y, Y, NY, Y, Y, Y

With a comma added after each stimulus item, it is possible to determine the number of attempts before a correct response is attained. It is also possible to see that there were only 12 original stimulus items. The client correctly responded on 8 of 12 stimulus items, or on 67% of the attempts.

Example B is provided to make an additional point about the inadequacy of a horizontal system.

Example B: NNY, NY, Y, Y, NY, Y, Y, Y, NY, Y, Y, Y

Again there were 12 stimulus items. The client's performance appears to be the same as that in the last example in that there were correct responses on 8 of the 12 stimulus items (67%). Assuming that the goal was the same and Example A was the result from the previous session and Example B the result from the present session, it appears that the client did not make progress. However, this is not the case when second, third, and fourth attempts are considered. In Example A, the client correctly responded on 1 of 4 second attempts (25%); however, in Example B, he made correct responses on 3 of 4 second attempts (75%). When third attempts are analyzed, progress is also evident (2 of 3 or 67% in Example A compared to 1 of 1 or 100% in Example B). In Example B, fourth attempts were not necessary, although one was needed in Example A. Therefore, by using a more thorough analysis, progress is evident.

This examination makes it clear why the horizontal system can be regarded as shallow. The data fall short of that necessary for complete, accurate records. Adaptations can offset, but not eliminate, these inherent problems. As you read about the vertical system, you will understand the benefits of vertical over horizontal systems.

Vertical Example

The same responses to the 12 stimulus items noted in horizontal Example B are recorded here using a vertical system:

1. NNY
2. NY
3. Y
4. Y
5. NY
6. Y
7. Y
8. Y
9. NY
10. Y
11. Y
12. Y

A quick analysis of the data enables one to immediately determine that the client responded correctly on 8 of 12 items, or in 67% of the attempts. Three of the 4 errors, or 75%, were corrected on the second attempt and 1 additional error was corrected on the third attempt.

With the data set up vertically, it is easier to quickly scan responses during the therapy session to determine whether a criterion was met. It is possible to further organize the response sheet to make scanning the data even easier:

	First Attempt	Second Attempt	Third Attempt
1.	N	N	Y
2.	N	Y	
3.	Y		
4.	Y		

	First Attempt	Second Attempt	Third Attempt
5.	N	Y	
6.	Y		
7.	Y		
8.	Y		
9.	N	Y	
10.	Y		
11.	Y		
12.	Y		

Using this method, data regarding first, second, and third attempts on a stimulus item are readily available. A tabular format like this is effective because all responses are recorded clearly, and even minimal progress can be detected by analyzing performance on second, third, and additional attempts on a stimulus item.

Completed Response Sheet—Vertical System

Figure 6.4 shows the client's responses or their outcomes recorded on the record sheet shown previously in Figure 6.2. The record uses a vertical format.

For objectives dealing with the use of language (as for Objective 3 in Figure 6.4), it is not adequate to simply note whether the client's response was correct or incorrect. If the response was incorrect, it is important to write verbatim what the client said so you can analyze the client's errors and use the results of this analysis to determine your therapeutic strategy. The documentation of the client's language can provide justification for continued therapy, progress, or carry-over. It is also important to indicate the type of cueing used, if any, to help obtain a correct response. In Figure 6.4, you can easily see that two of the correct responses were achieved through imitation.

Summary of Record Keeping

Clinicians can use either a horizontal system or a vertical system for record keeping. A horizontal system is not the best approach, however, even when it is made more useful through modifications, many of which are borrowed from the vertical system. Because the vertical system is better for measuring slight improvement, it is the better system for you to adopt early on in your career.

QUICK CHECK

Whether you are using a horizontal system or a vertical one, make certain you are recording the client's repeated attempts on a stimulus item.

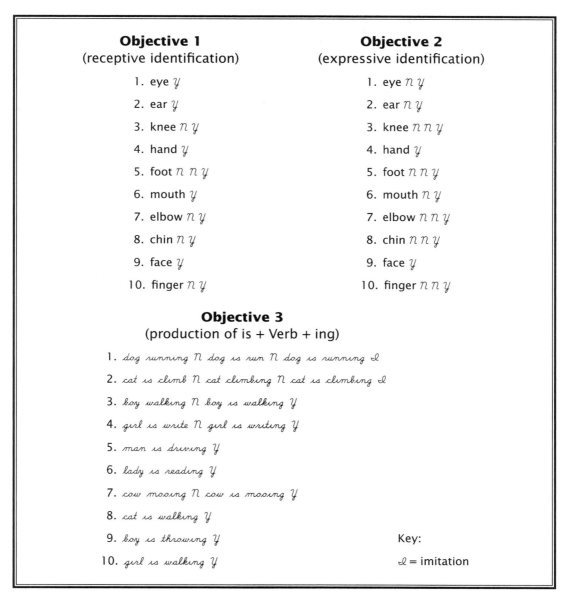

Objective 1
(receptive identification)

1. eye *y*
2. ear *y*
3. knee *n y*
4. hand *y*
5. foot *n n y*
6. mouth *y*
7. elbow *n y*
8. chin *n y*
9. face *y*
10. finger *n y*

Objective 2
(expressive identification)

1. eye *n y*
2. ear *n y*
3. knee *n n y*
4. hand *y*
5. foot *n n y*
6. mouth *n y*
7. elbow *n n y*
8. chin *n n y*
9. face *y*
10. finger *n n y*

Objective 3
(production of is + Verb + ing)

1. dog running *N* dog is run *N* dog is running *I*
2. cat is climb *N* cat climbing *N* cat is climbing *I*
3. boy walking *N* boy is walking *Y*
4. girl is write *N* girl is writing *Y*
5. man is driving *Y*
6. lady is reading *Y*
7. cow mooing *N* cow is mooing *Y*
8. cat is walking *Y*
9. boy is throwing *Y*
10. girl is walking *Y*

Key:

I = imitation

Figure 6.4. Completed response sheet.

Accountability

In addition to being necessary for effective therapy, accurate record keeping has another purpose that needs to be addressed. As in all allied health fields, professionals must be accountable for the decisions and actions taken in serving each client.

In its most elemental and nonlegal form, accountability is knowing what to do and doing what you know (assuming proficiency in both knowledge and practice and being able to document both). Records document that you knew the problem and provided appropriate services. Without records, or with inadequate records, other clinicians cannot review your work in preparation for taking on the client, and you cannot defend yourself against claims that you acted inappropriately in designing and executing a therapy program. Records are often the only resource to demonstrate that you acted responsibly and that you fulfilled your obligations to the client, to the profession, and to yourself.

In addition to keeping excellent records about therapy sessions, it is important to keep records of clinical hours and to be aware of requirements to stay current in the field. These topics are discussed in the following sections. Notice that the discussion of clinical hours is divided into two sections based on the date of a change in requirements.

Tracking Clinical Hours (If Applying for CCC Before December 31, 2004)

No set number of clinical hours is required for undergraduate students. Individual universities determine the number of clinical hours necessary for their own programs. The American Speech-Language-Hearing Association (ASHA, 2002b) currently requires a total of 375 clock hours to be obtained in supervised clinical observation (25 hours) and clinical practicum (350 hours) to be eligible to apply for a Certificate of Clinical Competence (CCC) after earning a master's degree. A maximum of 100 hours earned in practicum at the undergraduate level can count toward the hours necessary to obtain this certification. However, at this time, it is not possible to know *which* 100 hours will be counted. Therefore, it is necessary to keep track of *all* possible hours that can conceivably count toward certification. To do this, it is necessary to understand ASHA's observation and clinical practicum requirements. The basic requirements as given in ASHA's (2002b) *Certification & Membership Handbook: Speech–Language Pathology* are cited here to provide direction for pursuing CCC in speech–language pathology. (The author's commentary appears in brackets.) These requirements are as follows:

> Applicants ... must complete at least 25 clock hours of supervised observation prior to beginning the initial clinical practicum.... Those 25 clock hours must concern the evaluation and treatment of children and adults with disorders of speech, language, or hearing. (p. 21)

> No more than 25 of the clock hours may be obtained from participation in staffings in which evaluation, treatment, and/or recom-

mendations are discussed or formulated, with or without the client present. (p. 22) [Meetings with practicum supervisors may not be counted. Ample opportunity should be available to obtain these hours at the graduate level. Therefore, it is not necessary for undergraduates to track hours in this category.]

At least 250 of the 350 clock hours must be completed in the professional area for which the Certificate is sought while the applicant is engaged in graduate study. (p. 22) [All graduate coursework and graduate clinical practicum hours completed after January 1, 1994, must be started and finished at programs that are accredited by the Council on Academic Accreditation in Audiology and Speech–Language Pathology (CAA).]

At least 50 supervised clock hours must be completed in each of three types of clinical setting. (p. 22) [It is necessary to gain three diverse experiences. Each of these experiences must be unique as determined by your educational program. For example, if you provide services in two different rehabilitation hospitals but only receive experience with a stroke population, these settings would not be considered diverse. On the other hand, if you service a stroke population in one rehabilitation hospital and a brain-injured population in the other, these would serve as two of the three required diverse settings.]

The applicant must have experience in the evaluation and treatment of children and adults and with a variety of types and severities of disorders of speech [articulation, fluency, voice, dysphagia], language, and hearing. (p. 22) [This experience is supposed to include both individual and group client contact. However, ASHA does not specify the number of hours specifically needed in either group or individual therapy. Further, ASHA does not define or clarify "severities." To be safe, therefore, make certain that you conduct both individual and group therapy. Also make certain that the problems of your clients range in severity.]

At least 250 of the 350 supervised clock hours must be in speech–language pathology. At least 20 of those 250 clock hours must be completed in each of the eight categories listed below.
  1. Evaluation: Speech disorders in children
  2. Evaluation: Speech disorders in adults
  3. Evaluation: Language disorders in children
  4. Evaluation: Language disorders in adults ...
  5. Treatment: Speech disorders in children
  6. Treatment: Speech disorders in adults
  7. Treatment: Language disorders in children
  8. Treatment: Language disorders in adults (pp. 22–23)
[Evaluation consists of screening, assessment, and diagnosis accomplished before therapy begins. Formal reevaluations are also included in the evaluation category. Clock hours devoted to counseling associated with the evaluation and diagnostic process may be counted. Screening activities cannot make up the majority of evaluation hours in each category. Included under treatment is clinical

management (both direct and indirect services), progress in monitoring activities, and counseling. On the undergraduate level, it is best to track only direct clinical services. There should be ample opportunity to obtain hours in indirect services during graduate school.]

Up to 20 clock hours in the major professional area may be in related disorders.... Hours may be obtained for activities related to the prevention of communication disorders and the enhancement of speech, language, and communicative effectiveness. Similarly, activities implemented to prevent the onset of speech/language disorders and their causes as well as efforts to advance the development and conservation of optimal communication may be counted. (p. 23) [Hours earned in graduate school are usually counted in this category. It is not necessary to track these hours on the undergraduate level.]

At least 20 of the 350 clock hours must be in audiology. (p. 23) [These hours may involve the evaluation, screening, or treatment of individuals with hearing disorders.]

Treatment for hearing disorders refers to clinical management and counseling, including auditory training and speech reading, as well as speech and language services for those with hearing impairment. (p. 23)

Palmer and Mormer (1992) outlined the clinical observation and clinical practicum requirements in speech–language pathology. Their chart (Figure 6.5) provides a good summary of ASHA's certification requirements, which were previously presented in this section. Palmer and Mormer said, "This type of chart makes the needed hours apparent and assists in encouraging the students to take responsibility for accurate and precise record keeping" (p. 54). This chart will enable you to see at a glance exactly where you need to obtain hours.

Clinical Hours Tracking Sheets

The three forms provided in this section are included so you can have pertinent information regarding clinical requirements at your fingertips. Any one of these forms will assist with tracking clinical requirements in a painless fashion. Your choice of which form to use should be guided by your needs, as well as your personal preference. The first form appears in Figure 6.6. The form in Figure 6.7 was designed by Palmer and Mormer (1992). Their paper-and-pencil tracking sheet is designed for use each semester. Hegde and Davis's (1995) form, shown in Figure 6.8, will likewise assist you in keeping track of your clinical hours.

You will find one of these forms extremely helpful for recording your clinical practicum contacts, so make the choice, try it and, if you like it, stick with it. Should you not find it appropriate, switch to another. Be sure to transfer your hours, though.

Minimum 375 Clock Hours (c.h.)	25 c.h.	Clinical Observation			
	Min 350 c.h. Clinical Practicum (Max 25 c.h. Staffings) (Min 50 c.h. in each of three types of clinical settings)	**Speech–Language—Min 250 c.h.**		Min 20	1. Evaluation: Speech disorders in children
				Min 20	2. Evaluation: Speech disorders in adults
				Min 20	3. Evaluation: Language disorders in children
				Min 20	4. Evaluation: Language disorders in adults
				Min 20	5. Treatment: Speech disorders in children
				Min 20	6. Treatment: Speech disorders in adults
				Min 20	7. Treatment: Language disorders in children
				Min 20	8. Treatment: Language disorders in adults
				Min 20	9. Related disorders
		Audiology (Max 100, Min 35)	Min 35	Min 15	Evaluation or screening of individuals with hearing disorders
				Min 15	Habilitation/rehabilitation of individuals who have hearing impairment

Figure 6.5. Supervised clinical observation and clinical practicum requirements in speech–language pathology. *Note.* From "Tracking Clinical Learning Experience," by C. V. Palmer and E. A. Mormer, August 1992, *Asha*, p. 53. Copyright 1992 by the American Speech-Language-Hearing Association. Reprinted with permission.

Be sure to record hours in the appropriate slots on the form at the end of those days on which you have seen clients. Record your time using decimals—such as 0.5 for ½ hour, 1.0 for 1 hour, and 1.5 for 1½ hours—in the appropriate places. If your sessions are not in ½-hour increments, you might want to use Hegde and Davis's (1995) guidelines for reporting fractions of hours: 55 minutes = 0.9, 50 minutes =

(*text continues on p. 185*)

OBSERVATION AND PRACTICUM REQUIREMENTS

Name: _____   Dates: _____

Clinical Observation
(25 hours)

Evaluation		Treatment	
Children **Adults**		**Children** **Adults**	
Speech		Speech	
Language		Language	
Hearing		Hearing	

Clinical Settings
(3 types of settings)

1. _____

2. _____

3. _____

Clock Hours
(250 hours)*

Evaluation		Treatment	
Children **Adults**		**Children** **Adults**	
Speech		Speech	
Language		Language	

Audiology
(20 hours)

Evaluation or Screening
Treatment

---

*A minimum of 20 hours is necessary in each of the eight slots.

Figure 6.6. Observation and practicum requirements.

Clinic Practicum Contacts—Speech-Language Path. Student Name:
Student Clinician Record Log Student ID#:

| Date | Client Information | | Setting | Contact Hours by Evaluation Type | | | | | | | | | Init. |
	Last name	Age		1	2	3	4	5	6	7	8	9	
TOTALS													

Evaluation types: (1) Evaluation: Speech disorders in children, (2) Evaluation: Speech disorders in adults, (3) Evaluation: Language disorders in children, (4) Evaluation: Language disorders in adults, (5) Treatment: Speech disorders in children, (6) Treatment: Speech disorders in adults, (7) Treatment: Language disorders in children, (8) Treatment Language disorders in adults, (8) Treatment: Language disorders in adults, (9) Related disorders

Figure 6.7. Student worksheet for recording clinical practicum contacts in speech–language pathology. *Note.* From "Tracking Clinical Learning Experience," by C. V. Palmer and E. A. Mormer, August 1992, *Asha*, p. 54. Copyright 1992 by the American Speech-Language-Hearing Association. Reprinted with permission.

UNIVERSITY SPEECH AND HEARING CENTER
CLINICAL PRACTICUM HOURS

Student   Supervisor   Semester

Practicum Site   Circle one: Adults   Children

EVALUATION/DIAGNOSTIC HOURS

Date	Language	Articulation	Voice	Fluency	Other	Staffing	Supervisor Initials
Total							

TREATMENT HOURS

Date	Language	Articulation	Voice	Fluency	Other	Staffing	Supervisor Initials
Total							

Supervisor's signature   License #   ASHA CCC Account #

Figure 6.8. Worksheet for recording clinical practicum hours in speech–language pathology. *Note.* From *Clinical Methods and Practicum in Speech–Language Pathology* (2nd ed., p. 310), by M. N. Hegde and D. Davis, 1995, San Diego: Singular. Copyright 1995 by Singular Publishing Group. Reprinted with permission.

0.8, 45 minutes = 0.75, 40 minutes = 0.7, 35 minutes = 0.6, 25 minutes = 0.4, 20 minutes = 0.3, 15 minutes = 0.25, 10 minutes = 0.2, and 5 minutes = 0.1.

Use one tracking sheet per week. At the end of the week, compile the data. It is advantageous to make notes on the back, such as each client's last name and problem, and the session dates. At the end of the second week, compile the data from both sheets; at the end of the third week, compile the data from all three sheets; and so on. At the end of the semester, compile all the sheets onto one form and then immediately have your form signed by your supervisor. If your supervisor has any questions regarding your hours at this time, you should be able to easily find the answers by consulting all of your tracking sheets, especially the notes made on the back. Do not throw away any tracking sheets until your supervisor signs the composite tracking sheet covering the entire semester.

Tracking Clinical Hours (If Applying for CCC After January 1, 2005)

Although ASHA's new certification requirements for those applying for CCC are scheduled to take effect on January 1, 2005, changes may still be made to these preliminary published requirements established for the Certificate of Clinical Competence in Speech–Language Pathology (CCC-SLP). Therefore, if you will be earning your CCC in or after 2005, you will need to prepare yourself for meeting the new requirements. The first step is to obtain a copy of the *Certification & Membership Handbook* that addresses these 2005 requirements.

According to ASHA (2002a), the

> 2005 standards combine process and outcome measure of academic and clinical knowledge and skills. Process standards specify the experiences, such as course work or practicum hours; outcome standards require demonstration of specific knowledge and skills. The 2005 standards utilize a combination of formative and summative assessments for the purpose of improving and measuring student learning. (p. 1)

A tracking document, knowledge and skills acquisition (KASA) summary form for speech–language pathology, will be used. Entries will be made upon acquisition of knowledge or skill. KASA should be periodically reviewed "to assist students in determining knowledge and skills already acquired and those yet to be attained" (ASHA 2003, p. 2).

Students are required to complete a minimum of 400 clock hours (25 more hours than the pre-2005 requirements) of supervised clinical experience in speech–language pathology. Of these hours, 25 hours must be obtained through clinical observation (same as the pre-2005 requirement) and 375 hours must be obtained in direct client contact (compared to 350 hours previously required). Because at least 325 of the total 400 clock hours must be completed while engaged in a graduate program, only 75 clinical hours from an undergraduate program can count toward these certification requirements (compared to 100 hours in the pre-2005 requirements). Standard IV-F states that

> supervised practicum must include experience with client/patient populations across the life span and from culturally/linguistically diverse backgrounds. Practicum must include experience with client/patient populations with various types and severities of communication and/or related disorders, differences, and disabilities. (p. 9)

In the implementation of this standard, the applicant must have direct clinical experience with both children and adults. According to Standard III-C (p. 6),

> Specific knowledge must be demonstrated in the following areas:
> articulation
> fluency
> voice and resonance, including respiration and phonation
> receptive and expressive language (phonology, morphology, syntax, semantics, and pragmatics) in speaking, listening, reading, writing, and manual modalities
> hearing, including the impact on speech and language
> swallowing (oral, pharyngeal, esophageal, and related functions, including oral function for feeding; orofacial myofunction)
> cognitive aspects of communication (attention, memory, sequencing, problem-solving, executive functioning)
> social aspects of communication (including challenging behavior, ineffective social skills, lack of communication opportunities)
> communication modalities (including oral, manual, augmentative, and alternative communication techniques and assistive technologies)

Unlike in the pre-2005 certification requirements, the specific number of hours that must be obtained with adults and children is not specified. Likewise, the number of hours required in treatment and evaluation with various disorders and differences is not specified. Overall the number of hours has increased for certification requirements beginning with those obtaining their CCC in 2005, but there is more flexibility within these hours. Therefore, the best advice at this time is to keep track of your clinical hours by documenting all direct patient contact and to have your supervisor sign your organized documentation at the end of each semester. A worksheet similar to Figure 6.8

that reflects the differences and disorders listed in Standard III-C should be used to keep track of your evaluation and diagnostic hours. Also, worksheets similar to those illustrated in Figures 6.9 and 6.10 should be used to keep track of your clinical practicum hours.

QUICK CHECK

Know what ASHA's requirements are. Make certain you meet them.

Professional Accountability

It is extremely important for you to keep abreast of current developments in speech–language pathology, as well as in related professions that have an impact on speech–language pathology. You are responsible for providing the best assessments and therapy possible, and this is not always possible if your knowledge base is not current. You have a responsibility to all your clients, to your employer, and to your profession to keep current and to use this current information while servicing clients.

A new ASHA standard (Standard VII), which will go into effect with those obtaining CCC on January 1, 2005, mandates demonstration of continued professional development in order to maintain the CCC-SLP. This standard will apply to all certification holders regardless of the date of their initial certification. This standard states that, to renew your certification, you must earn 30 contact hours from either ASHA, continuing education providers approved by ASHA, an International Association for Continuing Education and Training authorized provider, or an employer-sponsored in-service, or you must earn 3 quarter hours from a college or university that holds regional accreditation or accreditation from an equivalent nationally recognized or governmental accreditation authority. The important thing to remember is that you need 30 contact hours of continuing education every 3 years to maintain your certification. If you earn your initial certification prior to December 31, 2004 (and back as far as January 1, 1990), you will have to accumulate your professional development hours between January 1, 2007 and December 31, 2009. If you earn your initial certification on or after January 1, 2005, you will have to accumulate your professional development hours between your certification date and 3 years after that date.

In addition to meeting ASHA's continuing education requirements, you will have to check your state's requirements. In Pennsylvania, for example, anyone holding a teaching certificate must comply with Act 48 (Public School Code of 1949–omnibus amendments), which requires

UNIVERSITY SPEECH AND HEARING CENTER
CLINICAL PRACTICUM EVALUATION/DIAGNOSTIC HOURS

_____   _____   _____
          Name   Supervisor   Semester

Evaluation/Diagnostic Hours

Date	Age*	1**	2	3	4	5	6	7	8	9	Other	Initials
Totals												

_____   _____   _____
    Supervisor's Signature   Supervisor's ASHA #   Date

*Age Codes

A (adult); **C** (child—5 years through 12 years); **P** (preschool—birth through 4 years 11 months); **T** (13 through 19 years)

**Evaluation/Diagnostic Hours

1. Articulation; 2. Fluency; 3. Voice and resonance (including respiration and phonation); 4. Receptive and expressive language (phonology, morphology, syntax, semantics, and pragmatics); 5. Hearing (including the impact on speech and language development); 6. Swallowing (oral, pharyngeal, esophageal, and related functions including oral function for feeding; orofacial myofunction); 7. Cognitive aspects of communication (attention, memory, sequencing, problem solving, executive functioning); 8. Social aspects of communication (including challenging behavior, ineffective social skills, lack of communication opportunities); 9. Communication modalities (including oral, manual, augmentative, and alternative communication techniques and assistive technologies)

Figure 6.9. Worksheet for recording evaluation and diagnostic hours in speech–language pathology.

UNIVERSITY SPEECH AND HEARING CENTER
CLINICAL PRACTICUM THERAPY HOURS

Name   Supervisor   Semester

Therapy Hours

Date	Age*	1**	2	3	4	5	6	7	8	9	Other	Initials
Totals												

Supervisor's Signature   Supervisor's ASHA #   Date

*Age Codes

A (adult); **C** (child—5 years through 12 years); **P** (preschool—birth through 4 years 11 months);
T (13 through 19 years)

**Therapy Hours

1. Articulation; 2. Fluency; 3. Voice and resonance (including respiration and phonation); 4. Receptive and expressive language (phonology, morphology, syntax, semantics, and pragmatics); 5. Hearing (including the impact on speech and language development); 6. Swallowing (oral, pharyngeal, esophageal, and related functions including oral function for feeding; orofacial myofunction); 7. Cognitive aspects of communication (attention, memory, sequencing, problem solving, executive functioning); 8. Social aspects of communication (including challenging behavior, ineffective social skills, lack of communication opportunities); 9. Communication modalities (including oral, manual, augmentative, and alternative communication techniques and assistive technologies)

Figure 6.10. Worksheet for recording therapy hours in speech–language pathology.

persons to complete continuing education requirements every 5 years to maintain their certificates as active. Speech–language clinicians working in the schools must hold a teaching certificate and therefore must meet the Act 48 requirements that went into effect on July 1, 2000. To remain in compliance with Act 48, one must either earn 6 collegiate credits or 6 Pennsylvania Department of Education–approved in-service credits or 180 continuing education hours or any combination of the above every 5 calendar years. Each collegiate or in-service credit is equal to 30 continuing education hours. This 5-year period began on July 1, 2000, for all persons issued certificates prior to and including July 2000. For those persons receiving certificates in August 2000 and after, the 5-year period becomes effective with the date on which the initial certificate is issued.

Additionally, some states require speech–language pathologists to be licensed. Forty-six states currently regulate speech–language pathology through either licensure or title registration. Of these 46 states, 41 have continuing education provisions built into their licensure renewal. These continuing education requirements are listed in Table 6.2.

According to ASHA (2002c), four states—Colorado, Idaho, Michigan, and South Dakota—and Washington, D.C., do not currently regulate speech–language pathologists. Six states—Alaska, Colorado, Connecticut, Hawaii, North Carolina, and Washington—currently have no provisions requiring continuing education for license renewal.

To be compliant, you need to be familiar with all of the requirements of your state. Your state's speech-language-hearing association will be able to provide you with these requirements.

QUICK CHECK

> Know what your continuing professional development requirements are. Be aware of both ASHA's and your state's requirements, as well as any other requirements affecting you.

Important Advice

Two pieces of advice should be followed at the appropriate points in your professional life. The first pertains to clinical hours: Upon completion of any practicum experience, have your immediate supervisor sign a record sheet of hours earned. Once it is signed, make two copies. Have the departmental secretary place one in your student file, and you place the other in your personal professional file.

TABLE 6.2

Continuing Education Requirements for State's Licensure Renewal

State	Continuing Education Requirement
Alabama	12 hours (1 CEU) in 1 year
Arizona	8 hours in 1 year
Arkansas	10 hours in 1 year
California	12 hours for licenses that expire in 2001; thereafter 24 hours in 2 years
Delaware	20 hours (2 CEUs) in 2 years
Florida	30 credit hours in 2 years
Georgia	25 hours in 2 years
Illinois	20 hours (2 CEUs) in 2 years
Indiana	36 clock hours in 2 years
Iowa	30 clock hours or 3 CEUs in 2 years
Kansas	20 hours (2 CEUs) in 2 years
Kentucky	15 hours in 1 year
Louisiana	10 hours (1 CEU) in 1 year
Maine	50 clock hours in 2 years
Maryland	20 hours (2 CEUs) in 2 years
Massachusetts	20 hours (2 CEUs) in 2 years
Minnesota	30 contact hours in 2 years
Mississippi	10 hours (1 CEU) in 1 year
Missouri	30 hours every 2 years (effective in 2000)
Montana	40 hours (4 CEUs) in 2 years
Nebraska	20 hours (2 CEUs) in 2 years
Nevada	15 hours in 1 year
New Hampshire (SLP only)	50 clock hours in 3 years
New Jersey	20 hours (2 CEUs) in 2 years
New Mexico	10 hours (1 CEU) in 1 year
New York	30 hours in 3 years
North Dakota	10 hours (1 CEU) in 1 year
Ohio	20 hours (2 CEUs) in 2 years
Oklahoma	20 hours every 2 years
Oregon	10 hours (1 CEU) in 1 year
Pennsylvania	20 hours in 2 years
Rhode Island	20 hours in 2 years (SLPs and Audiologists) 30 hours in 2 years (dual licenses)
South Carolina	32 hours in 2 years
South Dakota	12 hours in 1 year
Tennessee	10 hours (1 CEU) in 1 year
Texas	10 hours (1 CEU) in 1 year
Utah	20 hours (2 CEUs) in 2 years
Virginia	30 hours in 2 years
West Virginia	10 hours every 2 years
Wisconsin	20 hours (2 CEUs) in 2 years
Wyoming	20 hours in 1 year

Note. Retrieved September 29, 2003, from http://www.asha.org/about/legislation-advocacy/state/state_licensure.htm

If the signing of an hour sheet is part of the standard operating procedure of your clinical program, make certain the sheet is at least as detailed as those presented in this chapter. If it is not, then use one of the forms presented in this chapter and have your supervisor sign both of them. The supervisor's signature verifies that these are the number of hours you actually earned within the designated categories. Also obtain your supervisor's ASHA account number, as this information will be needed when you complete the paperwork for certification. If this advice is not followed, it could be time-consuming to reconstruct this information later. The supervisor may have taken a professional position elsewhere, and you may have difficulty locating him or her to verify practicum hours or to obtain his or her ASHA number. Also, the supervisor may no longer remember you and may not have a record of your clinical hours. Therefore, it is best to have your hour sheet designed as specifically as possible and to have your supervisor sign it in a timely fashion.

The second piece of advice pertains to certification requirements. It is your responsibility to be familiar with ASHA's certification requirements. Read ASHA's current *Certification & Membership Handbook: Speech–Language Pathology* at strategic points throughout your professional schooling. Make sure that you have the most current copy of this handbook at three strategic points in your professional career: before you begin your experience at student teaching on the undergraduate level, upon entering a graduate program, and during the semester preceding graduation. By doing this, you will stay on top of the number of hours needed to meet the current certification requirements.

The current certification standards have been in effect since January 1993. Major changes are currently being made and will go into effect on January 1, 2005. However, because of the significant impact that certification will have on your professional career, it is extremely important to consult the most current ASHA handbook to get on the right path and to stay on it so that you meet all the necessary requirements for certification.

KNOW IT,
USE IT!

After reading this chapter, you should be able to

1. describe all aspects of the system designed to streamline paperwork.
2. state four reasons why you might forget to record responses during a session.
3. explain a horizontal recording system in detail without error.
4. explain a vertical recording system in detail without error.
5. state and explain ASHA's current certification requirements (up until December 31, 2004).
6. state and explain ASHA's certification requirements that go into effect January 1, 2005.
7. explain why continuing education will be a part of your professional career.

References

American Speech-Language-Hearing Association. (2002a). *Background information and standards and implementation for the Certificate of Clinical Competence in Speech–Language Pathology* (effective date: January 1, 2005). Retrieved October 28, 2003, from http://www.asha.org/about/membership-certification/handbooks/slp/slp_standards_new.htm

American Speech-Language-Hearing Association. (2002b). *Certification & membership handbook: Speech–language pathology.* Rockville, MD: Author.

American Speech-Language-Hearing Association. (2002c). State licensure information. Retrieved September 29, 2003, from http://www.asha.org/about/legislation-advocacy/state/state_licensure.htm

American Speech-Language-Hearing Association. (2003). *Knowledge and skills acquisition (KASA) summary form for certification in speech–language pathology.* Retrieved October 29, 2003 from http://www.csd.jmu.edu/knowledge_skills_acquisition_slp.pdf

Hegde, M. N., & Davis, D. (1995). *Clinical methods and practicum in speech–language pathology* (2nd ed.). San Diego: Singular.

Kibbee, R., & Lilly, G. (1989). Outcome-oriented documentation in a psychiatric facility. *Journal of Quality Assurance, 10,* 16.

Leahy, M. (1995). *Disorders of communication: The science of intervention.* London: Whurr.

Palmer, C., & Mormer, E. (1992). Tracking clinical learning experience. *Asha, 34,* 53–55.

Swigert, N. B. (2002, February). Documenting what you do is as important as doing it. *The ASHA Leader,* pp. 1, 14, 17.

Chapter 7

Therapy Conferences

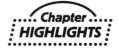 **Chapter HIGHLIGHTS**

- Purpose of therapy conferences
- Areas covered during therapy conferences
- Writing therapy conference reports
- Examples of therapy conference reports

Some university programs require student clinicians to conduct therapy conferences. This experience during training is beneficial because similar conferences are conducted in all employment settings where clients receive speech–language pathology services. Although these conferences are usually conducted toward the end of the semester in a university setting, they can occur at various points throughout the therapeutic process at the request of a parent, spouse, other family member, student clinician, or clinical supervisor. In settings not dictated by semesters, conferences may be held every 3 months. The purpose of the therapy conference differs depending on where the client is in the therapeutic process (e.g., starting therapy, involved in ongoing therapy, ending therapy). The length of time for a conference varies, but usually runs anywhere from 10 to 30 minutes.

One of the primary factors affecting the length of a conference is the comfort level of the student clinician in the role of conference facilitator, as well as the comfort level of the parent, spouse, or other family member. If all persons involved are comfortable, the conference tends to run longer. On the other hand, if the student clinician does not feel comfortable in this role, the conference tends to be shorter. Some student clinicians feel uncomfortable because they are not yet confident with their knowledge level or clinical ability. It is important for you to realize and believe that you are more knowledgeable in the area of communication problems than are most family members, unless

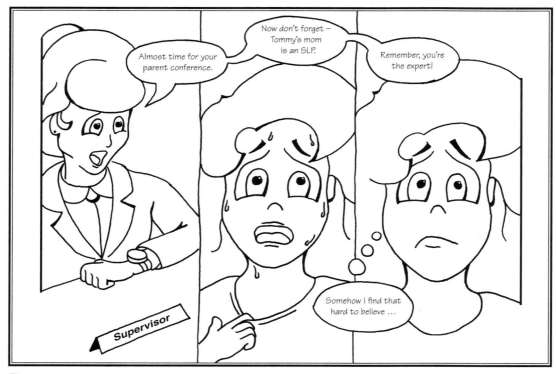

Figure 7.1. Anticipating the parent conference.

you have the pleasure of providing services to a family member of a speech–language pathologist. Any clinician would feel some initial uneasiness in this situation. (See Figure 7.1.)

Additional factors can influence the conference length. These include how much information you have prepared to present; how much time is available and has been set aside; how much information each attendee shares; how many questions the parent, spouse, or other family member asks; and how many interruptions occur particularly if any children are present.

The main purpose of a therapy conference is to provide information to, obtain information from, and share information with the client's family member. During this conference, you should inform the family member of the client's current functioning level. If results of formal and informal testing have not yet been discussed with the family member, you should present them at this time. Present the client's short- and long-range objectives, as well as the client's progress on each objective. Discuss any recommendations you have regarding needs that the client continues to have or any additional needs that may have arisen. For example, a recommendation concerning continued needs might be that the client should continue to receive therapy twice a week during the next semester, whereas a recommendation regarding additional needs might be that the client should be seen by an otolaryngologist. In addition, you should present the overall intervention plan, as well as the client's response to it. If the client's therapy program will be interrupted between semesters or over the summer, explain and demonstrate suggestions for a home program. Answer as completely as possible any questions that the family member asks. It is very important that the family member understands what he or she is expected to do, as well as how to do it and why he or she is doing it.

For this therapy conference to be most advantageous to everyone involved, it should be a two-way conference between you and the family member, with both involved as active participants. You should make certain that the family member feels free to add information or ask questions at any time during the conference. Provide several opportunities during the conference and at the end for the family member to ask questions. Perhaps the easiest way to do this is to ask if there are any questions after presenting and discussing each area. When a parent, spouse, or other family member does ask questions, it is your obligation to answer every question as thoroughly and correctly as possible in a manner that the family member can understand. If you are unable to answer a question or provide the requested information, you must immediately inform your supervisor and get guidance for a prompt, correct response. The old proverb, "better late than never," applies here.

Because it is impossible to know beforehand what will arise during therapy conferences, it is a good idea to have some knowledge of the counseling process and counseling procedures. Beginning student clinicians are encouraged to consult Luterman (2001) regarding the role of a speech–language pathologist as a counselor.

QUICK CHECK

The purpose of a therapy conference is to provide information to, obtain information from, and share information with the parent, spouse, or other family member. Address the following information: the client's current functioning level; test results that have not previously been shared with the parent, spouse, or other family member; short- and long-range objectives; and the client's progress in therapy. Provide suggestions regarding what the parent, spouse, or family member can do at home. Remember, you are the expert.

Therapy Conference Reports

When the therapy conference is over, a therapy conference report must be written. Four examples of such reports are presented in this chapter to give beginning clinicians a clearer idea of how to proceed. A conference with a grandparent is reflected in the first example, with a parent in the second and third examples, and with a spouse in the fourth example. These reports differ depending on the client's needs, as well as the parent's, spouse's, or other family member's needs. Before continuing with this text, read Therapy Conference Reports 1 and 2.

In the first two therapy conference reports, progress is evident. Progress of a general nature was addressed in the first report, whereas progress was specifically stated in the second report. A comparison was made in the second report between the client's functioning at the beginning of the semester and his current functioning. All persons attending a conference are different. Knowing that their child or grandchild is pro-gressing is enough information for some parents or grandparents. Other parents or grandparents have a desire to know how much their child or grandchild has progressed. Therefore, it is important to have this specific information at your fingertips. Before continuing with this text, read Therapy Conference Report 3.

The third therapy conference report had a different focus than the two preceding it. Mrs. Miller was in need of more counseling and education, as reflected in the content.

Therapy Report 4 features an adult rather than a child. Due to the client's speech problem, his wife served as the spokesperson.

QUICK CHECK

Therapy Conference Reports should accurately reflect what occurred during the conference. Information that was shared with the parent, spouse, or other family member should be reflected, as well as any concerns that the family member had.

(*text continues on p. 205*)

THERAPY CONFERENCE REPORT 1

Therapy Conference Report

[Identifying Information]

NAME:	Matthew Williams	FILE NUMBER:	
ADDRESS:	00 Broad Street	DATE:	October 28, [this year]
	Maintown, PA 00000	BIRTH DATE:	February 27, [3 years ago]
PHONE:	000-000-0000	AGE:	3 years 8 months
PARENTS:	Eli and Gina	CLINICIAN:	Nancy Crawford
		SEMESTER:	Fall [this year]

To discuss Matthew's progress during the fall semester, a conference with his grandmother, Shirley Williams, was held on Wednesday, October 28, because neither of Matthew's parents could attend. Matthew's evaluation, long-range goals, short-term objectives, and progress were discussed over the course of 10 minutes.

Mrs. Williams was informed that Matthew is progressing through the oral-motor objectives rapidly, and there has been improvement in his tongue control since the beginning of the semester. Mrs. Williams was pleased to hear that Matthew met the goal for auditory discrimination and that the next goal, correct production of /t/ in the initial position of words, would begin the next session. Matthew's grandmother said Matthew's parents were concerned about the lack of development of /ɚ/, /ð/, and blends in Matthew's speech. It was explained to her that these are later developing sounds, and the reason the focus was being placed on /t/ and eventually /d/ was because they were earlier developing sounds. Mrs. Williams also said that Matthew's parents were concerned about his communication skills, specifically his expressive language skills. She was told that therapy focusing on this aspect would also begin during the next session and that his expressive language would continue to be focused on and further evaluated throughout the next semester.

The clinician recommended that therapy continue twice a week for the next semester, and Mrs. Williams said Matthew's parents would agree. After questioning when therapy would begin for the spring semester, Mrs. Williams was informed that Matthew's parents would be contacted in early February for scheduling and that therapy activities to do at home with Matthew during the winter break would be given to him on his last day of therapy for this semester.

Nancy Crawford
_____
Nancy Crawford
Student Clinician

The above report was prepared by an undergraduate student.

Betty A. Brown
_____
Betty A. Brown, MS, CCC/SLP
Clinical Supervisor

THERAPY CONFERENCE REPORT 2

Therapy Conference Report

[Identifying Information]

NAME:	Evan Jones	FILE NUMBER:	
ADDRESS:	00 Main Street	DATE:	November 25, [this year]
	Maintown, PA 00000	BIRTH DATE:	December 2, [2 years ago]
PHONE:	000-000-0000	AGE:	2 years 11 months
PARENTS:	Ian and Helen	CLINICIAN:	Frances Carr
		SEMESTER:	Fall [this year]

On Monday, November 25, a conference was held with Evan's mother, Helen Jones, to discuss Evan's progress throughout the fall semester. During this 30-minute conference, Evan's long-range goals and short-term objectives were discussed, as well as his progress during this semester.

Evan's ability to follow one-step directions was discussed. It was explained that, to work on this goal, Evan was asked to point to an object or give an object to the clinician. Mrs. Jones was informed that Evan followed 20% of the one-step directions presented at the beginning of the semester compared with 78% currently. Another goal discussed was Evan's ability to establish eye contact when prompted by the clinician. It was noted that Evan looked at the clinician when prompted with "Look at me" 12 times during a recent session compared to 2 times during a session at the beginning of the semester. His last goal, ability to focus on an activity, gradually increased throughout the semester from 30 seconds to 6 minutes.

It was recommended that Mrs. Jones begin implementing behavior modification techniques with Evan. The use of time-out was discussed to decrease inappropriate behaviors such as hitting and kicking. Mrs. Jones stated that she previously used a similar technique with Evan. She put him in a chair in a corner for a period of 10 seconds following episodes of fighting with his brother. Mrs. Jones did not think the fighting episodes decreased. It was suggested that she try this method again but increase the amount of time Evan had to sit in the chair to 5 minutes to see if this had an impact on the number of fighting episodes.

Mrs. Jones agreed that therapy should continue next semester. The clinical supervisor recommended that Mrs. Jones contact her local school district for a full child study team evaluation to assess Evan's cognitive and behavioral functioning. Mrs. Jones expressed interest in enrolling Evan in a preschool program for disabled children in order to receive additional services.

Mrs. Jones expressed concern about her son's current language level. She stated that Evan exhibited a 1-year language delay when he was tested during the previous semester. She was advised that although formal testing was not administered this semester,

(continues)

his abilities could be informally assessed by comparing them to other children his age. She was informed that, based on observations during therapy sessions, Evan continued to exhibit about a 1-year delay. Mrs. Jones was informed that Evan is making progress, but not as rapidly as other children his age.

Frances Carr
_____
Frances Carr
Student Clinician

The above report was prepared by a graduate student.

Betty A. Brown
_____
Betty A. Brown, MS, CCC/SLP
Clinical Supervisor

THERAPY CONFERENCE REPORT 3

Therapy Conference Report

[Identifying Information]

NAME: Justin Miller
ADDRESS: 00 Long Road
Maintown, PA 00000
PHONE: 000-000-0000
PARENTS: John and Marie

FILE NUMBER:
DATE: April 30, [this year]
BIRTH DATE: March 28, [6 years ago]
AGE: 6 years 1 month
CLINICIAN: John B. Clemente
SEMESTER: Spring [this year]

On Thursday, April 28, a conference was held with Justin's mother, Marie Miller, to discuss his progress throughout the spring semester. During the half-hour conference, Justin's long-range and short-range goals were discussed, as well as his progress. Additional activities were also suggested to facilitate further improvement.

Mrs. Miller began the conference by stating that she is embarrassed by Justin's speech and often interprets what he says for others. She expressed concern over her son"s perceived lack of progress and attributed it to his "slowness." She was informed about the outcome of Justin's speech evaluation, which indicated multiple phonemes in error in varying positions. It was explained that the number of errors greatly impacts the ability of others to understand him and that it would be most beneficial to work on the sounds in error that are normally mastered at an earlier age. It was further explained that this reasoning was the basis for selecting Justin's long-range goals of producing /t/, /d/, and /m/ in the initial and final positions of words in sentences, and /p/ in the initial position of words in sentences. A short explanation and demonstration of a "routine" therapy session was given to illustrate the kind of feedback that Justin needs to enhance his success and progress. It was demonstrated, using picture articulation cards for the target sounds, how each sound is modeled at various levels, including isolation, syllable, word, phrase, and sentence, for Justin to imitate and ultimately produce. The role of delayed imitation to help him self-correct his errors was illustrated. Mrs. Miller was informed of Justin's current level of functioning: /t/ at the word level, /d/ and /m/ at the phrase level, and /p/ at the sentence level. It was explained that Justin was having more difficulty with production of /t/, probably due to the emergence of his permanent upper central incisors.

Mrs. Miller was receptive to suggestions given for carryover at home, including drill sheets for the /t/, /d/, /m/, and /p/ phonemes and a book list of familiar children's stories that address specific phonemes. She stated that Justin sometimes had difficulty attending when being read a story or practicing letter recognition. Mrs. Miller was assured that Justin's progress could be accelerated by having a continued positive attitude and increased practice at home. Mrs. Miller suggested setting time aside each night,

(continues)

possibly right before bedtime, to practice with Justin. She hoped that he would eventually anticipate this time and be more willing to focus on the task.

Mrs. Miller agreed that therapy should continue next semester. She gave permission for the clinician to send home a packet of activities for summer practice and stated that she would attempt to read to Justin more frequently.

John B. Clemente
_____
John B. Clemente
Student Clinician

The above report was prepared by an undergraduate student.

Betty A. Brown
_____
Betty A. Brown, MS, CCC/SLP
Clinical Supervisor

THERAPY CONFERENCE REPORT 4

Therapy Conference Report

[Identifying Information]

NAME: James Gregory

ADDRESS: 000 Smoke Street

                Maintown, PA 00000

PHONE: 000-000-0000

SPOUSE: Helen Gregory

FILE NUMBER:

DATE: April 28, [this year]

BIRTH DATE: March 28, [64 years ago]

AGE: 64 years

CLINICIAN: Bruce Carter

SEMESTER: Spring [this year]

On Thursday, April 28, a conference was held with Mr. Gregory and his spouse, Helen, to discuss his progress throughout the spring semester. During the 15-minute conference, Mr. Gregory did not attempt to speak but occassionally nodded his head in agreement with his wife's statements. Mr. Gregory's long-range and short-range goals were discussed.

Mrs. Gregory expressed concern over her husband's lack of speech clarity and questioned whether her husband would ever be understood by people outside the immediate family. Mrs. Gregory also stated how frustrated her husband was about not being able to be understood. Mr. Gregory nodded in agreement. Mrs. Gregory was reminded that it was only 2 months since her husband suffered his stroke and that progress was evident. She was also informed that initially Mr. Gregory had difficulty understanding language, although this no longer is an area of concern. The Gregory couple was also reminded that initially Mr. Gregory could not make any speech sounds but now he could put words together to form sentences. Further information on dysarthria was provided.

The Gregory couple was informed that Mr. Gregory's progress could be accelerated by practicing at home. Mrs. Gregory stated that they were both receptive to working on Mr. Gregory's speech at home, and he nodded in agreement. Therefore, additional oral exercises and activities were suggested to facilitate further improvement. The reason behind performing oral exercises was explained. New oral exercises were assigned, explained, and demonstrated. Two compensatory techniques (speaking slowly and over-exaggerating mouth movements) for improving intelligibility were likewise explained and demonstrated. Mr. Gregory was given a list of 20 common phrases to say while practicing these techniques.

(continues)

It was recommended that therapy continue twice a week. Mrs. Gregory stated that they would like sevices three times a week. This increase will be discussed with my supervisor and Mr. and Mrs. Gregory will learn the decision during the next session.

Bruce Carter
———————————————————
Bruce Carter
Student Clinician

The above report was prepared by an undergraduate student.

Betty A. Brown
———————————————————
Betty A. Brown, MS, CCC/SLP
Clinical Supervisor

Conclusion

It is important for you to feel comfortable or at least to convey the feeling of being comfortable while conducting therapy conferences. This helps to communicate a sense of competence and assures the parent, spouse, or other family member that you are an expert who knows what you are doing. Prepare for the conference and be organized. Have all items (i.e., test results, long- and short-range goals, therapy progress reports) that you plan to discuss at your fingertips. Anticipate some of the questions and concerns that the parent, spouse, or other family member may have. Think about how you will answer these questions and address these concerns in advance so you are not caught off guard. The more prepared you are, the more comfortable you will feel and the more competent you will come across. Preparation makes all the difference in the world.

KNOW IT, USE IT!

After reading this chapter, you should be able to

1. state the main purpose of a therapy conference.
2. state five areas covered in a therapy conference.
3. explain the importance of a two-way conference.
4. write a therapy conference report.

Reference

Luterman, D. M. (2001). *Counseling persons with communication disorders and their families.* Austin, TX: PRO-ED.

Chapter 8

Preparing for the Public Schools

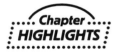

Chapter HIGHLIGHTS

- Impact of academic standards on school-based clinicians
- IDEA '97 and the effect on school-based clinicians
- Paperwork in the public schools
- Contents of an Individualized Education Program
- Contents of an evaluation report
- Samples of paperwork

Beginning speech–language clinicians are usually well prepared for providing hands-on speech and language services in the schools. However, they are rarely prepared for or knowledgeable about the extraordinary amount of paperwork required in the public school setting. Handling paperwork is typically the hardest, most difficult, and most frustrating part of working in the public school systems. Not only is there a lot of unique paperwork, but the regulations and mandates dictating this paperwork constantly undergo change. Therefore, it is unlikely that a school-based speech–language clinician will ever get to the point of feeling completely comfortable with the paperwork process.

A Word of ADVICE

To help you get a sense of what this chapter is discussing, review the appendixes now (simply glance through them—do not read them in depth at this point). When each form or report is discussed in text, take the time to carefully study each. Time spent on careful analysis at this point will pay big dividends to you later.

Brief Background

The Individuals with Disabilities Education Act of 1990 (IDEA; Public Law [P.L.] 101-476) regulates the delivery of services to children with disabilities in the schools. Decisions about services for children with speech, language, and hearing disabilities must be consistent with the requirements of IDEA. The IDEA Amendments of 1997 (P.L. 105-17), known as IDEA '97, changed the role of school-based speech–language pathologists in major ways. Two areas reflecting change involve therapy (the way it is done) and paperwork (what has to be done and how). Brannen et al. (2000) wrote, "The clinical model of exclusive pull-out therapy focusing on discrete speech or language skills should now be replaced by a comprehensive intervention program that supports students' involvement in academic, nonacademic, and extracurricular programs" (p. 6). Because of these mandates, changes became necessary in the traditional role of the school-based speech–language pathologist. IDEA '97 also resulted in measuring all student progress as related to the general education curriculum, further increasing the paperwork by requiring the speech–language clinician to prepare progress reports at least as often as traditional report cards are issued to regular education students. In most districts, progress reporting is done four times per year. The manner in which this is done is up to the school district. (See Appendix 8.A to get an idea of an optional progress report form used in Minnesota.) With passage of IDEA '97, school-based speech–language clinicians also had to become familiar with, knowledgeable about, and work within the general education curriculum. In an ASHA Telephone Seminar, Eger (2002) answered the question, "What does the general education curriculum mean?"

> It simply means all instruction is from regular courses at the regular grade level; all special education teachers have the regular courses for the age level of their students; all special education teachers use the same materials as other teachers; additional materials are used only after regular materials are not successful; and when using different materials, we continue to direct instruction to the regular course, the regular goals, objectives, and standards.

It has also become necessary for speech–language clinicians to write Individualized Education Programs (IEPs) differently. IEPs now have to be directly linked to the curriculum (thus, the name, "curriculum-linked IEP"). IEPs have to be aligned with the state standards, which are derived from the state regulations. See Appendix 8.B for an example of one set of standards in the language arts area (Mid-continent Research for Education and Learning [McRel], n.d.). The McRel Web site lists additional standards in the areas of writing, reading, listening, and speaking. The McRel standards specify the knowledge and skills students need to learn in each area by grade levels (K–2, 3–5, 6–8, and 9–12). McRel has been in the forefront of standards-based education for over 10 years. Many states have adopted these McRel standards, but other states have adopted their own standards. The academic standards used in a state can be found by looking up that state's department of education on the Internet.

According to Hock (2000), standards "are a gift for special educators. The frameworks provide an exceptional tool for planning IEPs" (p. 6). Standards also establish a framework of accountability for all students. Keep in mind, however, that academic standards used by states do not form a statewide curriculum, but instead serve as a baseline from which school districts develop their own standards that contain the district's goals and objectives. Each school district is responsible for designing and implementing its own curriculum based on its state's academic standards, as well as on its own standards, goals, and objectives. The state's standards must be considered when developing each child's IEP because his needs have to be matched with the general education curriculum and are consequently called curriculum-linked IEPs. All therapy provided by a speech–language clinician must then address the IEP. Because therapy addresses the IEP, it must also be based on the curriculum. Therefore, the type of therapy provided is referred to as curriculum-based therapy. Curriculum-based therapy is further addressed in Chapter 9.

Although speech–language clinicians in the schools were aware that IDEA '97 required changes in their functioning, they did not know the direction the changes were to take. The final Part B regulations that implement the statutory changes made by IDEA '97 were published in the Federal Register on March 12, 1999. School districts started providing in-services for their staffs regarding these 1997 changes during the 2001–2002 school year. Some districts started implementing these changes during the first half of the 2001 school year, whereas others did not begin implementation until the second half.

IDEA '97 was scheduled to be reviewed during the year 2002 as the amendments expired. "While Part B is permanently reauthorized, Parts C and D were up for reauthorization in 2002. The reauthorization process for Parts C and D provides an opportunity to review Part B as well" (ASHA, 2002a, p. 2). ASHA (2002b) stated, "IDEA was last reauthorized in 1997, and the current congressional authority for the law ends at the close of this federal fiscal year on Oct. 1 [2002]. This reauthorization process is expected to take at least two years" (p. 1). Thus, it appears that changes will be made on top of changes. However, on the basis of past practice, it will take a while for these changes to filter down to those having to implement them.

In March 2003, legislation to reauthorize IDEA was introduced in the U.S. House of Representatives. The bill, H.R. 1350, is known as Improving Education Results for Children with Disabilities Act of 2003. According to ASHA (2003), H.R. 1350 "would reauthorize, restructure, and extend programs under IDEA" (p. 1). Supposedly this bill "includes calls for stronger accountability and results for students, paperwork reduction, greater flexibility for school districts to improve early intervention, improved conflict resolution, and a reduction of the number of children wrongly placed in special education" (ASHA, 2003, p. 1).

According to K. R. Franklin (Director of ASHA's Capitol Hill Office) and C. D. Clarke (ASHA's Director of Education and Regulatory Advocacy) (personal communication, November 10, 2003), it does not appear that IDEA reauthorization will be finalized in calendar year 2003. They said "once reauthorization occurs, it will take at least one year, probably longer, for the regulations to be published." Therefore, it will not be known what the new IDEA reauthorization will mean to speech–language pathologists until long after this book is published.

QUICK CHECK

School-based public school clinicians need to be knowledgeable about the Individuals with Disabilities Education Act, the IDEA '97 Amendments, their state regulations and academic standards, their district's standards, and all new relevant legislation. Knowledge in all of these areas is necessary for the successful functioning of speech–language clinicians in a public school setting.

Required Paperwork

A school-based speech–language clinician must be knowledgeable about the paperwork that is mandated by IDEA '97. It is important to be familiar with eight forms that are a part of the multidisciplinary evaluation process, which is also referred to as the IEP process or the special education process. All of these processes fit under the rubric of Procedural Safeguards. The necessary forms, which vary slightly from state to state and school district to school district, and may be titled differently, are Permission to Evaluate; Procedural Safeguards Letter; Procedural Safeguards Notice; Evaluation Report; Invitation To Participate in the IEP Team Meeting or Other Meeting; Individualized Education Program (IEP); Notice of Recommended Educational Placement; and Permission to Reevaluate. In some states, for example, Minnesota, Permission to Evaluate and Permission to Reevaluate are both included on one form (Appendix 8.C). Blank examples of many of these eight forms can be found in Appendixes 8.C through 8.G. Completed examples of several forms appear in Appendixes 8.H through 8.J. Each of the eight pieces of paperwork within the multidisciplinary evaluation process is briefly addressed in the following sections.

Permission To Evaluate or Consent for Evaluation

The Permission to Evaluate Form may be called by a different name in other states. One possibility is Consent for Evaluation Form. (A sample copy of Oregon's Consent for Evaluation Form appears in Appendix 8.D.) This form is sent to the student's parent(s) or guardian(s) to gain consent to proceed. Tests and procedures that will be used during the evaluation must be stated. The parents are informed that their input is a part of the evaluation process and will be considered by the team. Additionally, some school districts send a Parent Input Form to the parents to give them an opportunity to provide information for the Evaluation Report. The parents are also informed that they are members of this team.

Procedural Safeguards Letter and Notice of Procedural Safeguards

Both the Procedural Safeguards Letter and the Notice of Procedural Safeguards must be made available to the student's parent(s) or guardian(s) at a minimum of four different times during the IEP process. Initially, the letter and notice are sent along with the Permission to Evaluate or Consent for Evaluation Form. The Procedural Safeguards Letter and Notice must also be made available to the parent(s) or guardian(s) upon each notification of an IEP meeting, upon reevaluation of the child, and upon receipt of a request for due process. Information for parents or guardians about state or local advocacy organizations is included. Phone numbers are provided for toll-free parental assistance, legal assistance, and free mediation services. The Notice of Procedural Safeguards describes the parents' rights and the procedures for safeguarding these rights. Impartial due process hearings are described. A copy of this notice, as used in Minnesota, appears in Appendix 8.E.

Evaluation Report

An Evaluation Report (ER) has two purposes. First, it is necessary to determine if a student has a disability. Second, it is necessary to determine if a student needs specially designed instruction. A copy of this ER must be presented to the parents no later than 60 school days after the written parental permission is received by the school. There are many essential parts of an ER (see Appendix 8.H). Some of the more relevant parts are addressed here.

Educational Levels of Performance and Educational Needs of the Child

The student's current functioning level, strengths, progress in the general education curriculum, response to the instructional program, and results of the instructional evaluation should be contained in the Educational Levels of Performance and Educational Needs of the Child section. The results of the speech and language evaluation are also recorded here. Questions posed in the referral statement should be addressed.

Evaluation Data Results of Direct Intervention

In the Evaluation Data Results of Direct Intervention section, three areas that affect the student's ability to access the general education curriculum are addressed. One area is physical, social, or cultural information relevant to the child's disability and need for special education. Only information that has relevance to eligibility or programming should be included. The other two areas are current classroom-based assessments and observations by teachers and related service providers. These observations should produce data that can be used to answer the referral question(s). Assessment data related to the student's functioning in the curriculum is included in this section.

Evaluations and Information Provided by the Parents of the Child

The intent of the Evaluations and Information Provided by the Parents of the Child portion is to use information provided by the parents to address the referral question(s). Parents can provide information pertaining to and results of any independent educational evaluations that the student has received. Parents may also provide information about instructional or behavioral strategies that they have implemented.

Summary of Findings/Interpretation of Assessment Results

The data collected throughout the evaluation process is analyzed in the Summary of Findings/Interpretation of Assessment Results section. The rationale for the determination of eligibility is explained. Any referral questions asked at the beginning of the evaluation are answered by the evaluation team. If the student is suspected of having a specific learning disability, additional documentation is necessary.

Conclusions

In the Conclusion section, an eligibility determination must be made. A student is either identified as having a disability and being in need of specially designed instruction, identified as having a disability but not being in need of specially designed instruction, or identified as not having a disability. According to the Code of Federal Regulations, disability categories include mental retardation, hearing impairment including deafness, speech or language impairment, visual impairment including blindness, emotional disturbance, orthopedic impairment, autism, traumatic brain injury, other health impairments, specific learning disability, deaf-blindness, or multiple disabilities [34 C.F.R. 300.7 (a)(1)]. Attention-deficit disorder (ADD) and attention-deficit/hyperactivity disorder (ADHD) are classified as "other health impairments." Secondary disabilities are also indicated in the conclusion section. Recommendations that will enable the student to meet his goals and participate in the general education curriculum are also provided in this section of the Evaluation Report.

Invitation To Participate in the IEP Team Meeting or Other Meeting

The Invitation to Participate invites the parent(s) or guardian(s) to attend and participate in the IEP meeting. If the invitation is for a meeting other than an IEP meeting, the nature of the meeting must be specified. The date, time, and location of this meeting must be provided. In case these arrangements are not convenient, a contact person and phone number should be given for calls to request changes. The names of the other people attending this meeting and their respective roles are given. An invitation to an IEP or placement meeting must be accompanied by a copy of the procedural safeguards notice. Several options regarding the meeting (attending, not attending, need alternative arrangements, need accommodations, etc.) may be listed. If this appears, the parent should check one of these options. A sample copy of this invitation from the state of Wisconsin appears in Appendix 8.F.

Individualized Education Program

The core sources for information about speech–language pathologists' legal obligations in developing IEPs for children with disabilities are IDEA '97 and the accompanying regulations issued by the U.S. Department of Education on March 12, 1999 (Brannen et al., 2000, Appendix A). The IEP must be developed within 30 calendar days from the date of the Evaluation Report. According to Arena (2001),

> The IEP is not a legal contract. It is formulated as a team effort, based on what the child needs—not what the school district (local educational agency) can provide. What the local district cannot provide must be obtained or contracted for. (p. 25)

The IEP process consists of four stages: development, implementation, review, and revision. Representatives of the local educational agency, the teacher, the parents, and the child, when appropriate, are all involved in developing the IEP. Arena (2001) wrote, "Simply stated, the IEP tells where the child is, where he should be going, how he'll get there, how long it will take, and how you will know he has arrived" (p. 25). The IEP form may vary somewhat from state to state or school district to school district because, according to Arena (2001), "There is no national form the written statement of the IEP must take. This decision is left entirely, in the law, to the local education agency" (p. 26). Although IEP forms may differ, they all must contain certain essential parts, some of which are addressed in the following text. Because of the complexity and the legal implications of the IEP, it is important that you become thoroughly familiar with its requirements. To help you in this regard, Appendix 8.I is a completed sample of an IEP form from Pennsylvania.

Present Levels of Educational Performance

The Present Levels of Educational Performance (PLEP) is a very important part of the IEP because it becomes the baseline. Every goal that is written must have its foundation somewhere in the PLEP; that is, every goal must be tied to a need specified in the PLEP. All information presented in this section must support the rest of the IEP and should be directly derived from the assessment results. A starting point for intervention should be clearly indicated. Another issue to be addressed in this section is how the student's disability affects involvement and progress in the general education curriculum. Both the student's strengths and needs should be discussed. Any needs identified must be addressed in the remainder of the IEP. This section may also include the student's performance in response to changes in instruction or other supports, instructional accommodations, or adaptations.

Measurable Annual Goal

The IEP needs to list goals that can realistically be accomplished in a 12-month time frame and that are measurable. These goals need to directly evolve from the PLEP. Annual goals must relate to general curriculum areas in which the student's disability affects his ability to be involved and to progress.

These annual goals include either benchmarks or short-term objectives that enable assessment of the child's progress within the general curriculum. According to Lucas (2000), "Benchmarks are statements about reference points along the path toward learning a new skill or set of skills. They are identified sub-skills that are required to meet the desired standard" (p. 5). Benchmarks are general statements that represent milestones to goals. Short-term objectives (or short-range objectives) were addressed in Chapter 1. Brannen et al. (2000, Appendix B, p. 2) explained that "short-term objectives are measurable, intermediate steps between a student's present level of educational performance and the annual goals established for the student." Short-term objectives comprise specific statements that contain conditions, behaviors (performance), and criteria. (For a review of this information, consult Chapter 1.) The expected level of achievement and method of evaluation must be indicated on the IEP. Specially designed instruction is flexible in that it can appear in one of two places on the IEP. It can be listed (a) with each goal or objective or (b) in a section on special education/related services.

Special Education/Related Services

In the IEP, special education, which is specially designed instruction, and related services need to be addressed. Related services include but are not limited to the following: audiology, counseling services, early identification, medical services, occupational therapy, parent counseling and training, physical therapy, psychological services, recreation, school health services, social work services, speech pathology, and transportation. This list is not exhaustive, because the law states that "each public agency shall take whatever steps are necessary to provide nonacademic and extracurricular services and activities so that handicapped children are afforded an equal opportunity for participation in such services" (Arena, 2001, p. 23). Also included in this section are supplementary aids and services that are provided to the student or on the student's behalf and program modifications or supports for school personnel.

Participation in State and District-Wide Assessments

States require that students with disabilities participate in state and district-wide assessment programs. If accommodations or modifications are necessary for the student to participate, they must be stated in this section of the IEP. If the IEP team determines that the student will not participate in this assessment or part of this assessment, reasons why the assessment is not appropriate for the student must be presented. The alternative assessment that will be used must be stated.

Least Restrictive Environment

Because a student must be placed in the least restrictive environment, an explanation must be provided in the IEP addressing why a student will not be educated with nondisabled peers in the regular classroom and in extracurricular and other nonacademic activities. The percentage of time that a student receives special education out of the regular education classroom must be indicated. The categories are less than 21%, 21% to 60%, and 61% or more outside of the regular education classroom in regular schools with nondisabled students.

Notice of Recommended Educational Placement

The Notice of Recommended Educational Placement (NOREP) summarizes recommendations for the student's educational program. It addresses many areas, such as what action was proposed or refused, as well as the reasons. It includes a description of other options that were considered and why they were rejected, items that formed the basis for the proposed action or the refusal of the action, and the educational placement recommended for the student. Parents or guardians either approve or disapprove this placement. If they disapprove, they provide a reason. At this point, the parents or guardians may request a prehearing conference, mediation, or a due-process hearing. If a due-process hearing is requested, it must be held within 30 days of the request, and the decision must be forthcoming within 45 days of receipt of the request. The form must be signed by the parent or guardian and returned. The NOREP should be implemented as soon as possible, but no later than 10 days after its completion. To better understand the NOREP, consult Appendix 8.J to see a completed sample. An example of a form with the same intent, Nebraska's Notice and Consent for Placement in Special Education Services, is in Appendix 8.G.

Permission To Reevaluate

As stated previously, the Permission to Reevaluate notice may be titled differently in various states, but the intent remains the same. This permission notice informs the parent(s) or guardian(s) that the student will be reevaluated and why, indicates the tests and procedures that will be used, and gives the proposed date for the reevaluation. Another copy of the Procedural Safeguards Notice is sent with the Permission to Reevaluate. If reasonable attempts are made to obtain parental or guardian consent and a response is not received, the school district is permitted by law to proceed with the reevaluation. The reevaluation report is to be completed and the parents have to be presented with a copy no later than 60 school days after the school district receives the signed Permission to Reevaluate form. A school-age student is to be reevaluated every 3 years. The form in Appendix 8.C is Minnesota's permission form for both evaluation and reevaluation.

Conclusion

All parts of the multidisciplinary evaluation process are important. To perform the duties of a speech–language clinician in the public schools, you must become thoroughly familiar with and comply with all parts of this process. Be aware of all changes required by law, and implement them in a timely fashion.

Thoroughly familiarize yourself with each aspect of the paperwork process. Know what information must be included and where it should be included. Find out the designated time frame and work within it.

After reading this chapter, you should be able to

1. explain the main problem confronting speech–language clinicians employed in the public schools.
2. state at least 10 of the disability categories acknowledged in the Code of Federal Regulations.
3. name eight pieces of paperwork encountered by school-based clinicians.
4. state at least three higher level influences (outside of the school) that dictate the functioning of school-based speech–language clinicians.
5. state at least three areas that must be covered in an IEP.
6. explain the impact of IDEA '97 on speech–language clinicians employed in the public schools.

Appendix 8.A

Example of Progress Report Form

	PROGRESS REPORT (Optional Form)

Student Name: _____ Report Date: _____

School: _____ Grade: _____ Date of IEP: _____

Progress toward the annual goals and the extent to which annual goals can be achieved by the end of the IEP year:

#: [ ]	**Goal:**	
[ ] insufficient progress [ ] adequate progress [ ] goal met	Comments:	

#: [ ]	**Goal:**	
[ ] insufficient progress [ ] adequate progress [ ] goal met	Comments:	

#: [ ]	**Goal:**	
[ ] insufficient progress [ ] adequate progress [ ] goal met	Comments:	

#: [ ]	**Goal:**	
[ ] insufficient progress [ ] adequate progress [ ] goal met	Comments:	

Note to Parents: You are entitled to request a meeting to discuss this review.

Note. This document is included in this book only as an example and is not intended to be copied and used. Reprinted with permission from Minnesota Department of Children, Families & Learning, Minnesota Special Education. Retrieved October 31, 2003, from http://education.state.mn.us/stellent/groups/public/documents/translatedcontent/pub_053132.pdf

Appendix 8.B

Example of Language Arts Standards

Language Arts Standards

Writing

1. Uses the general skills and strategies of the writing process

2. Uses the stylistic and rhetorical aspects of writing

3. Uses grammatical and mechanical conventions in written compositions

4. Gathers and uses information for research purposes

Reading

5. Uses the general skills and strategies of the reading process

6. Uses reading skills and strategies to understand and interpret a variety of literary texts

7. Uses reading skills and strategies to understand and interpret a variety of informational texts

Listening and Speaking

8. Uses listening and speaking strategies for different purposes

Note. Reprinted with permission from Mid-continent Research for Education and Learning. Retrieved October 31, 2003, from http://www.mcrel.org/compendium/SubjectTopics.asp?subjectID=7

Appendix 8.C

Example of Notice of Educational Evaluation/Reevaluation Plan

<table>
<tr>
<td></td>
<td>NOTICE OF EDUCATIONAL
EVALUATION/REEVALUATION PLAN
(Page 1 of 2)</td>
</tr>
</table>

Student Name: _____ Date: _____

School: _____ Grade: _____ DOB: _____

Dear _____:

a. ☐ This notice is for an initial evaluation to determine your child's eligibility for special education. The school district must receive your signed permission before it can begin the evaluation.

b. ☐ This notice is for a reevaluation. (Select one of the boxes below.)

    ☐ Based on a review of existing data regarding your child, additional testing is needed to determine if your child continues to have a disability and needs special education services.

    ☐ Based on a review of existing data as described below, additional testing is <u>not</u> needed to determine whether your child continues to have a disability and continues to be in need of special education services.

Describe other options or factors that were considered relevant to this evaluation such as behavior, blindness or visual impairment, deafness or hard of hearing, assistive technology, race, culture, or language:

Following is a statement of adaptations needed to conduct this evaluation:

Area(s)	Materials and Procedures	Evaluator's Title
Intellectual Functioning		
Academic Performance		
Social, Emotional, Behavioral		
Communication		
Motor Ability		
Functional Skills		
Physical Status		
Sensory Status		
Transition, including Vocational		
Other procedures:		

(continues)

Page 2 **Evaluation Notice** Student Name: _____

The evaluation will be conducted at _____
and is provided at no cost to you. Location(s)

Note to parent(s): If you have questions please contact:

_____
Name   Position   Telephone

Resources you may contact for further information about parent rights and procedural safeguards:

ARC Minnesota (Advocacy for Persons with Developmental Disabilities): 651-523-0823, 1-800-582-5256

Family Service Inc., Learning Disabilities Program: 651-222-0311, 1-800-982-2303, TTY: 651-222-0175

MN Disability Law Center: 612-332-1441, 1-800-292-4150, TTY: 612-332-4668

MN Department of Education: 651-582-8689, TTY: 651-582-8201

PACER (Parent Advocacy Coalition for Education Rights): 952-838-9000, 1-800-53-PACER, TTY: 952-838-0190

PARENT ACTION

Parent(s): If "box a" is checked on page 1, select one of the options below, sign and date this form, and return this right away. The school district must receive your signed permission before it can begin the evaluation.

☐ **I give permission** to the school district to proceed with the evaluation as proposed.

☐ **I do not give permission** for the school to proceed with the evaluation as proposed. I understand that you will contact me to offer a conciliation conference or mediation. I understand that I (or the district) have the right to proceed directly to a due process hearing.

Parent(s): If "box b" is checked on page 1, select one of the following options, sign and date this form, and return this right away. If your signed permission is not received, the district will wait 14 calendar days before beginning. If you object in writing within 14 calendar days after receiving this notice, the district will not begin the evaluation.

(continues)

☐ **I agree** with the evaluation plan. I understand that an evaluation report will be written within 30 school days (age 3–21) or 45 calendar days (birth through age 2).

☐ **I do not agree** with the group's decision. I request that further evaluation be done.

_____   _____
Parent Signature (Student if age 18 or older)   Date

Enclosure: Notice of Procedural Safeguards

Date received by district	(for district use only)	Evaluation completion due:

[30 school days (age 3–21)]
[45 calendar days (birth through age 2)]

This form is available in several languages, Braille, or other formats.
Contact the IEP manager for an alternate format.

Note. This document is included in this book only as an example and is not intended to be copied and used. Reprinted with permission from Minnesota Department of Children, Families & Learning, Minnesota Special Education. Retrieved April 14, 2003, from http://education.state.mn.us/stellent/groups/publicdocuments/translatedcontent/pub_053127.pdf

Appendix 8.D

Example of Prior Notice About Evaluation/Consent for Evaluation

---

Date: _____
MM/DD/YY

PRIOR NOTICE ABOUT EVALUATION/CONSENT FOR EVALUATION

Dear _____

_____ has been referred for an evaluation. The Team is proposing the following:

☐ To evaluate your child's need for special education services.	☐ To reevaluate your child's needs for special education services.	☐ No additional evaluation data are needed to determine that your child needs or continues to need special education. The reason(s) why are: _____ If you disagree, you may request an assessment to determine whether your child continues to be a child with a disability.
Because:		

This proposal is based on the following evaluation procedures, tests, records or reports:

Other options we considered were:

We decided against these options because:

Any other factors considered by the team:

Sincerely, _____
Name and Title   Phone

(continues)

CONSENT FOR EVALUATION

We request your consent because:

☐ This is an initial evaluation and will be used to determine whether your child is a child with a disability and to determine special education needs.

☐ This evaluation will include intelligence or personality testing.

☐ This is a reevaluation and will be used to decide your child's continued eligibility and/or education needs. Except for tests of intelligence and personality, if you don't respond, the evaluation can be conducted without your consent.

The evaluation procedure(s), assessment and/or test(s) we plan to use include the following:

If the evaluation includes release of student educational records requiring parent consent, the "Records Release Form(s)" identifies the records to be released, and to whom; see Record Release dated: _____

☐ I give my permission for the evaluation. I understand my consent is voluntary and may be revoked any time before the evaluation process begins.

☐ I refuse permission for the evaluation.

_____   _____
    Signature (Parent/Guardian/Surrogate Parent)   (mm/dd/yy)

Parents of a child with a disability have protection under the procedural safeguards, which are enclosed. For assistance in understanding this information you may contact:

_____   _____   _____
          NAME   TITLE   PHONE

Note. This document is included in this book only as an example and is not intended to be copied and used. Reprinted with permission from Oregon Department of Education, Office of Special Education. Retrieved April 14, 2003, from http://www.ode.state.or.us/sped/doc.pub/forms/schoolage/

Appendix 8.E

Example of Notice of Procedural Safeguards

NOTICE OF PROCEDURAL SAFEGUARDS
PARENTAL RIGHTS FOR SPECIAL EDUCATION

March 2000

INTRODUCTION

This brochure provides an overview of special education rights, sometimes called procedural safeguards. These same procedural safeguards are also available for students with disabilities who have reached the age of 18. This **Notice of Procedural Safeguards** must be given to you when you ask for a copy. It must also be given to you:

1. the first time your child is referred for a special education evaluation;
2. each time an annual individual education program (IEP) or an annual individual family service plan (IFSP) meeting is scheduled for your child;
3. each time your child is reevaluated;
4. if you request a due process hearing;
5. if the district suspends your child for more than ten (10) consecutive days; or,
6. if the district places your child in an interim alternative education setting for up to 45 days for certain drug and weapons-related misconduct.

PRIOR WRITTEN NOTICE

The district must provide you with prior written notice each time it proposes to initiate or change, or refuses to initiate or change the identification, evaluation, or education placement of your child.

This written notice must include:

1. A description of the action proposed or refused;
2. An explanation of why the district proposes or refuses to take the action;
3. A description of any other options the school considered and the reasons why those options were rejected;
4. A description of each evaluation procedure, test, record, or report the school used as a basis for its proposal or refusal;
5. A description of any other factors relevant to the school's proposal or refusal;
6. A statement that your child has protection under these procedural safeguards and information about how you can get a copy of the brochure; and
7. Sources for you to contact to obtain assistance in understanding these procedural safeguards.

FOR MORE INFORMATION

If you need help in understanding any of your procedural rights or anything about your child's education, please contact the principal or the person listed below. This notice must be provided in your native language or other mode of

(continues)

communication you may be using, like a sign language interpreter.

If you have any questions or would like further information, please contact:

Name _____

Phone _____

You may also contact a statewide Minnesota advocacy organization to explain the notice to you:

ARC Minnesota (advocacy for persons
　with developmental disabilities):
　651-523-0823, 1-800-582-5256
Family Service Inc., Learning Disabilities
　Program: 651-222-0311, 651-222-0175
　(TTY), 1-800-982-2303
MN Association for Children's Mental Health:
　651-644-7333, 1-800-528-4511
MN Brain Injury Association: 612-378-2742,
　1-800-444-6443
MN Department of Children, Families &
　Learning: 651-582-8689, 651-582-8201
　(TTY)
MN Disability Law Center: 612-322-1441,
　612-332-4668 (TTY), 1-800-292-4150
MN Special Education Mediation Service:
　651-297-4635, 651-297-5353,
　1-800-627-3529 (TTY)
PACER (Parent Advocacy Coalition for
　Educational Rights): 612-827-2966
　(Voice), 612-827-7770 (TTY),
　1-800-53-PACER

PARENTAL CONSENT

The district must obtain your **written consent** before conducting its initial evaluation with your child and before the first time it provides special education and related services to your child. Giving consent for an initial evaluation does not mean that you have given consent for an initial placement.

The district can do a reevaluation without your consent if it can show that reasonable steps have been taken to get your written consent. After reasonable efforts have been made to obtain your consent, the district can proceed with the proposed reevaluation if you do not object in writing within ten days.

You have a right **to object in writing** to any action the district proposes. Upon receipt of your written objection, the district will ask you to attend a conciliation conference, mediation, or other mutually agreed upon method of alternative dispute resolution.

If you object to a proposed service or evaluation, the district may not deny your child any other service or activity. The district must continue to provide an appropriate education to your child.

If you do object in writing, the district cannot evaluate your child without your consent unless authorized by a hearing officer. The district can proceed with its proposal if you fail to object in **writing.**

1. Schools cannot give information to a medical agency without parental consent.
2. The district can request but not require you to utilize your private health insurance to help pay for services.

INDEPENDENT EDUCATIONAL EVALUATIONS

An independent educational evaluation (IEE) is an evaluation by a qualified person(s) who is not an employee of your district. You may ask for an IEE at school district expense if you disagree with the district's evaluation. **Your request must be in writing.** A hearing officer may also order an independent evaluation of your child at school district expense during a due process hearing.

Upon request, the district must give you information regarding its criteria for selection of

(continues)

an independent examiner and information about where an independent education evaluation may be obtained.

If the district does not believe an IEE is necessary, the district must ask a hearing officer to determine the appropriateness of its evaluation. If the hearing officer determines the district's evaluation is appropriate, you still have the right to an independent evaluation, but not at public expense.

If you obtain an IEE, the results of the evaluation must be considered by the IEP/IFSP team and may be presented as evidence at a due process hearing regarding your child.

EDUCATION RECORDS

Access to Records

If you want to look at your child's records, ask the principal to provide you with access to those education records you want to review. These records include all information that is collected, maintained, or used by staff. The district must let you review the records without unnecessary delay and before any IEP/IFSP meeting or any hearing about your child. The district has ten (10) business days to respond to your request.

Your right to inspect and review records includes the right to:

1. An explanation or interpretation of your child's records upon request;
2. An opportunity to have someone of your choice inspect and review the records; and
3. Request that the district provide copies of your child's educational records to you. A fee may be charged for the copies.

Record of Access

The district must keep a record of any individual other than authorized district employees who has reviewed your child's education rec-

ords. This record of access must include the name of the person, the date when he/she reviewed the records, and his/her purpose for reviewing the records.

Consent to Release Records

Parent consent is required before personally identifiable information is released to unauthorized persons or agencies.

Fees for Searching, Retrieving, and Copying Records

The district may not charge a fee to search or retrieve records, but may charge a reasonable fee for making copies of these records, unless you cannot afford to pay the fee.

Amendment of Records at Parent's Request

1. The district is obligated to inform you of the type and location of its education records on your child.
2. If you believe that information in your child's records is inaccurate, misleading, or violates the privacy or other rights of your child, you may request in writing that the district amend or remove the information. The district must decide if it will change the records. If the district decides not to make the changes, the district must inform you in writing that you have the right to a hearing to challenge the district's position. The hearing officer decides whether the information is accurate.

Destruction of Records

Before the district destroys any education records pertaining to your child, you will be informed. However, the school will always maintain permanent information on your child, including: name, address, phone number, and transcripts with grades and classes.

(continues)

MEDIATION

Mediation is a voluntary process. You or your district may request mediation from the Minnesota Special Education Mediation Service (MNSEMS) at 651.297.4635. Mediation uses a neutral third party trained in mediation techniques. Mediation may not be used to deny or delay your right to a due process hearing. Both you and district staff must agree to try mediation before a mediator can be assigned. At any time during the mediation, you or the district may withdraw.

If your child is age birth to 3, you may request mediation and all public agencies involved in the dispute must participate in the process. Mediations for children birth to 3 must be completed within 30 days. Mediation proceedings for older children have no time restrictions.

WRITTEN COMPLAINTS

Any organization or individual may file a complaint with the Minnesota Department of Children, Families & Learning (CFL). Complaints sent to CFL must:

1. Be **in writing** and be signed by the individual or organization registering the complaint;
2. Allege violations of state or federal special education law or rule which have occurred within the last year unless a longer period is reasonable because the violation is continuing;
3. State the facts upon which the allegation is based; and
4. Include the name, address, and telephone number of the person or organization registering the complaint.

The complaint should be mailed to:

Minnesota Department of Children,
Families & Learning
Division of Accountability and Compliance
Complaint System Supervisor
1500 West Highway 36
Roseville, MN 55113-4266
651.582.8689 Phone   651.582.8725 Fax

IMPARTIAL DUE PROCESS HEARING

Both you and the district have a right to request **in writing** an impartial due process hearing. A due process hearing may address any matter related to identification, evaluation, education placement, or provision of a free appropriate public education.

If you request a hearing in writing, the district must inform you of the availability of mediation. The district must provide you with information regarding free or low-cost legal services available in your area.

Procedures for Initiation of a Due Process Hearing

Upon your written request to the district for a hearing, the district must give you a copy of your rights. Your **written request** must include:

1. The name of your child;
2. The address of your child;
3. The name of school your child is attending;
4. A description of the problem(s) related to the proposed or refused initiation or change of special education or related services. Include as many facts as possible, and
5. A proposed resolution of the problem to the extent known to you at the time.

(continues)

The district directly responsible for your child's education must arrange for the hearing to be conducted. The rights list below is an outline and not a complete guide to a due process hearing.

Both you and the district have certain rights in a hearing, including the right to:

1. One opportunity to remove a hearing officer within 48 hours of their appointment (does not apply to "expedited hearings");
2. Have an attorney and one or more individuals who have knowledge or training about children with disabilities represent and advise you prior to and at the hearing;
3. Present evidence, including expert medical, psychological, and education testimony, records, tests, reports and/or other information;
4. Compel the attendance of witnesses and to confront and cross-examine witnesses;
5. Participate in a pre-hearing conference held within ten (10) calendar days of the appointment of the hearing officer;
6. Stop the introduction of any evidence that was not given to either party at least five (5) business days before the hearing;
7. Be told that the hearing officer has the authority to subpoena any person or paper necessary to adequately understand the issues of the hearing;
8. Have your child, who is the subject of the hearing, present at the hearing;
9. A closed hearing unless you specifically request an open hearing; and
10. Receive a written copy or, at your option, an electronic verbatim record of the hearing at no cost to you.

The hearing decision is final unless you or the district appeal the decision.

Disclosure of Additional Evidence Before a Hearing

At least five (5) business days before a hearing, you and the district must disclose to each other all evaluations of your child completed by that date and recommendations based on those evaluations that are intended to be used at the hearing. A hearing officer may refuse to allow you to introduce any undisclosed evaluations or recommendations at the hearing without consent of the other party. All evidence must be limited to the specific issues described to the hearing officer.

Administrative Hearing Appeal Process

If you decide to appeal the final decision of a hearing officer, the appeal must be made **in writing** to CFL within 30 calendar days of the receipt of the written decision. CFL will then appoint a hearing review officer and ensure that a final decision is mailed within 30 calendar days after the filing of the appeal, unless the reviewing official has granted an extension at the request of either party. You may appeal the findings and decision made in a hearing review by appealing the decision to state or federal court.

CIVIL ACTION

When either you or the district disagree with the findings or decisions made by a hearing review officer, either party may file a court action. The action may be brought in state or federal district court. In any civil action, the court will:

1. Receive the records of the administrative proceedings;
2. Hear additional evidence at the request of a party;
3. Base its decision on the preponderance of the evidence; and
4. Grant such relief as the court determines is appropriate.

(continues)

PLACEMENT DURING A HEARING OR CIVIL ACTION

During a hearing or judicial action, unless the district and the parent agree otherwise, your child remains in the education placement where he/she is currently placed, commonly referred to as the "stay-put" rule.

Two exceptions to the "stay-put" rule exist:

1. For students who have been removed from their educational setting to an interim alternative educational placement for certain weapon or drug violations, "stay-put" would be the interim alternative educational placement, not the current educational setting; and
2. After a hearing officer's decision is issued agreeing with the parents that a change in placement is appropriate, the hearing officer's decision would be the "stay-put" placement during subsequent appeals.

EXPEDITED HEARINGS

Hearings must be expedited in the following situations:

1. Whenever you request a hearing to dispute the district's determination that your child's behavior was not a result of his/her disability;
2. Whenever you request a hearing to dispute a 45 day interim alternative education placement order by school personnel; or
3. When a district requests an expedited hearing to establish that it is dangerous for your child to remain in the current placement.

Placement by a Hearing Officer

A hearing officer may decide to move your child to an interim alternative educational setting for up to 45 calendar days:

1. When the district has demonstrated that your child is substantially likely to injure self or others if he/she remains in the current placement; and
2. When the district has made reasonable efforts to minimize the risk of harm in the current placement.

INTERIM ALTERNATIVE EDUCATIONAL PLACEMENT

The district may change your child's educational placement for up to 45 calendar days, if your child:

1. Possesses a weapon at school or a school function; or
2. Knowingly possesses or uses illegal drugs, or sells or solicits the sale of a controlled substance while at school or a school function.

The interim alternative educational setting is determined by the IEP team. Even though this is a temporary change, it must allow your child:

1. To continue to progress in the general curriculum, although in a different setting;
2. To continue to receive those services and modifications, including those described in your child's IEP, that will help your child meet his/her IEP goals; and
3. Include services and modifications designed to prevent the behavior from recurring.

If your child is placed in an interim alternative educational setting, an IEP meeting must be convened within ten (10) school days of the decision. At this meeting, the team must discuss the behavior and its relationship to your child's disability, review evaluation information regarding the behavior, and determine the ap-

(continues)

propriateness of your child's IEP and behavior plan.

ATTORNEY'S FEES FOR HEARINGS

You may be able to recover attorney fees if you prevail in a due process hearing. A petition for fees must be filed in a court of competent jurisdiction. A judge may make an award of attorney's fees based on prevailing rates in your community. The court may reduce an award of attorney's fees if it finds that you unreasonably delayed the settlement or decision in the case.

PRIVATE SCHOOL PLACEMENT

You may be able to recover tuition expenses for a private school placement if:

1. You inform the district either at an IEP/IFSP meeting or give written notice to the district of at least 10 business days of your intent to enroll your child in the private school; and

2. You state why you disagree with the district's proposed IEP/IFSP or placement.

3. A hearing officer finds that the district failed to provide or is unable to provide your child with an appropriate education and that the private placement is appropriate.

If the district gave you written notice of its intent to evaluate your child before you removed your child from the public school, you must make your child available to the district for evaluation.

Failure to tell the school of your intent to enroll your child in a private school at public expense, failure to make your child available for evaluation, or other unreasonable delay on your part could result in a reduction or denial of reimbursement for the private school placement. If the district prevented you from providing this notice or you cannot write in English, the hearing officer may not reduce the reimbursement.

Note. Reprinted with permission from Minnesota Department of Children, Families & Learning, Minnesota Special Education. Retrieved April 14, 2003, from http://education.state.mn.us/stellent/groups/publicdocuments/translatedcontent/pub_035725.pdf

Appendix 8.F

Example of Invitation to a Meeting of the Individualized Education Program (IEP) Team

---

Invitation sent with statement of
parental rights _____
(Initials)

INVITATION TO A MEETING OF THE
INDIVIDUALIZED EDUCATION PROGRAM (IEP) TEAM (A-9)

CESA #7, _____ SCHOOL DISTRICT

[If you need this invitation in a different language or communicated in a different way, or have questions about this invitation, please contact _____ at _____.]

Dear _____   Date _____

You are a participant on the IEP Team which will meet to address the educational needs of your child, _____. IEP team meetings must be held at a mutually agreeable time and place. An IEP team meeting has tentatively been scheduled for the following date _____, time _____ and location _____. If these meeting arrangements are not agreeable to you, please call _____ at _____. You may bring other people who have knowledge or special expertise about your child to the meeting with you. The purpose of this IEP team meeting is (check all that apply):

EVALUATION AND REEVALUATION
(if this section is the only one checked, it is not necessary to send a parent rights statement)
☐ Determine initial eligibility for special education
☐ Determine continuing eligibility for special education

(continues)

INDIVIDUALIZED EDUCATION PROGRAM (IEP) *if student is eligible*

☐ Develop an initial IEP   ☐ Transition _____ (age 14)   _____ (age 16)

☐ Develop an annual IEP   ☐ Transition _____ (age 14)   _____ (age 16)

☐ Review/revise IEP   ☐ Transition _____ (age 14)   _____ (age 16)

PLACEMENT *if student is eligible*

(*if this section is the only one checked, it is not necessary to send a parent rights statement*)

☐ Determine initial placement

☐ Determine continuing placement

OTHER

☐ Specify: _____

☐ Review existing information to determine need for additional tests or other evalua-tion materials (*meeting optional; if this box is the only one checked, it is not necessary to send a parent rights statement*)

☐ Conduct a manifestation determination (*must also check appropriate boxes under IEP & placement*)

☐ Determine an interim alternative educational setting (IAES) (*must also check appro-priate boxes under IEP & placement*)

If transition is checked above as one of the purposes of this meeting, your child is invited to attend. We are also inviting representatives from the following agencies: ☐ None

_____   _____
Agency   Title/Position   Agency   Title/Position

If at any point during this meeting you or other IEP team participants believe that additional time is needed to permit your meaningful involvement, additional time will be provided. Deci-sions related to the purpose(s) checked above may be made in one meeting or may require more than one meeting, depending on individual circumstances.

At the beginning of the meeting, the school district will discuss with you your right to have additional time as described above and of your right to have a copy of the IEP team's evalua-tion report prior to developing an IEP and placement. Upon request you and the other IEP team participants may receive a copy of the team's evaluation report prior to continuing with the development of your child's IEP and placement. If you have not requested a copy of the team's evaluation report and a purpose of this meeting is to determine whether your child is or continues to be a child with a disability (impairment and need for special education), the school district will give you a copy of the IEP team's evaluation report when you receive a no-tice of your child's placement or notice that your child is not a child with a disability.

(continues)

The following IEP team participants will attend the meeting:

_____ , Regular ed. teacher   _____ , Special ed. Teacher
                (Title)   (Title)

_____ , LEA Representative   _____
                (Title)   (Title)

_____   _____
                                          (Title)   (Title)

_____   _____
                                          (Title)   (Title)

_____   _____
                                          (Title)   (Title)

You and your child have protection under the procedural safeguards (rights) of special education law. A statement of parent and child rights will be enclosed with this notice if the purpose of the meeting includes developing or reviewing/revising the Individualized Education Program (IEP). A statement of parent and child rights will not be included if the purpose of the meeting is only for evaluation and reevaluation, only for placement, or only for determining the need for additional tests or other evaluation materials. The purposes of the meeting are checked on the first page of this invitation. If a statement of parent and child rights is not enclosed and you would like another copy, please contact the district at the telephone number above.

Sincerely,

_____
(Name and Title of District Contact Person)

Note. This document is included in this book only as an example and is not intended to be copied and used. Reprinted with permission of Wisconsin Cooperative Service Unit 10, Special Education Department. Retrieved April 25, 2003, from http://www.cesa.7.k12.wi.us/sped/1999spedforms/A-9.pdf

Appendix 8.G

Example of Notice and Consent for Placement in Special Education Services

---

EDUCATIONAL SERVICE UNIT 10

**NOTICE AND CONSENT FOR PLACEMENT IN
SPECIAL EDUCATION SERVICES**

STUDENT: _____   DATE: _____

SCHOOL: _____   GRADE: _____

Dear Parent/Guardian:

It is the intent of the _____ Public Schools to work with you as a team in providing appropriate educational and related services for your child. To the maximum extent appropriate, your child is to be educated with other students in the general education curriculum. Based on the Individual Education Program that was developed for your child, the IEP placement team, of which you are a member, will consider various options and determine the appropriate program(s).

The team considered the following option(s) prior to reaching the placement decision and rejected those option(s) because: _____

_____

_____

_____

The team proposes to serve your child within the following program(s) and/or related service(s):

_____

_____

_____

(continues)

The proposed placement is based upon the following evaluation procedures, tests, records or reports:

_____

_____

_____

Other factors which are relevant to the school's proposal, if any: _____

_____

Parental Procedural Safeguards

Parents of children with a disability have protection under the procedural safeguards of the Individuals with Disabilities Education Act. If you do not have your copy and would like another, you may contact your child's case manager. If you have any questions regarding your rights or need help in understanding the federal and state laws for educating children with disabilities and parental rights granted by those laws contact: ESU 10 Special Education Dept. (308-237-5927), or the Nebraska Department of Education–Lincoln Office: (402) 471-2471.

PARENTAL CONSENT/DENIAL FOR PROPOSED PLACEMENT

I/we have received a copy and understand the content of this Notice and:

☐ I/We **give consent** for the proposed placement specified in this notice.
   I/We understand that this consent is voluntary and may be revoked at any time by notifying the school district.

☐ I/We have received a copy and understand the content of this Notice and **do not give consent** for the proposed placement specified in this notice. The reason for not giving consent for the placement is:

Signature of Parents/Guardians/Surrogate _____

Date: _____

Parent's Address: _____ City: _____

NE Zip: _____ Home Phone: _____ Work Phone: _____

District Representative Signature: _____

Date: _____

Appendix 8.H

Completed Example of Evaluation Report

EVALUATION REPORT (ER) Format
School Age

☒ Initial Referral (Complete all following components excluding Reevaluation Only section)

☐ Reevaluation (Complete Demographic component, Reason for Referral and Reevaluation Only section first. Complete all other components only if additional data is determined as needed under the Reevaluation component.)

Demographics

Student Name: Eddie Carlson   **Date of Report:** October 29, 2001

School District: Universal School District

School: Universal Elementary School

Student Birth Date: 5/1/93   **Grade:** 3

Current Educational Program: regular 3rd grade class

Other Demographic Data, As Needed: none

Reason(s) For Referral:

Eddie was referred for an evaluation by Mrs. Jones, his third grade teacher, because he is having great difficulties in reading and language arts in the third grade. After extensive intervention provided by the remedial reading teacher and through direct interventions by his classroom teacher, his abilities in decoding and sight vocabulary remain at the first grade level. He has difficulty following directions in all instructional areas. The referral question was, "Why is Eddie not making sufficient progress in reading?"

EDUCATIONAL LEVELS OF PERFORMANCE AND EDUCATIONAL NEEDS OF THE CHILD:

Eddie demonstrates average intellectual functioning (WISC–III Full Scale IQ of 97).

(continues)

In reading and language arts, the difficulties reported by his teacher and mother were confirmed by norm-referenced testing. On the Woodcock-Johnson Psychoeducational Battery, Eddie achieved an overall standard score of 72 in reading and 50 in written language. These scores indicated a K–grade 1 level of achievement.

The *Clinical Evaluation of Language Fundamentals–3 (CELF–3)* was administered to assess overall language skills in a variety of receptive and expressive language areas. Eddie's performance on this measure indicated overall language skills are below average. Receptive skills are within the low average range. Receptively, Eddie demonstrated low average performance when following directions, identifying associated words, assessing semantic relationships within sentences and responding to questions about paragraphs. Expressive skills are below average due to weaknesses in the sentence assembly task. Eddie demonstrated average performance on the remaining expressive tasks including sentence formulation, sentence repetition and generating category members. Findings indicated that Eddie has difficulties in language comprehension, vocabulary, direction following, event-sequencing and working memory. Articulation skills appeared to be normal.

Clinical Evaluation of Language Fundamentals–3 (CELF–3):

Receptive Subtests	Standard Score
Concepts and Directions	6
Word Classes	3
Semantic Relationships	5
Receptive Language Quotient:	61 (85–115 = average)

Expressive Subtests	Standard Score
Formulated Sentences	3
Recalling Sentences	8
Sentence Assembly	5
Expressive Language Quotient	69 (85–115 = average)

Supplemental Subtests	Standard Score
Listening to Paragraphs	9
Word Associations	9
Total Language Quotient	63

The CTOPP (an assessment of phonemic skills) indicated an inability to segment two-syllable words, to identify final sounds in words and to identify and produce rhymes, all skills that are necessary in learning to read. Eddie was able to identify words that began with the same sound.

(continues)

Informal assessments (Rapid Letter Naming test and a Phonics Screening Survey) of Eddie's reading skills indicated that: He was able to rapidly name all the letters of the alphabet; his decoding skills were limited to identification of some initial letter sounds; and he had a sight vocabulary of approximately thirty words.

Results of norm-referenced testing indicated that Eddie is at a third grade level in math (Key Math Standard Score of 98). This finding is supported by results of the informal assessment and classroom observations (see Evaluation Data Results of Direct Intervention). Eddie performed well in social studies and science activities and assignments when materials were read to him.

Student's needs:

- Eddie needs systematic, intensive, and direct instruction in reading using multisensory techniques in order to develop phonological, decoding, automaticity and fluency skills.
- Eddie needs to have directions and instructions broken down into sequential units with visual cues, modeling and guided practice.

EVALUATION DATA RESULTS OF DIRECT INTERVENTION—The team will include information on the following areas that impact the student's ability to access the general curriculum:

- **Physical, social or cultural background information relevant to the child's disability and need for special education.**

   Mrs. Carlson reported that Eddie's medical history was typical except he didn't speak until well past the age of 3. He achieved other developmental milestones at the appropriate time. He has many friends and is generally liked by adults and older children. Eddie lives with his mother and one other younger brother. English is his native language.

- **Current classroom based assessments and observations and observations by teachers and related service providers.**

   Eddie was observed on a number of occasions by the school psychologist and speech therapist.

   During math he needed to be given instructions for a paired activity two or three times. He then quickly completed the assignment with an 85% accuracy and went to a math learning center while others completed the assignment.

   Classroom based assessments: Prior to third grade Eddie received strategic and intensive instruction from the classroom teacher. He received support in reading, writing and following directions. He received instruction using the first grade reading series; he retained 60% of the sight words he was taught. Although he could match letters to sounds, he had difficulty blending sounds to read simple decodable words (e.g. "cvc" patterns). After repeated readings, he was able to decode "cvc" words with 100% accuracy, but could not demonstrate this skill two days later. When grade level text was read to him, he was

(continues)

able to retell all the important story elements. A number of phonics interventions were tried at the end of last year; the multi-sensory approaches (sky-writing, sand writing) were the only ones that yielded any retention.

This year the teacher has used an informal reading inventory and curriculum based oral reading measures; Eddie's instructional level for decoding and fluency are at a grade one level. He relies primarily on initial sounds along with picture and context clues to guess at unknown words. He knows 30 sight words on a first grade list.

Eddie was able to experience success in following directions when instructions were broken down and accompanied by modeling. His 3rd grade teacher reported that if she used this approach with Eddie, he was more successful (only if the task was in his skill repertoire).

EVALUATIONS AND INFORMATION PROVIDED BY THE PARENTS OF THE CHILD:

Eddie's mother, Ms. Lois Carlson, reported that he has always had difficulty with his schoolwork, especially reading. She has trouble getting him to do his homework. He does not read on his own at home. He doesn't follow directions very well and seems to forget what he is asked to do. Mrs. Carlson reports that Eddie has many friends and has not had behavior problems at home or in the community. With the exception of arguments over his homework, Eddie appears to be a happy child.

IF AN ASSESSMENT IS NOT CONDUCTED UNDER STANDARD CONDITIONS, DESCRIBE THE EXTENT TO WHICH IT VARIED FROM STANDARD CONDITIONS:

No assessment was conducted under nonstandard conditions.

SUMMARY OF FINDINGS/INTERPRETATION OF ASSESSMENT RESULTS:

Despite a variety of intensive interventions, Eddie continues to experience difficulty learning to read. He will benefit from specially designed instruction in the areas of reading as well as using an explicit, systematic, multisensory structured language approach.

For a child suspected of having a specific learning disability, the documentation of the team's determination of eligibility must include a statement of: 1) whether the child has a specific learning disability; 2) the basis for making the determination; 3) the relevant behavior noted during the observation of the child; 4) the relationship of that behavior to the child's academic functioning; 5) the educationally relevant medical findings, if any; 6) whether there is a severe discrepancy between achievement and ability that is not correctable without special education and related services; and 7) the determination of the team concerning the effects of environmental, cultural, or economic disadvantage.

(continues)

1. Eddie has a specific learning disability in reading and language comprehension.

2. This has been determined through norm referenced and classroom-based assessments as well as through classroom observations.

3. No medical condition was discovered during routine doctor's examinations that would cause any educational difficulties. Eddie's hearing acuity and vision are normal and his attendance is excellent.

4. Eddie's cognitive abilities supported by his intelligence assessments, classroom assessments and during informal testing indicate that Eddie has the ability to work within the general third grade education curriculum. However, his reading levels are at early first grade. Special education support using specially designed instruction will be necessary to give him the intensity of instruction he needs to allow him to achieve.

5. Environmental, cultural and economic factors are not a significant contributing factor to his educational achievement.

CONCLUSIONS

☒ **Student is a child with a disability.**

> **Disability category:** Specific learning disability in reading
>
> **(If appropriate) Secondary Disability category:** Speech and Language Impairment

☒ **Student is in need of specially designed instruction**

Recommendations regarding special education and related services needed to enable the child to meet goals and to participate as appropriate in the general curriculum:

It is recommended that Eddie receive direct, systematic, intensive reading instruction. It is also recommended that he receive speech and language support to assist with the development of phonological awareness and listening skills.

OR

☐ **Student is not a child with a disability, or is a child with a disability but does not need specially designed instruction.**

(continues)

COMPLETE FOR REEVALUATIONS ONLY:

DATE IEP TEAM* REVIEWED EXISTING EVALUATION DATA:

INFORMATION REVIEWED:

- Existing evaluation data
- Evaluations and information provided by the parents
- Current classroom based assessments and observations
- Observations by teachers and service providers
- Whether any additions or modifications to the special education and related services are needed to enable the child to meet the measurable annual goals in the IEP and to participate as appropriate in the general curriculum

*IEP Team must include a school psychologist when evaluating a child with Autism, Emotional Disturbance, Mental Retardation, Multiple Disabilities, Other Health Impairment, Specific Learning Disability and Traumatic Brain Injury

For a child suspected of having a specific learning disability, the documentation of the team's determination of eligibility must include a statement of: 1) whether the child has a specific learning disability; 2) the basis for making the determination; 3) the relevant behavior noted during the observation of the child; 4) the relationship of that behavior to the child's academic functioning; 5) the educationally relevant medical findings, if any; 6) whether there is a severe discrepancy between achievement and ability that is not correctable without special education and related services; and 7) the determination of the team concerning the effects of environmental, cultural, or economic disadvantage.

CONCLUSION (Select one)

☐ **The IEP Team determined that no additional data is required.**

    Reason(s) no additional data is required: Progress reports on IEP goals, classroom assessments, and standardized district test data indicate that no additional data is needed in order to determine new IEP goals, objectives and specially designed instruction.

    _____ **The student continues to be eligible for and in need of special education, or**

    _____ **The student no longer is eligible for special education. (The parent may request an assessment to determine whether the student continues to be a child with a disability)**

OR

(continues)

☐ **The IEP Team determined that there is a need for additional data. The LEA shall issue the permission to reevaluate and administer tests and other evaluation materials as may be needed to produce the following data:**

Review of existing evaluation data
- Evaluations and information provided by the parents
- Current classroom based assessments and observations
- Observations by teachers and service providers
- Present levels of performance and educational needs
- Determination of continued eligibility for special education

Upon completion of the reevaluation, the district will complete the ER and issue the report to the required members of the evaluation team.

EVALUATION REPORT—SIGNATURES

SIGNATURE	TITLE	YES	NO
(Only applicable for evaluating children with specific learning disabilities)			
Mrs. Barbara Carlson	Mother	X	
Dr. Leslie Rogers	Psychologist*	X	
Miss Charlene Jones	Regular Education Teacher	X	
Mr. Mark Flynn	Speech Pathologist	X	
Miss Betty Smith	Reading Teacher	X	

*Required when evaluating a child with Autism, Emotional Disturbance, Mental Retardation, Multiple Disabilities, Other Health Impairment, Specific Learning Disability and Traumatic Brain Injury. Not mandated for Deaf/Blind, Hearing Impaired, Speech/Language, Visual Impairment and Orthopedic Impairment.

Copies to:
  Parent
  Teacher
  Building Principal
  Others:

Note. Reprinted with permission of Pennsylvania Department of Education, Bureau of Special Education. Retrieved April 13, 2003, from www.pde.state.pa.us/special_edu/site

Appendix 8.I

Example of a Completed Individualized Education Program

INDIVIDUALIZED EDUCATION PROGRAM (IEP) Format

SAMPLE FOR TRAINING PURPOSES
School Age

IEP Team Meeting Date: November 18, 2001

IEP Implementation Date (Projected Date when Services and Programs Will Begin):

11 / 26 / 01
Mo   Day   Yr

Anticipated Duration of Services and Programs: 11 / 17 / 02
Mo   Day   Yr

Student Name: Josh Anderson   DOB: 1/9/89   Age: 12 years 10 months

Grade: 7   Anticipated Year of Graduation: 2006

School District: City School District

Parent Name: Margaret Anderson

Address: 350 North Beaver Lane   Phone: (H) 333-555-2222
Likonia, PA 19046   (W) 333-555-1111

County of Residence: Montgomery   Other Information: None

IEP TEAM/SIGNATURES*

The Individualized Education Program (IEP) Team makes the decisions about the student's program and placement. The student's parent(s), the student's regular teacher and a representative from the local education agency are required members of this team. A regular education teacher must also be included if the student participates, or may be participating in regular education. Signature on this IEP documents attendance, not agreement.

(continues)

NAME (typed or printed)	POSITION (typed or printed)	SIGNATURE
Ms. Margaret Anderson	Parent	Margaret Anderson
	Parent	
	Student*	
Mr. Al Paxton	Regular Education Teacher	Al Paxton
Ms. Carrie Leeds	Special Education Teacher	Carrie Leeds
Dr. Lavinia Hughes	Local Ed. Agency Rep. (Chair)	Lavinia Hughes
	Community Agency Rep.**	
	Vocational Teacher (if appropriate)	
Mr. David Cole	Guidance Counselor	David Cole
Dr. Rachel Johnson	School Psychologist	Rachel Johnson
Mrs. Helen Smith	Behavior Analyst	Helen Smith

*The IEP team must invite the student if transition services are being planned or if the parents choose to have the student participate.
**As determined by the LEA as needed for transition services.

PROCEDURAL SAFEGUARDS NOTICE

I have received a copy of the Procedural Safeguards Notice. The District has informed me whom I may contact if I need more information.

Signature: _Margaret Anderson_   Date Received: 11/11/01

I. SPECIAL CONSIDERATIONS THE IEP TEAM MUST CONSIDER BEFORE DEVELOPING THE IEP. ANY FACTORS CHECKED MUST BE ADDRESSED IN THE IEP.

Is the Student Blind or Visually Impaired?

___X___ No

_____ Yes—Team must provide for instruction in Braille and the use of Braille unless the IEP Team determines, after an evaluation of the child's reading and writing skills, needs and appropriate reading and writing media (including an evaluation of the child's future needs for instruction in Braille or the use of Braille), that instruction in Braille or the use of Braille is not appropriate.

(continues)

Is the Student Deaf or Hearing Impaired?

__X__ No

_____ Yes—Team must consider the child's language and communication needs, opportunities for direct communications with peers and professional personnel in the child's language and communication mode, academic level, and full range of needs, including opportunities for direct instruction in the child's language and communication mode in the development of the IEP.

_____ Communication Needs

_____ Assistive Technology, Devices and/or Services

_____ Limited English Proficiency

__X__ Behaviors that impede his/her learning or that of others

_____ Transition Services

_____ Other (Specify) _____

II. PRESENT LEVELS OF EDUCATIONAL PERFORMANCE

An Informal Phonics Screening Survey, done by his special education teacher as part of the IEP progress report in May, indicated that Josh has the ability to: (1) rapidly name all the letters of the alphabet, (2) automatically read single syllable words and nonsense words at an 80% level, (3) read the first syllable of a multi-syllabic word at a 70% level. An informal phonological assessment indicates that Josh has no difficulty separating one syllable words into sounds or combining sounds together to form one syllable words.

Curriculum based assessments were also performed in September as part of the weekly IEP progress report, using Josh's science and social studies texts. He read at an accuracy level of less than 50% and was unable to decode any of the new technical vocabulary and guessed at words using context clues such as pictures and personal experiences. When the social studies text was read to him orally, he was able to answer questions that pertained to direct recall of fact and main ideas. He could not create definitions of new vocabulary or make predictions. It was not until he was asked to read from a third grade literature book that his oral reading accuracy level reached 90% (instructional level). While he stumbled over two syllable words, he was able to laboriously decode them. His fluency level was at 45 words per minute and consequently his comprehension was poor. When asked to retell the story just read, Josh was only able to tell the main idea and one supporting detail. Out of a possible score of 10, he scored a 2.

(continues)

His science and social studies teacher reported that when Josh is given an opportunity to draw or create a model to demonstrate proficiency in a unit of study, he does quite well. The teacher found that Josh does learn content from lectures, through videos, and from group projects. He participates in class discussions.

This school year Josh has had a significant increase in the amount and intensity of verbal threats and bullying behavior. His verbal acts of aggression include threats to hit, smack, hurt or fight with other students.

HOW THE STUDENT'S DISABILITY AFFECTS INVOLVEMENT AND PROGRESS IN GENERAL EDUCATION CURRICULUM (Include the child's strengths and needs which will effect the student's involvement and progress in the general curriculum.):

Based on Josh's educational levels of performance, he demonstrates extensive difficulties in decoding, automaticity and comprehension. Now that he is in Middle School, his reading difficulties prevent him from using the texts and other print materials that are used extensively in his content area classes. Adaptations that were identified in his previous IEPs such as word lists for pre-teaching of new vocabulary, information organizers and highlighted copies of assigned reading materials have not enabled Josh to perform successfully in the seventh grade. He needs to learn strategies on how to use these adaptations. His teachers suggest that accommodations such as reading texts materials to him, having a peer work with him, and using recorded materials as learning tools may also help Josh be successful. He is successful academically when involved in multisensory instruction and discussions that are not heavily dependent upon print.

Based on results of a Functional Behavior Assessment, Josh engages in offtask behaviors and bullying when expected to read independently in his content area classes. In contrast, Josh does not display these behaviors when involved in discussions, group work and hands-on activities. Josh has many friends and is well liked by his peers.

Student's needs:

- Josh needs systematic, intense, and direct instruction in reading in order to develop decoding, automaticity, and comprehension skills.
- Multisensory techniques need to be used during reading instruction.
- Josh needs to be taught strategies so that he can use adaptive tools in his content area classes.
- Josh needs to receive print materials in a variety of ways such as discussion, recordings, through work with a buddy, and using videos.
- Josh needs to be directly taught other appropriate options when he is unable to meet the demands of written assignments.

(continues)

III. GOALS AND OBJECTIVES:

(Use as many copies of this page as needed to plan appropriately)

MEASURABLE ANNUAL GOAL: <u>Josh will fluently (125 wpm) and accurately (90%) orally read the texts</u>

<u>provided by the leveled materials from the reading program.</u>

SHORT TERM OBJECTIVE/BENCHMARK	EXPECTED LEVEL OF ACHIEVEMENT	METHOD OF EVALUATION
Josh will orally decode a list of two syllable words taken from a 4th grade text at a rate of less than two seconds per word.	80% accuracy	Word list Teacher probe
Josh will orally read a list of two syllable words taken from a 4th grade text at a rate of one second or less per word.	80% accuracy	Word list Teacher probe
Josh will correctly read a list of three syllable words taken from a 4th grade text at a rate of one second or less per word.	80% accuracy	Word list Teacher probe
Josh will read a selection of a 4th grade text at 75 words per minute.	85% accuracy	Text selection Teacher probe
Josh will read a selection of a 4th grade text at 100 words per minute.	90% accuracy	Text selection Teacher probe

REPORT OF PROGRESS ON ANNUAL GOALS

How goals will be measured: <u>Reading probes teacher takes from the text materials that are part of the</u>

<u>reading program used to instruct Josh and from 4th grade textbooks used in the school district.</u>

How progress will be reported: <u>Reading accuracy scores will be summarized and data will be entered on</u>

<u>this form and attached to report card.</u>

1ST	2ND	3RD	4TH	OTHER IF APPLICABLE

(continues)

MEASURABLE ANNUAL GOAL: Josh will use adaptive materials and techniques to complete reading assignments in science and socials studies at an accuracy rate of 75%.

SHORT TERM OBJECTIVE/BENCHMARK	EXPECTED LEVEL OF ACHIEVEMENT	METHOD OF EVALUATION
Josh will describe and apply a learned strategy in order to complete a study guide in science or social studies	80% accuracy	Teacher prepared study guide, teacher evaluation
Josh will describe and apply a learned strategy in order to read and understand new vocabulary using a pre-teaching vocabulary guide that accompanies a social studies assignment	80% accuracy	Teacher evaluation
Josh will apply a learned strategy to complete an information organizer that accompanies a science reading assignment	80% of the time	Teacher prepared information organizer Teacher evaluation

REPORT OF PROGRESS ON ANNUAL GOALS

How goals will be measured: Josh will be able to describe the learning strategies needed to complete teacher made study guides, pre-lesson vocabulary guides and information organizers and will then complete them at an accuracy rate of 75%.

How progress will be reported: Scores of Josh's description of strategies and samples of completed adaptive materials will be attached to the report card.

1ST	2ND	3RD	4TH	OTHER IF APPLICABLE

(continues)

MEASURABLE ANNUAL GOAL:

Behavior: <u>Josh will eliminate all threatening behaviors, both verbal and physical, by using learned behavioral</u>

<u>strategies.</u>

SHORT TERM OBJECTIVE/BENCHMARK	EXPECTED LEVEL OF ACHIEVEMENT	METHOD OF EVALUATION
When confronted with academic demands that frustrate Josh, he will mark, then skip over the difficult sections, completing what he can independently.	100% accuracy	Permanent product check and counts
When experiencing frustration from academic work, Josh will ask for help from the classroom or special education teacher.	100% accuracy	Teacher behavior evaluation form Student self-monitoring tool
Josh will recognize when he is beginning to become frustrated and will signal teacher that he needs time to regain control before behaviors start.	100% accuracy	Frequency counts Student self-monitoring tool

REPORT OF PROGRESS ON ANNUAL GOALS

How goals will be measured: <u>Information gathered from teacher reports, student self-monitoring tools,</u>

<u>permanent products.</u>

How progress will be reported: <u>Data will be summarized, entered on this form and attached to report</u>

<u>card.</u>

1ST	2ND	3RD	4TH	OTHER IF APPLICABLE

(continues)

IV. SPECIAL EDUCATION/RELATED SERVICES:
A. PROGRAM MODIFICATIONS AND SPECIALLY DESIGNED INSTRUCTION:
(*Specially designed instruction may be listed with each goal/objectives.*)

1. A systematic reading program that use direct instruction, decodable texts and multisensory techniques such as Corrective Reading or Wilson Reading Program.
2. Computer Assisted Instruction for phonics reinforcement.
3. Adapted science and social studies materials (study guides, modified directions, information organizers and pre-teaching vocabulary guides) that will accompany reading assignments. Explicit strategies must accompany each adaptive material and must be taught directly and explicitly with allowance for guided practice.
4. Science, social studies and literature tests that are read to him.
5. Text and other print materials that are recorded, provided through discussion or through working with a buddy.
6. Peer buddy to work with Josh when demands for completion of tasks that require extensive reading are frustrating.
7. Direct, explicit and systematic instruction in alternative behaviors to use when frustrated.

B. RELATED SERVICES: List the services that the student needs in order to benefit from or access his/her special education program:

Service	Location	Projected* Beginning Date	Frequency	Anticipated* Duration
none				

*Include only if differs from IEP beginning and/or duration dates.

C. SUPPORTS FOR THE CHILD PROVIDED FOR SCHOOL PERSONNEL:

The special education teacher will provide the strategies for using the adaptive materials along with formats and suggested methods for creating them. She will work with the Science and Social Studies teachers.

The guidance counselor will work with Josh's content area teachers to develop a consistent set of responses to his behavior and how to do frequency counts for progress reporting.

(*continues*)

D. EXTENDED SCHOOL YEAR: The IEP Team has considered and discussed ESY services, and determined that:

Josh is not in need of ESY programming.

V. PARTICIPATION IN STATE AND DISTRICT-WIDE ASSESSMENTS

STUDENT PARTICIPATION—STATE ASSESSMENTS
This section applies to student's age/grade eligible for the PSSA/PASA
(Reading, Math–grades 5, 8, 11; Writing–grades 6, 9, 11)

_____ Student will participate in the PSSA without accommodations.

OR

_____ Student will participate in the PSSA with the following accommodations:

PSSA Reading (grades 5, 8, 11)

PSSA Math (grades 5, 8, 11)

PSSA Writing (grades 6,9, 11)

OR

_____ Student will participate in the Pennsylvania Alternate System of Assessment (PASA). (Effective beginning the 2000–01 school year, the alternate assessment in Pennsylvania is PASA).

If the IEP Team has determined it is not appropriate for the student to participate in the PSSA, the team must explain why the PSSA is not appropriate:

Choose how the student's performance on the PASA will be documented:

_____ Videotape (which will be kept confidential as all other school records)

_____ Written Narrative (which will be kept confidential as all other school records)

(continues)

STUDENT PARTICIPATION—DISTRICT ASSESSMENT

_____ Student will participate in the District assessments without accommodations.

OR

___X___ Student will participate in the District assessments with the following accommodations:
- Science and social studies tests read to him
- Allowance for dictation when extensive writing responses are required

OR

_____ If the IEP Team has determined that it is not appropriate for the student to participate in the district-wide assessment they must explain why the assessment is not appropriate for the student and how the student will be assessed

VI. LEAST RESTRICTIVE ENVIRONMENT (LRE)

EDUCATIONAL PLACEMENT (Type of Service, Type of Support, ex: Full-time learning support)

Resource Room Learning Support _____

Explanation of the extent, if any, the student **will not participate** with non-disabled children in the regular class and in the general education curriculum:

Josh will participate in all aspects of the general education program in the regular classroom except during the time that English literature is being taught. He will, at this time, receive his reading instruction in the Resource Room.

Percentage of time the student receives special education <u>outside</u> of the regular education classroom:

___X___ Less than 21% outside of the regular education classroom

_____ 21–60% outside of the regular education classroom

_____ 61% or more outside of the regular education classroom

Location of Program: ___Urban Middle School_____

(continues)

VII. TRANSITION PLANNING

1. Will the student be 14 years of age or older during the term of this IEP?

    __X__ No—(Not necessary to complete this Section)

    _____ Yes—Team must address the student's courses of study and how the course of study applies to components of the IEP.

Student's courses of study:

_____

_____

_____

2. Will the student be 16 years of age or older during the term of this IEP or is the student younger and in need of transition services as determined by the IEP Team?

    __X__ No—(Not necessary to complete this Section)

    _____ Yes—Team must address and complete this Section

DESIRED POST-SCHOOL OUTCOMES: Define and project the desired post-school outcomes as identified by the student, parent and IEP team in the following areas. State how the services will be provided and person(s) responsible for coordinating these services.

SERVICE	HOW SERVICE IS PROVIDED	PERSON RESPONSIBLE
Post Secondary Education/Training		
Employment		
Community Living		
a) Residential		
b) Participation		
c) Recreation/Leisure		

(continues)

STATEMENT OF COORDINATED TRANSITIONAL SERVICES AND ACTIVITIES NEEDED TO SUPPORT DESIRED POST-SCHOOL OUTCOMES: (Instructional areas should support the desired post-school outcomes for the student. Examples such as Instruction and Related Services, Community Experiences, Acquisition of Daily Living Skills, Functional Vocational Evaluation, and Adult Living may appear as annual goals, short-term instructional objectives or benchmarks, and/or specially designed instruction, based on the student's needs.)

_____

_____

_____

_____

_____

_____

LINKAGES

List the agencies, which may provide services/support (before the student leaves the school setting):

_____
Agency Name   Phone Number

_____
Responsibilities/Linkages

_____
Agency Name   Phone Number

_____
Responsibilities/Linkages

_____
Agency Name   Phone Number

_____
Responsibilities/Linkages

Note. Reprinted with permission from Pennsylvania Department of Education, Bureau of Special Education. Retrieved April 13, 2003, from www.pde.state.pa.us/special_edu/site

Appendix 8.J

Example of a Completed Notice of Recommended Educational Placement

NOTICE OF RECOMMENDED EDUCATIONAL PLACEMENT
School Age

Date: 11/12/01

Name and Address of Parent: Ms. Barbara Carlson
200 North Brighton Street
New Chasm, PA 19050

Student's Name: Eddie Carlson

Dear Ms. Carslon:

This notice summarizes recommendations for your child's education program.

This notice is to be given to the parent of a child with a disability a reasonable time before the school district proposes to initiate or change, or refuses to initiate or change the identification, evaluation or educational placement of the child or the provision of a free appropriate public education to the child.

1. **Action proposed or refused:**

   Eddie will begin receiving special education and related services beginning 11/17/01.

2. **Why the action is proposed or refused:**

   This placement is proposed based upon the results of multidisciplinary evaluation (ER 10/29/01) that indicate that Eddie is in need of special education services.

3. **A. Description of any other options that were considered:**

   Continued placement in regular education.

   B. Reasons why these options were rejected:

   Results of the multidisciplinary evaluation (ER 10/20/01) reveal that Eddie has educational needs that cannot be adequately met in the regular education classroom.

   (continues)

4. **Evaluation procedure(s), test(s), record(s) or report(s) used as a basis for the proposed action or action refused:**

WISC–III, Woodcock-Johnson Psychoeducational Battery, Clinical Evaluation of Language Fundamental–3 (CELF–3), Comprehensive Test of Phonological Processing (CTOPP), Key Math, informal assessments of early literacy skills, classroom-based assessments in reading and mathematics, and classroom observations.

5. **Other factor(s) relevant to proposal or refusal:**

NONE

The educational placement recommended for your child is: (Type of service, type of support, ex: full time learning support)

Resource Learning Support

Dr. Thomas B. Goodwin	*Dr. Thomas B. Goodwin*	11/12/01
School District Superintendent	Signature	Date

You have certain rights and protections under law that is described in a document titled ***Procedural Safeguards Notice.*** If you need more information or want a copy of the ***Procedural Safeguards Notice,*** you may contact:

Carolyn Stevens	Director, Pupil Personnel Services	(814) 878-4646
Name	Position	Phone Number

DIRECTIONS FOR PARENTS: Please check one of the options, sign this form, and return it within **10 days** to the person listed above.

☐ I **approve** this recommendation
☐ I **do not approve** this recommendation

My reason for **disapproval is:**

_____

I request:
☐ Pre-hearing Conference
☐ Mediation
☐ Due-process Hearing

I will need the following accommodations to be made so that I may attend the above.

_____

_____	_____	_____
Parent's Signature	Date	Daytime Phone

References

American Speech-Language-Hearing Association. (2002a, February). ASHA Comments to ED on IDEA Reauthorization. *ASHA Government Relations and Public Policy Update*. Rockville, MD: Author.

American Speech-Language-Hearing Association. (2002b, February 5). ASHA releases 2002 public policy agenda. *The ASHA Leader, 7*(2), 1.

American Speech-Language-Hearing Association. (2003, April 15). IDEA Bill Introduced. *the ASHA leader, 8*(7), 1.

Arena, J. (2001). *How to write an IEP* (3rd ed.). Novato, CA: Academic Therapy Publications.

Brannen, S. J., Cooper, E. B., Dellegrotto, J. T., Disney, S. T., Eger, D. L., Ehren, B. J., Ganley, K. A., Isakson, C. W., Montgomery, J. K., Ralabate, P. K., Secord, W. A., & Whitmire, K. A. (2000). *Developing educationally relevant IEPs: A technical assistance document for speech–language pathologists*. Rockville, MD: American Speech-Language-Hearing Association.

Eger, D. L. (2002, February 1). Designing curriculum-linked IEPs: Strategies for speech–language pathologists, ASHA Telephone Seminar.

Hock, M. (2000, July–August). Ten reasons why we should use standards in IEPs. *In CASE*.

Individuals with Disabilities Education Act of 1990, 20 U.S.C. § 1400 *et seq*.

Individuals with Disabilities Education Act Amendments of 1997, 20 U.S.C. § 1400 *et seq*.

Lucas, S. (2000). *The SLP's IDEA companion*. East Moline, IL: LinguiSystems.

Mid-continent Research for Education and Learning (n.d.). *Language arts standards* (4th ed.). Retrieved October 31, 2003, from http://www.mcrel.org/compendium/SubjectTopics.asp?subjectID=7

Minnesota Department of Education. (2003a). *Notice of educational evaluation/re-evaluation plan*. Retrieved October 31, 2003, from http://education.state.mn.us/stellent/groups/public/documents/translatedcontent/pub_053127.pdf

Minnesota Department of Children, Families & Learning, Minnesota Special Education. (2003b). *Notice of procedural safeguards—Parental rights for special education*. Retrieved October 31, 2003, from http://education.state.mn.us/stellent/groups/publicdocuments/translatedcontent/pub_035725.pdf

Minnesota Department of Children, Families & Learning, Minnesota Special Education. (2003c). *Progress report form*. Retrieved October 31, 2003, from http://education.state.mn.us/stellent/groups/public/documents/translatedcontent/pub_053132.pdf

Nebraska Educational Service Unit 10, Special Education Department. (2001). *Notice and consent for placement in special education services*. Retrieved April 25, 2003, from http://userweb.esu10.k12.ne.us/~sped/PDF/placementconsent.pdf

Oregon Department of Education, Office of Special Education. (2000). *Prior notice about evaluation/consent for evaluation*. Retrieved November 1, 2003, from http://www.ode.state.or.us/sped/docpub/forms/schoolage/5150b-P.doc

Pennsylvania Department of Education, Bureau of Special Education. (2001a). *Evaluation report (ER) format*. Retrieved April 13, 2003, from www.pde.state.pa.us/special_edu/site

Pennsylvania Department of Education, Bureau of Special Education. (2001b). *Individualized education program (IEP) format.* Retrieved April 13, 2003, from www.pde.state.pa.us/special_edu/site

Pennsylvania Department of Education, Bureau of Special Education. (2001c). *Recommended educational placement.* Retrieved April 13, 2003, from www.pde.state.pa.us/special_edu/site

Wisconsin Cooperative Service Unit 10, Special Education Department. (2003). *Invitation to a meeting of the Individualized Education Program (IEP) Team.* Retrieved November 1, 2003, from http://www.cesa7.k12.wi.us/sped/1999spedforms/A-9.pdf

Chapter 9

Beyond Basic Therapy

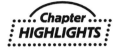

Chapter HIGHLIGHTS

- Group therapy versus therapy in a group
- Types of interaction in group therapy
- Problems to avoid when conducting group therapy
- Misconceptions about play therapy
- Background on curriculum-based therapy
- Using curriculum-based therapy

Individual therapy—which is considered "basic therapy" in this chapter—seems to be the easiest type of therapy for beginning clinicians to conduct. The personal comfort level of clinicians seems highest while involved in this type of therapy, probably because individual therapy was emphasized during their coursework and because of the less threatening 1:1 clinician–client ratio. Additionally, the focus of individual therapy is on one diagnosis and usually one objective at a time, whereas the focus in group therapy may be on several diagnoses and several objectives at a time as a factor of the number of clients in the group. The clinician–client ratio in group therapy may increase to as much as 1:5. With special populations in the public schools (e.g., students working on life skills, students with autism), one clinician might work with a small group of 6 to 8 students. When conducting play therapy, the favorable 1:1 ratio might be maintained, but beginning clinicians do not seem as prepared or as comfortable conducting play therapy due to the nature of its spontaneity and seeming lack of structure. This chapter discusses group and play therapy. Curriculum-based therapy is also addressed, and background information regarding its usage in public schools is presented.

Group Therapy

Because beginning clinicians tend to transfer what they know about and what they do during individual therapy to their group therapy sessions, beginning clinicians working with groups of clients rarely perform actual group therapy. There is a definite distinction between "therapy in a group" and "group therapy." Actual group therapy is harder to plan and execute than individual therapy or therapy in a group. Most beginning clinicians start out doing therapy in a group, which boils down to providing individual therapy in a group setting. The following dialogue is an example of this type of therapy involving two clients. The goal of the session is for Johnny to produce the /s/ phoneme correctly in the initial position of individual words and for Billy to produce the /s/ phoneme correctly in the initial position of words in sentences.

CLINICIAN:	(showing the client a picture) What's this?
JOHNNY:	/θʌn/
CLINICIAN:	Was /s/ good?
JOHNNY:	No.
CLINICIAN:	What do you need to do to make it correctly?
JOHNNY:	Keep my front teeth together.
CLINICIAN:	Yes, say it again. (shows picture)
JOHNNY:	sun
CLINICIAN:	Good sound! This one? (shows picture)
JOHNNY:	soap
CLINICIAN:	Nice! Here's another. (shows picture)
JOHNNY:	soup
CLINICIAN:	Good job! It's Billy's turn now. (shows picture) Make a sentence.
BILLY:	The /θɪŋk/ is dirty.
CLINICIAN:	Was /s/ right?
BILLY:	No. I forgot to put my teeth together.
CLINICIAN:	Try again!
BILLY:	(concentrating) The sink is dirty. That was good!
CLINICIAN:	Yes, good sound. This one? (shows picture)
BILLY:	The sailboat is pretty.
CLINICIAN:	Super! One more. (shows picture)
BILLY:	The soda is cold.
CLINICIAN:	Nice work! It's Johnny's turn.

If you role-play this scenario in your head, you can see that the beginning clinician was providing individual therapy to each client within the context of a group setting. There was absolutely no interaction between the clients. Therefore, it might be more advantageous for each client to be seen for 15 minutes of individual therapy instead of 30 minutes of so-called group therapy. Although the clinician gave each client an equal number of turns and the turns were alternated, the time was divided in half and each client received approximately 15 minutes of therapy. The clinician worked on a single objective and with one client at a time. Thus, *therapy in a group* was conducted rather than *group therapy*.

Interaction

Non–Goal-Related Interaction

Two types of interaction can occur during group therapy sessions. The first is that which occurs on non–goal-related activities (e.g., one child presents pictures for the other child to say, one child monitors the other child's production). The second type of interaction requires students to work together on their therapy goals. When clinicians are instructed to perform "group therapy," they are expected to incorporate interaction into their sessions. However, it is the first type of interaction, the easier type, that is most frequently implemented. An example of this type of interaction between Billy and Johnny (the same clients and goals as in the previous example) follows:

CLINICIAN:	Johnny, here are Billy's cards. Billy, here are Johnny's cards. Billy, show Johnny a card.
BILLY:	(shows a picture of a sun)
JOHNNY:	<u>s</u>un
CLINICIAN:	Billy, was his sound good?
BILLY:	(nods head yes)
CLINICIAN:	Good work, boys! Johnny, show Billy a card.
JOHNNY:	(shows a picture of a saddle)
BILLY:	The <u>s</u>addle is new.
CLINICIAN:	(looks at Johnny). Well?
JOHNNY:	It was good.
CLINICIAN:	Nice job, boys!

Interaction was not observed on the actual goals of the session, but it occurred in non–goal-related areas. Each client was actively involved throughout the entire session. When it was not the one client's turn to respond, he showed pictures to the other client and listened to his responses in order to state whether or not they were correct. Another way clinicians frequently try to accomplish this first type of interaction is through the use of activity boards. They feel that interaction is obtained because the clients are moving various spaces on the same board. This type of interaction is better than none, but it leaves a lot to be desired in the actual implementation of effective and efficient group therapy.

Goal-Related Interaction

The second, more desirable type of interaction involves blending the actual therapy goals of the students. This type of interaction requires more planning and is harder to achieve. Most beginning clinicians think this type of interaction is possible only if the clients are working on identical goals. This is not necessarily so. In the following dialogue, the previous non–goal-related example has been redesigned to portray the idea of group therapy. (Mentally role-play this scenario.)

CLINICIAN:	(showing the client a picture) What's this?
JOHNNY:	<u>s</u>un
CLINICIAN:	Good sound! (looking at Billy) Use Johnny's word in a sentence.
BILLY:	The <u>s</u>un is yellow.
CLINICIAN:	Good job! What's this? (looking at Johnny)
JOHNNY:	<u>s</u>oap
CLINICIAN:	Sounds good! Make a sentence (looking at Billy).
BILLY:	I wash with <u>s</u>oap.
CLINICIAN:	Nice!

Interaction was obtained on the goals of the session. Billy's responses were derived from Johnny's responses and built on them. This procedure could also be reversed. Another example (to mentally role-play) follows:

CLINICIAN:	(showing Billy a picture) Make a sentence!
BILLY:	The <u>s</u>un is yellow.
CLINICIAN:	Good! (looking at Johnny) What word has your sound?
JOHNNY:	<u>s</u>un
CLINICIAN:	How was it?
JOHNNY:	It sounded good.
CLINICIAN:	Right!

Interaction was again obtained on the goals of the session. In this example, Johnny's responses were derived from Billy's sentences.

Non–Goal-Related and Goal-Related Combination

It is possible to obtain both non–goal-related and goal-related interaction in the same session, as shown in the next example. (Keep on mentally role-playing that you are the clinician.)

CLINICIAN:	Billy, here are some pictures. Johnny, here are some pictures. Billy, show Johnny a card.
BILLY:	(shows a picture of a seal)
JOHNNY:	s̲eal
CLINICIAN:	(looks at Billy) Well?
BILLY:	It was good.
CLINICIAN:	You're both right! Your turn. (looks at Billy)
BILLY:	The s̲eal is black.
JOHNNY:	Sounded good! Show me another card. (looks at Billy, who then shows him a can of soup)
JOHNNY:	s̲oup
BILLY:	Sounds good! I don't like s̲oup.
CLINICIAN:	(looking at Johnny) Well?
JOHNNY:	It was good.
CLINICIAN:	Johnny, show Billy a card.
JOHNNY:	(holds up a bar of soap)
BILLY:	We use s̲oap to get clean.
JOHNNY:	Good sound! My turn. s̲oap
BILLY:	Good sound, too!

Non–goal-related interaction is evident when the clients show each other picture cards to elicit responses and also when each client monitors the other client's responses. Goal-related interaction is evident when interaction occurs on the goals of the session. For example, when Billy presents a sentence, Johnny extracts his target word and produces it. When Johnny says a target word, Billy builds on it by putting the word into a sentence.

After studying these examples, beginning clinicians can see not only that group therapy can be done, but also that interaction on the goals can be accomplished. One question that might still need answering, however, is whether group therapy can realistically be done if the clients do not all have the same type of problem. To demonstrate, the next scenario involves three clients, Ian, Matt, and Ali. One client presents with an articulation problem, and the other two clients present with different mild expressive language problems. Ian has an articulation problem on the phoneme /r/. Matt has a problem with use of plurals, and Ali has a problem with use of irregular past tense. Specifically, their respective goals are correct production of /r/ in the initial position of words in sentences; correct use of regular plurals at the word level; and correct use of irregular past tense in sentences.

| CLINICIAN: | (divides a pile of picture cards and gives half to Matt and half to Ali) Matt, listen for nouns, and Ali, listen for verbs in Ian's sentence. Matt, show Ian a card. |
| MATT: | (holds up a picture of a robot) |

IAN:	The <u>r</u>obot sings a song.
CLINICIAN:	Matt, was that a good /r/ sound?
MATT:	Yes.
CLINICIAN:	Good job, both of you. Ali, what is the verb?
ALI:	sings
CLINICIAN:	Use the past tense in Ian's sentence.
ALI:	The robot <u>sang</u> a song.
CLINICIAN:	(looking at Ian) Is Ali right?
IAN:	(nods)
CLINICIAN:	Matt, were there any nouns?
MATT:	Yeah, robot and song.
CLINICIAN:	Make each plural.
MATT:	<u>robots</u>, <u>songs</u>
CLINICIAN:	Ali, is Matt right?
ALI:	Yes.
CLINICIAN:	Ali, show Ian a card.
ALI:	(holds up a picture of a river)
IAN:	The <u>r</u>iver <u>r</u>uns into the island.
CLINICIAN:	Ali, did Ian use a good /r/ sound?
ALI:	He used two good /r/ sounds.
CLINICIAN:	Good going both of you! Matt, make the nouns plural.
MATT:	<u>rivers</u>, <u>islands</u>
CLINICIAN:	Is Matt right? (looking at Ian)
IAN:	(nods)
CLINICIAN:	Ali, your turn. What do you need to do?
ALI:	Make the verb past tense and use it in Ian's sentence.
CLINICIAN:	Right! Go ahead.
ALI:	The river <u>ran</u> into the island.
CLINICIAN:	Matt, is Ali right?
MATT:	Yeah.
CLINICIAN:	Way to go, group!

This scenario portrays the achievement of goal-related interaction when working with three clients on three different goals. Goal-related interaction occurs because all of the clients are using the same stimulus sentence, and in this case, extracting from it to meet their individual goals. For example, at the beginning of the scenario, Ian constructed a sentence. He met his goal by correctly producing /r/ in the word *robot*. Ali extracted the verb and changed it to irregular past tense (*sang*) and used it in Ian's sentence to meet her goal. Matt extracted the nouns from Ian's sentence and put them into their plural forms (*robots, songs*).

Summary of Interaction

Strive to incorporate interaction, particularly goal-related interaction, into your therapy sessions. Accept the challenge of providing group therapy rather than therapy in a group.

QUICK CHECK

Analyze the dynamics of your group therapy. Are you really conducting group therapy or is it therapy in a group? Are you achieving goal-related interaction? Now is the time to learn mental role playing to put you in the picture.

Play Therapy

Play therapy or nondirective therapy is usually the preferred method when working with young children or with children who are functioning on a low cognitive level. Beginning clinicians must realize that this type of therapy should be productive and not merely a free-for-all. Frequently, beginning clinicians are under the impression that all they need to do is *play* with the child and that they do not need to plan for this type of therapy session; however, this is not the case. Planning and preparation by the clinician are essential in order for play therapy to be effective. The session must have real structure, some of which is imposed prior to the beginning of the child's therapy session.

Before the session, you can do several things to facilitate play therapy. Structure the environment by determining what materials will be available for the child to interact with and then place these materials strategically around the therapy area. Eliminate distractions (e.g., toys, puzzles, books) by removing them from the room if possible, or at least by placing them out of the child's line of vision. Try to encourage the child's attraction to the desired items by strategic placement around the therapy area and by taking his interests into consideration when planning the item selection for the session. For the session to be productive, you need to know the child's current level of speech, language, and cognitive functioning. Based on this information, you can establish realistic goals prior to the start of the session. Progress toward these goals must be evident throughout the session.

One of the most salient elements of play therapy is following the lead of the child. The focus of therapy should reflect the child's attention. Whatever the child attends to at the moment becomes the immediate focus. If the child is not yet speaking, you should provide a model of and label for the item or event to which the child is attending.

If the child verbalizes, you should provide additional language that is linguistically and contextually appropriate, or help the child say words better by providing a correct articulatory model or by expanding his utterance. Another key element of play therapy is that the session must be fun for the child. In essence, during play therapy, you need to structure the unstructured by mapping goals onto the session. It is also important that you keep an accurate record of the child's responses during each session.

Some examples of mapping goals onto the session are presented. If Child A is not yet using real words to communicate, a realistic goal to be achieved during play therapy may be "to imitate consonant–vowel (CV) combinations three times during the session." If Child B is starting to imitate real words, a realistic goal may be "to imitate five words during the session." If Child C is starting to spontaneously produce words when stimulated, a possible goal may be "to spontaneously produce six words during the session." If Child D is producing single-word utterances and is ready to move to two-word utterances, a suitable goal may be "to imitate three agent + action utterances." A realistic goal for Child E may be "to correctly produce /b/ in the initial position of words in 90% of his attempts."

Always check your records from the previous session and use the data to plan and determine what is realistic for the client to accomplish during the next session. If the child met the previous goal(s), expect more from him during his next session. For example, if Children A through E accomplished the goals stated previously, expect either a greater number of responses or a higher level response from each child during his or her next session. For example, Child A may be able "to imitate CV combinations eight times during the session along with being able to spontaneously produce one CV combination." It may be realistic for Child B "to imitate eight words and also spontaneously produce one word during the session." Child C may be able "to spontaneously produce 10 words during the session." Child D may be able "to imitate six agent + action utterances along with being able to spontaneously produce one agent + action utterance." Perhaps a suitable goal for Child E is "to correctly imitate /b/ in the final position of 10 words." By looking at the child's performance from the previous session, it is possible to see that a greater number of responses is expected from Child A (increasing from three to eight CV imitations), Child B (increasing from imitating five to eight words), Child C (increasing spontaneous production from 6 to 10 words), and Child D (increasing from three to six imitations of agent + action) in their upcoming sessions. A higher level response is being required of Child A (spontaneously produce one CV combination), Child B (spontaneously produce one word during the session), Child D (spontaneously produce one agent + action utterance), and Child E (correctly imitate /b/ in the final position of 10 words). The point is that when a child meets a goal, the goal needs to be increased in complexity. This new goal needs to be harder but still obtainable for the child.

To help you understand how to orchestrate play therapy sessions, two examples are provided. In both examples, the child has access to a jar of bubbles, a book, a barn with farmyard animals in it, and a ball. (Now you are set to really get into mental role playing.)

Example 1

The clinician's established goals for this session are that the client will

1. correctly imitate /b/ in the initial position of six words.
2. spontaneously produce 10 words during the session.

For the child to be successful, he must be given opportunities to attempt words beginning with /b/. Therefore, when planning the session, the clinician must select materials that will enable the child to produce words beginning with /b/. Note that the first goal was considered when selecting the materials (bubbles, book, barn, and ball).

The child enters the therapy area and looks at the available materials. He sits down on the floor by the book and starts looking at it.

CLINICIAN:	(stimulates) book ... book ... big book ... book ... (The dots indicate that the clinician pauses between each stimulation to give the child an opportunity to process and eventually respond.)
CLIENT:	(points to a picture of a dog and looks at the clinician)
CLINICIAN:	(mindful of the goals, points to the dog) Bingo ... Bingo. (The clinician just named the dog "Bingo" to enable the child another opportunity to imitate a word beginning with /b/.)
CLIENT:	(points to a picture of a boy and looks at the clinician)
CLINICIAN:	boy ... boy ... big boy ... boy
CLIENT:	/ɔɪ/
CLINICIAN:	/b/ /b/ /bɔɪ/
CLIENT:	/bɔɪ/
CLINICIAN:	(as she points to the boy) Yes, boy ... boy.
CLIENT:	(loses interest in the book and goes over to the bubbles, sits down, and gives the jar of bubbles to the clinician)
CLINICIAN:	(takes the bubbles, looks at the child, and waits)
CLIENT:	open

CLINICIAN:	open bubbles (she removes the lid and then blows some bubbles). (stimulates) bubble ... bubble ... big bubble ... bubble (the child is popping bubbles; the clinician starts doing it also) bop ... bop ... bop ... (The clinician is ever mindful of the goal and stimulates another word beginning with /b/.)
CLIENT:	(looks at clinician) more
CLINICIAN:	more bubble ... more bubble ... more what?
CLIENT:	/bʌəl/
CLINICIAN:	(immediately blows more bubbles and starts popping them) bop (as one is popped) ... bop
CLIENT:	(imitates) bop
CLINICIAN:	All gone. (she looks at the child and waits.)
CLIENT:	/bʌəl/
CLINICIAN:	bubble. Here's more (blows bubbles). More bubble. Big bubble.
CLIENT:	bop (as he pops bubbles) (When all the bubbles are popped, the child gets the barn and begins playing; the child takes animals—horse, sheep, pig—out of the barn.)
CLINICIAN:	(models) barn ... barn ... big barn
CLIENT:	(picks up horse)
CLINICIAN:	(when child does not verbalize, the clinician models) horse ... horse
CLIENT:	(puts horse in barn)
CLINICIAN:	(models) horse in ... horse barn ... horse in ... in barn ... barn
CLIENT:	/bɔn/
CLINICIAN:	/baɚn/

This excerpt should give you a better understanding of the orchestration of play therapy. Although only a part of the session appeared, there is evidence that work toward accomplishing goals was being performed. There were two instances of imitation of /b/ ("boy" and "bop"), two instances of delayed imitation of the phoneme /b/ ("bubble" and "barn"), and five spontaneous productions of words ("open," "more," "bubble" [twice], and "bop"). Therefore the child, with the clinician's planning and guidance, is making progress toward meeting his goals.

Example 2

The clinician's goals for this session are that the client will

1. imitate 10 two-word utterances during the session.
2. spontaneously produce two two-word utterances during the session.

Again, the child has access to a jar of bubbles, a book, a barn, and a ball. The child enters the therapy area (mentally visualize this as it unfolds), sits down by the barn, and starts playing with it.

CLIENT:	(opens the barn door)
CLINICIAN:	(remains silent; when the child does not verbalize, the clinician models the language) open door … barn door … open door
CLIENT:	(removing pig from barn) pig
CLINICIAN:	pig out … pig floor
CLIENT:	(drops pig)
CLINICIAN:	pig fall … ouch …
CLIENT:	(making pig walk)
CLINICIAN:	pig walk
CLIENT:	(bringing sheep out of the barn) sheep
CLINICIAN:	sheep out … sheep floor … (pretends to feed the sheep) sheep eat
CLIENT:	sheep eat (pretending to feed the sheep)
CLINICIAN:	(pretends to feed the pig)
CLIENT:	pig eat
CLINICIAN:	pig eat apple
CLIENT:	(removes horse from barn) horse … out
CLINICIAN:	yes, horse out
CLIENT:	horse out
CLINICIAN:	horse out barn
CLIENT:	horse out (pretends to feed the horse) horse eat
CLINICIAN:	horse eat apple … eat apple
CLIENT:	eat apple
CLINICIAN:	horse eat apple
CLIENT:	(tires of playing with the barn and starts putting animals away; puts pig in)
CLINICIAN:	pig in … pig in barn … pig in (looks at child expectantly)
CLIENT:	pig in (picks up sheep, puts in barn, and remains silent)
CLINICIAN:	sheep in
CLIENT:	sheep in (picks up horse and remains silent)
CLINICIAN:	horse in (looks at child expectantly)
CLIENT:	horse in
CLINICIAN:	horse in barn

In the excerpt above, the child imitated a total of seven two-word utterances ("sheep eat," "horse out" (twice), "eat apple," "pig in," "sheep in," and "horse in"). Of these seven utterances, six of them were different. The child also spontaneously produced two two-word utterances ("pig eat" and "horse eat") and already met his session goal, which implies that the clinician's expectation for the child was lower than what the child was capable of accomplishing as more time remained in the actual session. This information will prove to be useful to the clinician when planning the goals for the next session.

QUICK CHECK

> When implementing play therapy, make certain you follow the child's lead, make the session fun, and structure the unstructured. Always keep an accurate record of the child's responses. Make certain you have determined goals, have a plan for the session, and are guiding the client toward meeting his specific goals. Before each session, you will need to mentally visualize situations that may occur.

Curriculum-Based Therapy

Curriculum-based therapy or curriculum-relevant therapy has become more prevalent since the passage of the Individuals with Disabilities Education Act Amendments of 1997. As explained in Chapter 8, Individualized Education Programs (IEPs) must be aligned with the state's academic standards, which are derived from the state regulations. If a student qualifies for specially designed instruction, all his needs must be based on the general education curriculum. Therefore, an IEP that is linked to the general curriculum has to be designed. Because all therapy provided addresses the IEP, therapy also must be based on the general curriculum. According to Ehren (2002),

> Curriculum-relevant therapy is an approach calling for SLPs to address curriculum in a unique way, making use of their special competencies in language and its disorders. It does not mean that SLPs will become responsible directly for mastery of subjects such as chemistry, American history, or algebra, but rather contribute to the acquisition of this content by teaching the language underpinnings, as applied directly to the content. (p. 72)

Therapy Excerpt 1

Pennsylvania's academic Standard 1.1 for reading, writing, speaking, and listening is learning to read independently. Part of this standard (1.1.3.E) for third grade is to acquire a reading vocabulary by identifying and correctly using words (e.g., antonyms, synonyms, categories of words). If a student is having difficulty in these areas, or some of these areas, the problem areas need to appear on the IEP. In the following scenario, Sally, Jenna, Joe, and Ethan are four students who have the same IEP goal derived from this standard. They are seen together in a group. The IEP goal is "(Name) will identify and correctly use antonyms (taken from his or her reading book) in sentences in 90% of his or her attempts." At the last therapy session, antonyms were explained and then the students found additional examples in their reading books and constructed a list to be used in their next therapy session.

CLINICIAN:	What did you work on last time?
STUDENTS:	(all eagerly raise and wave their hands)
CLINICIAN:	Sally
SALLY:	antonyms
CLINICIAN:	Super! Ethan, what is an antonym?
ETHAN:	It's a word that means the same as another word.
CLINICIAN:	Is Ethan correct?
STUDENTS:	(silence)
CLINICIAN:	Jenna, what is an antonym?
JENNA:	It's a word that means the opposite of another word.
CLINICIAN:	Good! An antonym is the opposite of another word. What's a word called when it means the same as another word?
SALLY:	Is it a synonym?
CLINICIAN:	Yes. It is a synonym.
CLINICIAN:	Ethan, look at your list. Pick a word and put it in a sentence. Then Jenna will give an antonym for your word. Remember, an antonym is the opposite.
ETHAN:	All right. *Solid.* A rock is *solid.* (looking at Jenna)
JENNA:	*Liquid* is an antonym for *solid.* Water is a *liquid.*
CLINICIAN:	Group, say the two antonyms.
ALL:	(in unison) *solid* and *liquid*
CLINICIAN:	Good going! Sally, select a word from your list and put it in a sentence. Then Joe will give an antonym.
SALLY:	*finish.* I will *finish* all of my homework. (looking at Joe)
JOE:	*end.* I am almost at the *end* of the book.
CLINICIAN:	Group, is Joe correct?.
GROUP:	(in unison) No!
CLINICIAN:	Why not, Jenna?
JENNA:	*End* means the same as *finish,* so they are synonyms.
CLINICIAN:	Good, Jenna. Joe, try again.
JOE:	*start.* I will *start* my homework after school.
CLINICIAN:	Yes! Say the antonyms, group.
GROUP:	*finish* and *start*

CLINICIAN:	This time Ethan will select a word from his list and Jenna will put it in a sentence. Sally will give the antonym and Joe will put it in a sentence. Start, Ethan.
ETHAN:	*cloudy* (looking at Jenna)
JENNA:	It is *cloudy* outside.
CLINICIAN:	Sally, what's an antonym for *cloudy*?
SALLY:	*sunny*
CLINICIAN:	Joe, is *sunny* an antonym for *cloudy*?
JOE:	Yes.
CLINICIAN:	Use *sunny* in a sentence. (looking at Joe)
JOE:	I like *sunny* weather.
CLINICIAN:	Group, say the two antonyms.
ALL:	(in unison) *cloudy* and *sunny*

The session continues with the students taking turns and working on other antonym pairs, such as *giant* and *small, lost* and *found,* and *kind* and *mean.* This session addresses the curriculum in that the antonyms came from selections in their reading books. This session also reflects some of the principles of group therapy that were presented earlier in this chapter.

Therapy Excerpt 2

Pennsylvania's academic Standard 1.6 focuses on speaking and listening. Part of this standard (1.6.5.C) for fifth graders is to speak using skills appropriate to formal speech situations. A subpart consists of being able to pronounce words correctly. If a student has difficulty in this area, and if it becomes a focus, it must be indicated on the IEP. An IEP goal derived from this standard appears on the IEPs of two students, Michael and Bryce, who will be seen together in a group. The IEP goal is "(Name) will correctly use /s/ and /z/ in all contexts in vocabulary related to school subjects in 90% of his attempts." The SLP was aware that the students were studying states and capitals in social studies. Therefore, vocabulary relating to this subject matter was used during the following session dialogue. Each student received a pack of index cards with the state on one side and its capital on the other side.

CLINICIAN:	Today's focus is on states and capitals from your social studies class. What sounds are you working on?
BRYCE:	S
CLINICIAN:	Well, that's the letter. What sound does it make?
STUDENTS:	(in unison) /s/

CLINICIAN:	That's right. When you see the letter S in print, it sometimes makes another sound. Michael, do you remember this other sound?
MICHAEL:	/z/
CLINICIAN:	Good! Remember to make good /s/ and /z/ sounds. What do you need to do to make good sounds, Bryce?
BRYCE:	I need to put my front teeth together.
CLINICIAN:	Michael, is this what you need to do?
MICHAEL:	Yeah.
CLINICIAN:	Make *all* your /s/ and /z/ sounds correctly. Michael, ask Bryce your first card.
MICHAEL:	What'/θ/ the capital of West Virginia, Bryce?
BRYCE:	Charleston
MICHAEL:	That's right!
CLINICIAN:	Michael, how was your sound?
MICHAEL:	It was good.
CLINICIAN:	Which sound was good?
MICHAEL:	/s/ in West Virginia
CLINICIAN:	Yes, but you used your old sound in *what's*. Try it again. Say, "What's the capital?"
MICHAEL:	What'sss (prolonging it) the capital.
CLINICIAN:	Good sound! Bryce, what capital did you say and how was your sound?
BRYCE:	Charleston and it was good.
CLINICIAN:	Bryce, select a card.
BRYCE:	(looking at Michael) Uh oh. This i/ð/ a hard one. Whoops, i/z/. What's the capital of Mississippi?
MICHAEL:	Jackson and my /s/ was good.
BRYCE:	You're right. Your turn.
CLINICIAN:	Bryce, how were your sounds in *Mississippi*?
BRYCE:	They were OK.
CLINICIAN:	(looking at Michael)
MICHAEL:	What's the capital of Minnesota?
BRYCE:	Boise. My sound was good.
CLINICIAN:	What sound was it, Bryce?
BRYCE:	It was /z/.
MICHAEL:	Wait! That's not the capital.
BRYCE:	How about St. Paul? My /s/ was good.
MICHAEL:	You got it that time.
BRYCE:	(looking at his cards) I'm in trouble (anticipating two target sounds). Wisconsin. I got them both!
MICHAEL:	Madison. My sound was good.
MICHAEL:	My turn. Missouri, my sound was good.
BRYCE:	Jefferson City. I got both sounds right!

The session continues with practice on /s/ and /z/ in the state names Kansas, South Dakota, Nebraska, Arkansas, and South Carolina, and in the capital names Annapolis, Tallahassee, Indianapolis, Columbus, and Lansing. The students continue to monitor their productions of their target sounds. This session addresses the curriculum as the students work on the phonemes /s/ and /z/ using words from social studies. Principles of group therapy that were previously presented are also reflected in this excerpt.

Therapy in the public schools must be curriculum based. Know your state department of education's as well as your school district's academic standards. Each IEP must address these standards. Therapy sessions must address the IEP, which also has to be based on the general education curriculum. Measure all students' progress as it relates to the general education curriculum.

Hopefully reading this chapter will help you to move beyond basic, individualized therapy and become comfortable conducting genuine group therapy and play therapy sessions. If you are student teaching or performing an externship in the public schools, become familiar with the general education curriculum and your state's standards. IEPs must be aligned with these standards, and therapy must address the IEP and be based on the curriculum. It is also a good idea to start anticipating how you will act in these therapy sessions. Use mental role playing to imagine yourself as the clinician. You may be one before you know it!

After reading this chapter, you should be able to

1. explain the difference between "therapy in a group" and "group therapy."
2. design a group therapy session where there is non–goal-related interaction.
3. design a group therapy session where there is goal-related interaction.
4. design a play therapy session.
5. state at least three things you will incorporate into a play therapy session.
6. design a curriculum-based therapy session.

References

Ehren, B. (2002). Speech–language pathologists contributing significantly to the academic success of high school students: A vision for professional growth. *Topics in Language Disorders, 22*(2), 60–80.

Individuals with Disabilities Education Act Amendments of 1997, 20 U.S.C. § 1400 *et seq.*

Pennsylvania Department of Education. (n.d.). *Academic standards for reading, writing, speaking and listening.* Retrieved November 2, 2003, from http://www.pde.state .pa.us/k12/lib/k12/RWSLStan.doc

Chapter 10

Enhancing Performance

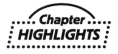
Chapter HIGHLIGHTS

- Problems encountered during the therapy process
- Solutions to problems encountered during the therapy process
- Refining the beginning clinician's performance during the therapy session
- Usefulness of mental role playing

This chapter provides suggestions to make your sessions run more smoothly and to enable you to perform more efficiently and effectively during the therapeutic process. This chapter does not provide general therapeutic techniques or theories, which should have been studied previously, although I may occasionally remind you of some of this information by providing examples that show how classroom knowledge is incorporated into the therapeutic process. When you complete this chapter, you should be able to deal with many of the common problems experienced as you commence providing clinical services.

Before reading further, however, you should think back to those cues I provided in Chapter 9 for you to use mental role playing. I cannot stress enough that now is the time for you to employ what sociologists term "anticipatory socialization." Simply, this means that you think through or mentally visualize yourself performing the roles expected of you before you occupy that professional position. How will you act? What should you say? How will others see you?

Although you may have information from students, professors, or other professionals about the organizational expectations and climate you can expect, you need to become confident, poised, and prepared. Therefore, imagine yourself in the role of a clinician before you find yourself fearful and trembling in the actual therapy situation. As you review the following problems and solutions, imagine yourself in the equation. Doing so will make the reality easier (and more pleasant) when you face it.

Problem and Solution 1: Seating Arrangement

Record Keeping

Beginning clinicians frequently use suboptimum seating arrangements. Rather than being assigned to a room where the furniture is nailed to the floor and the clinician is told where to sit and where to seat the client(s), the clinician is usually responsible for arranging the seating and preparing the room prior to the client's arrival. Although the task may seem simple, problems with the seating arrangement have often been encountered. Fortunately, solutions are available to alleviate these problems.

Because most people are right-handed, I use right-handed clinicians as an example. Right-handed clinicians naturally tend to seat clients to their right at a table. However, this seating arrangement results in the session's records being kept directly under a client's eyes. The record keeping is a constant fascination and distraction to the client. Furthermore, when the client watches the clinician mark the record sheet of a formal test, the client may gain some knowledge that affects how he responds. This may bias the testing results.

It may appear that a suitable solution is to place the client across the table from the clinician. This arrangement will rectify the problem of viewing records, but it creates others. It becomes difficult to reach across the table when, for example, the client needs to feel the vibration of the clinician's vocal cords or the clinician's air stream against his hand.

Another problem resulting from the seating arrangement arises when the right-handed clinician, for example, has the client sit to her left at the table and then moves the record-keeping sheet to the left, probably because of a need to turn and maintain eye contact with the client. This position proves difficult because the clinician must twist and turn to record a response (see Figure 10.1).

The problems that result from these seating arrangements can easily be rectified by placing the record-keeping sheet on the side of the clinician's writing hand. If the clinician is right-handed, records should be kept on the right side. If the clinician is left-handed, the records should be kept on the left side. The client should be on the side farthest from the clinician's writing hand. For the right-handed clinician,

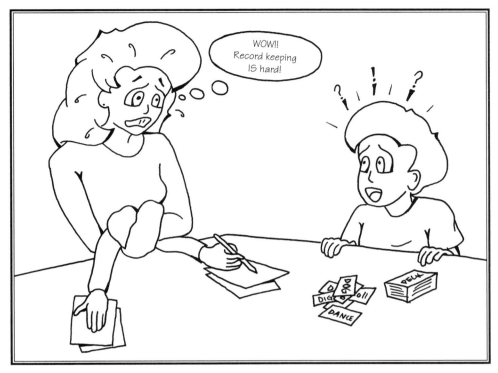

Figure 10.1. Tied in knots!

the client should be on the clinician's left. If the clinician is left-handed, the client should be on the clinician's right. These adjustments will minimize the client's distraction by keeping records out of immediate sight and eliminate the clinician's gyrations. These changes should result in smoother running sessions.

These more effective seating arrangements allow the clinician's dominant hand to be free to keep records while the other hand manipulates the clinical materials (turning pages, flipping cards, etc.). In this manner, the flow of the session is not interrupted while responses are recorded. Consider the consequences of an alternative approach. At a session I observed, a right-handed clinician seated the client on her left and placed her record response sheet on her right. This clinician appeared to be off to a good start. Instead of "reserving" her right hand for record-keeping purposes, however, the clinician sometimes selected a card with her left hand, put the pen (held in her right hand) down on the table, and transferred the card from her left to her right hand. After the client responded, the clinician transferred the card back to her left hand. When this happened, the clinician either forgot to record responses or stopped the flow of the session to record responses.

However, when the clinician continued to hold the pen in her dominant hand, she consistently recorded the client's responses. Merely holding the pen served as a reminder and played a role in consistent record keeping, which improved the clinician's overall accountability.

Although other seating arrangements are possible, different problems result. For example, when only chairs without tables are used, clinicians have to balance therapy materials and record sheets on their laps. Manipulating materials and recording responses become a juggling act. Typically, whenever anything becomes an effort, it either does not get done or gets done inconsistently, which is not acceptable for therapy or accountability. To remediate this problem, using a lapboard or sitting on the floor with the tablet on the floor can eliminate the juggling act.

Client Access

The best clinician cannot "help" a client if she has no access to the client. When working with preschool children with problems adjusting to the newness and unfamiliarity of the therapeutic situation and clinician or separating from a significant other, it may be necessary for the clinician to be seated between the child and the door in case interception becomes necessary. These children have not yet become acclimated and may try to remove themselves from the new and unfamiliar situation or they may try to find the familiar person waiting for them by making a dash for the door (see Figure 10.2). Advantageous seating arrangements can prevent the clinician from having to chase the child or coax the child to return to the therapy room. Avoiding these interferences can make therapy more productive.

QUICK CHECK

Prior to starting each session, make certain your seating arrangement is efficient for both record keeping and client access.

Problem and Solution 2: Reinforcement

To be effective during various aspects of the therapeutic process, the clinician must understand and appropriately apply reinforcement. Non–goal-directed behaviors must not be *accidentally* reinforced, and goal-directed behaviors must not be *inappropriately* reinforced. The manner

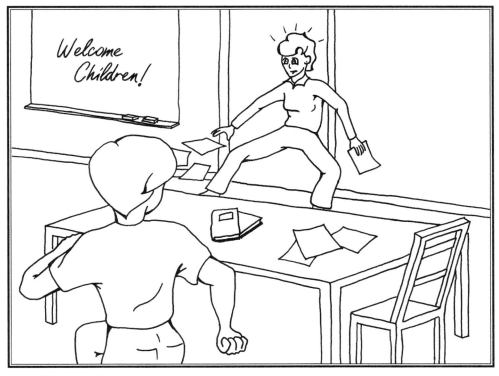

Figure 10.2. Blocking the runaway.

in which reinforcement is used differs depending on the task. Reinforcement techniques are not the same during therapy and testing.

Therapy

Reinforcement is frequently used during therapy sessions. Properly employed, it can be instrumental in establishing or maintaining certain behaviors. When reinforcement is not used appropriately, detrimental results can occur.

Accidental or Inappropriate Usage

Clinicians have a tendency to use a select word or a few select words when providing verbal reinforcement. For example, "good" is frequently chosen to perform this function. Although variety is preferred, there is nothing wrong with using the word "good" during the session if it is used *only* for the purpose of reinforcement. However, this is usually not the case. "Good" is also frequently used as a casual comment or a conversational filler.

The following example occurred in a session when the client's goal was to correctly produce the /r/ phoneme in the initial position of words. The clinician's use of "good" as a casual comment followed the client's extraneous response. The client was shown a picture of a robe, which happened to be blue, in an attempt to elicit the word *robe*. The following occurred:

CLIENT: I like blue.
CLINICIAN: You like blue? Good.

The clinician's intent was not to reinforce the client but simply to acknowledge his comment. Thus, the word "good," if typically used to reinforce session goals, should not be used for unrelated purposes because its *reinforcing effect* will be weakened or lost. It is important to note that the same dialogue might occur if the session's goals were initiating conversation or spontaneously commenting. Then the clinician's use of "good" would be justified immediately following the client's response. A more appropriate way of dealing with the client's extraneous comment would be to briefly respond to the content. Responses such as, "I like blue, too," or "Blue is my favorite color, too," would be more appropriate.

Next is an example showing inappropriate usage of "OK":

CLINICIAN: (models for client) Say /s/.
CLIENT: (produces a distorted /s/)
CLINICIAN: OK. That wasn't right.

The client was immediately reinforced for producing a distortion of the /s/ phoneme. This unintentional reinforcement occurred when the clinician said "OK" immediately following the client's response. This beginning clinician knew the client's production was not correct and had no intention of reinforcing this incorrect production. The clinician used "OK" as a filler to give herself an extra moment to think of another therapeutic technique to implement. Reinforcement is a powerful tool and must always be used appropriately. When mixed feedback signals are given to the client, it not only disrupts the learning process but is frustrating for both the client and the beginning clinician. The best solution to this problem is to decrease overall "OK" usage.

Less obvious instances of inappropriate and accidental reinforcement also occur. In one example, the beginning clinician was working with a client who was functioning at a low cognitive level. This client tended to mouth objects, which is not considered desirable behavior. The clinician gave objects to the client one at a time and said, "What do you do with _____?" When a car was presented, the client immediately put the car in her mouth. The clinician removed the car, said "no" to indicate that the response was not appropriate, and modeled both the correct action and suitable language. Then a ball was presented, and the client mouthed the ball. The clinician responded as she did previously. Next, a cup was presented, and the obvious happened. The client mouthed the cup, and the clinician reinforced the client for this behavior. In essence, the clinician was reinforcing the same behavior that she had tried to extinguish in the first two trials. In anticipation of the child's extremely predictable response, the clinician should not have presented an object that could be mouthed.

In another example, a clinician reminded a client to swallow because one of the goals was to eliminate drooling. At one point in the session, the clinician sat on the floor and placed the client across her lap in a supine position with the client's head tilted posteriorly. After a period of time, the clinician reinforced the client for not drooling. Reinforcement in this case was not deserved because the laws of gravity made it impossible to drool in that position. A client should not receive reinforcement under circumstances in which he is not in control of the behavior.

Continuous Reinforcement

Continuous reinforcement is most effective for establishing a new skill or behavior. Initially, each correct response should be reinforced, and this reinforcement should immediately follow the client's correct response. In the following excerpt, from a session where the goal was correct imitation of the /t/ phoneme in the initial position of words, every correct response was immediately reinforced.

CLINICIAN:	Say "ten."
CLIENT:	ken
CLINICIAN:	Raise your tongue tip. Say "ten."
CLIENT:	ten
CLINICIAN:	Good! Say "top."
CLIENT:	top
CLINICIAN:	Super! Say "to."
CLIENT:	to
CLINICIAN:	Very nice!

Intermittent Reinforcement

Once a new skill is established, the reinforcement schedule should be changed to an intermittent one. This schedule type reduces the possibility of satiation during therapy and also produces greater resistance to extinction. One type of intermittent reinforcement, called fixed ratio, occurs after a fixed number of responses. Reinforcement may occur after every third or fifth response, or whatever number is considered appropriate when taking into account the client, his ability, his needs, and the type of therapy. The client's goal in this example is to correctly produce the /p/ phoneme in all positions of words in sentences.

CLIENT:	(looking at pictures) The p̲illow is big.
CLINICIAN:	This one.
CLIENT:	The p̲ot fell.
CLINICIAN:	Next!
CLIENT:	The p̲ie is good.
CLINICIAN:	This one.
CLIENT:	The cup̲ broke.
CLINICIAN:	Nice work! Keep going!
CLIENT:	The cup̲ is colorful.
	His name is P̲ete.
	The p̲an is rusty.
	Take a p̲ill.
CLINICIAN:	Super! Try some more.

This example shows reinforcement being given after every fourth correct response.

Specific and Varied Reinforcement

Reinforcement should be both specific (directly related) to the task performed and varied. In this manner, the client knows exactly what behavior is being reinforced and does not become bored hearing the clinician say the same thing repeatedly. In the following three examples, reinforcement is neither specific nor varied.

CLINICIAN:	Point to *chair*.
CLIENT:	(points to chair)
CLINICIAN:	Good!

CLINICIAN:	Say /s/.
CLIENT:	/s/
CLINICIAN:	Good!

CLINICIAN:	(points to picture to elicit regular plural) one cat, TWO _____
CLIENT:	cats
CLINICIAN:	Good!

In all three examples, the clinician's reinforcement consisted solely of using the word *good*. Not only was the reinforcement not varied, but it was not specific to the task. Reinforcement makes more of an impact when the client knows why he is being reinforced. It also makes more of an impact when the reinforcing words are changed to best fit the client's response.

The following examples demonstrate usage of specific as well as varied reinforcement.

CLINICIAN:	Point to *chair*.
CLIENT:	(points to chair)
CLINICIAN:	Good pointing!

CLINICIAN:	Say /s/.
CLIENT:	/s/
CLINICIAN:	Great sound!

CLINICIAN:	(trying to elicit regular plural) (points to picture) one cat, TWO _____
CLIENT:	cats
CLINICIAN:	Super! You said "cats."

In these examples, the clinician's reinforcement was not always the same. It was varied and, more important, specific to each task. In this way, the client is reminded of why he was reinforced. Because the reinforcement is varied, the clinician appears to be more involved in the therapy session.

Tangible Reinforcement

Tangible reinforcement should follow the same rules as verbal reinforcement: Goal-directed behaviors should be reinforced, and non–goal-directed behaviors should not be reinforced. For example, one client's goals were to correctly produce the /s/ phoneme in isolation and to correctly produce the /l/ phoneme in the initial position of words. At the end of the session, the beginning clinician said, "Because you were good, you get a sticker." The implication is that the client earned a sticker because he behaved. Nowhere in the goals for the session was behavior mentioned. Also, whether or not a client behaved requires subjective judgment. The awarding of a sticker was not in any way based on the client's performance on the goals.

For reinforcement to be effective, the client should be aware of his exact requirements at the start of the session. The explanation must be presented in a manner that the client can understand. Some suggestions follow:

CLINICIAN:	If you get 100 good responses, you can connect the dots from 1 to 30.

CLINICIAN: Every time you produce a good /s/, put a chip in the cup. If the cup is full at the end of the session, you'll earn a sticker.

CLINICIAN: If 90% of your responses are correct, you can color three leaves at the end of the session.

CLINICIAN: When you produce a good /l/, cross off one of these balloons. If all the balloons are crossed off at the end of the session, you'll earn a sticker. (The page contained 100 balloons.)

The first and third examples are more complex than the second and fourth. It is important that directions are presented at a level that the client understands.

If the clinician actually wants to reinforce the client's behavior, it must be stated in a goal. For example, if a client has interrupted each session by getting out of his chair an average of five times, the clinician cannot expect the client to eliminate the disruptive behavior completely as soon as the goal is instituted. Therefore, the goal cannot be set so high that the client cannot experience success. Also, earning a sticker is rewarding to the client only if he wants one. If it is not rewarding, find something that is. An example of reinforcement based on behavior follows:

CLINICIAN: Here are four chips. (points) Every time you get out of your chair, you'll lose a chip. At the end of the session, if any chips are still here (points), you will earn a sticker. If there are no chips, you will not earn a sticker.

The client has been made aware of the expectations. He now knows that earning the sticker depends on his performance on the goals of the session. He knows exactly what has to be done to earn the tangible reinforcement. A goal should not be set so high that the client becomes discouraged or so low that the client reaches it long before the session is over. Records regarding the client's performance from the previous session should be consulted to help establish realistic expectations for the next session.

Naturalistic Versus Artificial Reinforcement

Naturalistic reinforcement is powerful. Because this type of reinforcement is concrete, it is useful with young children or those functioning on a low cognitive level. Naturalistic reinforcement normally occurs in the environment and may include common events such as gaining and sustaining an adult's attention, getting desires and needs met, and engaging in pleasurable human interaction (Reed, 1994, p. 449). This type of reinforcement is not used as much as it should be. For example, a session goal for an 18-month-old client who does not use words spontaneously is to imitate names of things that are functional to him. The following excerpts from the therapy session show that the clinician used artificial reinforcers instead of naturalistic reinforcers.

CLINICIAN:	(shows a cookie and models) Cookie … cookie.
CLIENT:	/ʊ/
CLINICIAN:	(knows the client can get a better approximation) Say "cookie."
CLIENT:	/ʊi/
CLINICIAN:	Nice talking!

CLINICIAN:	(shows a jar of bubbles) Bubble … bubble.
CLIENT:	/ʌbl̩/
CLINICIAN:	Super!

CLINICIAN:	(shows a jar of juice and pours a small amount of juice into a cup; holds cup toward child) Juice … juice.
CLIENT:	/u/
CLINICIAN:	Good talking!

Note that the use of verbal praise in these examples is not going to make much of an impact on this child. The substitution of clapping, hugging, and the dispensing of tokens also would be artificial reinforcement. The use of these artificial reinforcers will not teach the client the "power of communication"—that is, that he can manipulate his environment by talking.

On the other hand, with natural reinforcement, the client will learn the power of communication and that he can manipulate the environment. Examples showing usage of natural reinforcement follow:

CLINICIAN:	(shows a cookie) Cookie … cookie.
CLIENT:	/ʊ/
CLINICIAN:	(knows the client can get a better approximation) Say "cookie."
CLIENT:	/ʊi/
CLINICIAN:	(gives the child a piece of the cookie to eat)
CLIENT:	(eagerly eats the cookie piece)

CLINICIAN:	(shows the child a jar of bubbles) Bubble … bubble.
CLIENT:	/ʌbl̩/

CLINICIAN:	(blows bubbles)
CLIENT:	(squeals in delight and "pops" bubbles)
CLINICIAN:	(shows client a jar of juice and pours a small amount of juice into a cup; holds cup toward child) Juice … juice.
CLIENT:	/u/
CLINICIAN:	(extends the cup toward the client)
CLIENT:	(takes the cup and drinks the juice)

Naturalistic reinforcers make the most impact when trying to establish behaviors. In addition, they tend to facilitate generalization. Therefore, it is important to use this type of reinforcement whenever possible because its effects are far-reaching.

Testing

Reinforcement given during formal testing differs from that given during therapy. Because the purposes behind these professional tasks differ, it follows that reinforcement procedures should also differ. The overall goal of therapy is to enable the client to succeed. Initially, the client becomes aware of his success through the clinician's specific feedback for correct responses. Given specific feedback, the client either repeats or changes his response.

The purpose of the testing situation is to determine how the client is currently functioning. The client should not be made aware of the correctness or incorrectness of any response and should not be given the opportunity to produce a better response. Therefore, reinforcement should not be contingent on the correctness of a response but instead should reflect the fact that the client is performing the task.

For the testing situation, it might be more accurate and specific to think in terms of *praise* and *encouragement* instead of reinforcement. Words of praise or encouragement are not necessary after each response but should be provided as needed. Many beginning clinicians administering evaluations have been observed using the extremes of praise and encouragement. In one instance, a beginning clinician was observed administering the 101-item *Test for Auditory Comprehension of Language* without providing any praise or encouragement.[1] When questioned, she explained that she was not supposed to reinforce the client during

---

[1]The test mentioned has been revised and is now the *Test for Auditory Comprehension of Language–Third Edition* (Carrow-Woolfolk, 1999). This edition contains only 48 items.

testing. At the other extreme, another beginning clinician was observed saying "good" after each of the 101 items. When questioned, this clinician responded that she thought each response had to be reinforced. Note how easily information can be taken out of context and inappropriately applied.

An example portraying correct usage of praise and encouragement during administration of the *Peabody Picture Vocabulary Test–Third Edition* (Dunn & Dunn, 1997) follows:

CLINICIAN:	Show me "bus."
CLIENT:	(points to correct response)
CLINICIAN:	Show me "drinking."
CLIENT:	(points to correct response)
CLINICIAN:	Show me "hand."
CLIENT:	(points to correct response)
CLINICIAN:	Show me "climbing."
CLIENT:	(points to correct response)
CLINICIAN:	You're working hard! Show me "key."
CLIENT:	(points to correct response)
CLINICIAN:	Show me "reading."
CLIENT:	(points to correct response)
CLINICIAN:	Show me "closet."
CLIENT:	(points to correct response)
CLINICIAN:	Show me "jumping."
CLIENT:	(points to incorrect response)
CLINICIAN:	You're looking at all the pictures. Show me "lamp."

This example shows praise and encouragement given whenever the clinician feels it is necessary. The particular response provided is not contingent on the correctness of the response, but instead is given to the client for performing the task, which, in this case, is pointing. It is important to keep this in mind to prevent the invalidation of results.

QUICK CHECK

Ask yourself whether you are using reinforcement appropriate to the nature of the task. Is it specific and varied? Are you using naturalistic reinforcement when possible?

Problem and Solution 3: Verbal Models

The profession of speech–language pathology emphasizes speech, language, and communication; therefore, it stands to reason that all persons preparing to become clinicians should demonstrate skills in these areas. Unfortunately, this is not always the case. Behaviors that do not provide good models need to be eliminated soon after they are identified.

The "OK" Syndrome

The overuse of "OK," or the "OK" syndrome, is evident during many therapy sessions of beginning clinicians. These clinicians appear to use "OK" to serve five functions. The first function is using "OK" as a conversational filler. In this instance, they say "OK" for no apparent reason throughout the session. Many beginning clinicians do not seem comfortable with pauses or silence occurring within a session. When these moments occur, there is a tendency to interject "OK," although it serves no apparent purpose.

A second usage of "OK" is that of a tag question. The clinician makes a statement into a nonauthoritative request.

> CLINICIAN: Say it again, OK?

A third function of "OK" is to provide feedback. Often, beginning clinicians do not directly distinguish between correct or incorrect responses. They say "OK" after an incorrect response instead of providing specific feedback.

> CLINICIAN: Say /s/.
> CLIENT: /θ/
> CLINICIAN: OK. This time, close your teeth. Say /s/.

Beginning clinicians also tend to use "OK" as a positive reinforcer after a client gives a correct response. When "OK" is used in this fourth manner, the clinician is not making a firm commitment to the client's response.

> CLINICIAN: Say /s/.
> CLIENT: /s/
> CLINICIAN: OK. Say it again.

Using "OK" as a positive reinforcer is too vague, especially by clinicians who use "OK" with other meanings. Stronger reinforcing words, such

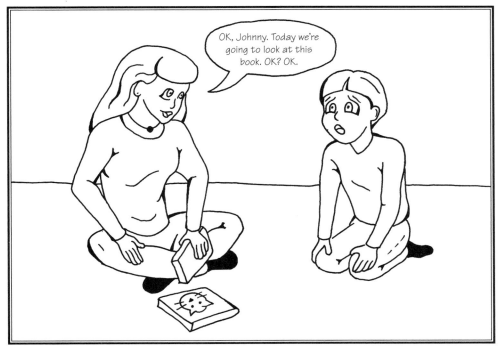

Figure 10.3. The "OK" syndrome.

as "Great sound!" and "Super /s/!" should be used. These more meaningful words will make more of an impact on the client, and the client will strive harder to consistently achieve that good production.

The fifth function of "OK" is as an answer to a question that is followed by the tag question, "OK?" (see Figure 10.3). In other words, the clinician responds to her own question.

CLINICIAN: Let's work on /tʃ/, OK? OK.

Overusing any particular word is monotonous for the listener. Because "OK" does not contribute to providing good language and communication models, excessive usage of "OK" should be eliminated. Breaking the habit of overusing "OK," however, is easier said than done. Your initial response will be disbelief when you are informed that you used "OK," for example, 22 times in 3 minutes. Until you are made aware of the frequency with which you use "OK," it is not possible to understand the need for elimination.

The first step, then, is to become aware of overusing "OK." Rather than relying on the supervisor's constant reminder, *you* must recognize and accept responsibility for your frequent usage. This can be done by audiotaping a session (with your client's or a family member's permission obtained on an appropriate release form) and counting the number of times you said "OK," and determining the number of minutes you were involved in speaking. Then, calculate the number of times you said "OK" per minute. Review the tape and write down the context in which all usages occurred. Analyze why each instance occurred and determine its function. The five functions described previously can serve as the framework for this analysis. If an "OK" does not fit this framework, place it in an "other" category. Then further analyze all occurrences in this "other" category and determine whether you can identify any additional functions. Once you are aware of your increased usage, you will start to catch yourself as you say "OK," which is the second step to breaking this habit. Soon thereafter, you will move to the third step, awareness that you are about to say "OK." However, instead of saying "OK," you will quickly shift to either saying something more appropriate or remaining silent. In this manner, you can break the "OK" habit.

Unnatural Production

Beginning clinicians often unconsciously use unnatural presentation (emphasis or overexaggeration) of words for clients to imitate or receptively identify pictures or objects. Rather than making the task easier for the client, the clinician complicates the task by presenting words in an unnatural and incorrect manner. For example, one beginning clinician pronounced the word *button* as /ˈbʌt ˈtən/ instead of using the more frequent productions of /ˈbʌtn̩/ or /ˈbʌʔn̩/. Her pronunciation was both unnatural and incorrect in that /t/ should only arrest the first syllable and not also release the second syllable. In addition, she stressed both syllables equally instead of giving primary emphasis to only the first syllable. Due to the unnaturalness of this production, the word takes longer to say because a deliberate effort must be made. Similarly, this beginning clinician pronounced *eating* as /ˈit ˈtɪŋ/ instead of /ˈit ɪŋ/. Again, the clinician incorrectly used the /t/ phoneme to arrest the first syllable and to release the second syllable, and she incorrectly placed equal emphasis on both syllables. The clinician also mispronounced *letter* as /ˈlɛt ˈtɚ/. The same problems discussed with regard to the first two examples are again evident; additionally, however, in the word *letter*, the /t/ phoneme should be heard as /d/, presented phonemically as /ˈlɛdɚ/.

Instances of unnatural production seem to occur when emphasis is placed on an individual word or when a word is pronounced out of the context of running speech. It is not possible to present clients with correct and accurate models if words are spoken in an unnatural and incorrect manner. Therefore, it is essential that words, regardless of the situation, be presented naturally.

Ungrammatical Utterances

It is important for beginning clinicians to both *use* and *model* grammatical utterances. Examples of ungrammatical usage are "You listened good," "Listen close," and "You're pointing so nice today." Correct grammatical usage would be "You listened well," "Listen closely," and "You're pointing so nicely today" (see Figure 10.4). Simply put, if clinicians do not "practice what they preach," their clients will lose respect for and form an unfavorable impression of them.

The clinician needs to model utterances when those initiated by a client are not grammatically correct, even if they do not fall under the jurisdiction of a therapeutic objective. This modeling should be done consistently and in a noncondescending manner. For example, if the client says, "How much do I got?" the clinician should casually say, "How much do you have? You have ...." If the client says, "What that

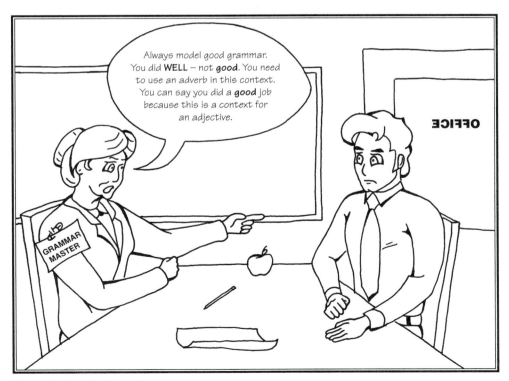

Figure 10.4. Grammar master.

is in there?" the clinician should say, "What is that in there? It's a ...."
If the client says, "If it ain't ...," the clinician should model, "If it isn't
...." The point is that ungrammatical utterances should not be overlooked and the client should not receive ridicule, reinforcement, or pun-
ishment for this usage. The clinician should casually state the client's
utterance in a corrected fashion and then respond to the client's question or statement.

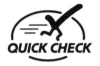

> Audiotape one of your sessions (with your client's or a family member's
> permission on an appropriate release form). Listen to your verbal models.
> Make certain you are not guilty of using the "OK" syndrome, unnatural
> production, or ungrammatical utterances.

Problem and Solution 4: Loquaciousness

Loquaciousness refers to excessive talking. Constant talking on the
clinician's part is problematic because when the clinician is talking, the
client is not responding, not working toward the goal(s) of the session,
and consequently not correcting his problem. The logical solution is
for the clinician to stay focused on the goal(s) of the session and make
certain that all of her talking is necessary and relevant (e.g., giving directions, modeling, giving feedback, providing reinforcement).

> Audiotape a session (with your client's or a family member's permission
> on an appropriate release form). Listen to the tape and determine if all
> your talking is necessary and relevant.

Problem and Solution 5: Smothering the Client

"Smothering the client" refers to the clinician's use of language beyond
the client's expressive linguistic ability. For example, during an observation of a client who was not yet producing single words, a doll accidentally fell off the table. The beginning clinician modeled, "The doll
fell off the table." This clinician was modeling language that was far
beyond the client's linguistic ability. Modeling is more effective when

it is at a level either commensurate with or only a step or two above the client's current linguistic ability, depending on the situation. A more effective way to model in this situation is to say the single words "doll" (while pointing to the object) and "fall" (while gesturing or reenacting the action), followed by production of the two-word utterance "doll fall." Longer or more complex utterances should not be presented because this client is not yet producing single words.

QUICK CHECK

When working with clients who have expressive language problems, analyze your language. Make certain you are modeling language at a level either commensurate with or a step or two above the client's current linguistic ability, depending on the situation. Do not model beyond the client's level.

Problem and Solution 6: Fostering Dependency

It appears that speech–language pathologists who promote independence are able to legitimately discharge their clients more quickly than those who encourage dependency. Successful clinicians encourage their clients to take responsibility for both their problems and their therapeutic programs. Leahy (1995) stated, "experience has shown that successful speakers are those able to take over their own therapy" (p. 225). A logical question to ask at this point is "Who would ever encourage dependency?" Dependency is unconsciously encouraged in the therapeutic situation in something as basic as verbal interaction. Some clinicians subconsciously foster the client's dependency by sharing the client's problem and behaviors, by encouraging the client to perform tasks for the benefit of the clinician and not for his own betterment, and by being authoritarian. According to Leahy (1995), "therapy which is ever dependent on the clinician is of limited or no value" (p. 225).

Two examples of sharing the problem and behaviors during verbal interaction are as follows: "Keep our hands out of our mouth" and "We're going to start our lesson now." The clinician must remember that she is speaking of the client's hands, the client's mouth, and the client's lesson. Examples of encouraging the client to perform tasks for the benefit of the clinician are as follows: "Say it for me," "Read them again for me," and "Can you read this aloud for me, Bill?" The client should be performing the tasks out of his desire to correct his problem and not out of desire to please the clinician. Examples depicting an authoritarian role are as follows: "I want you to listen to me," "I want you

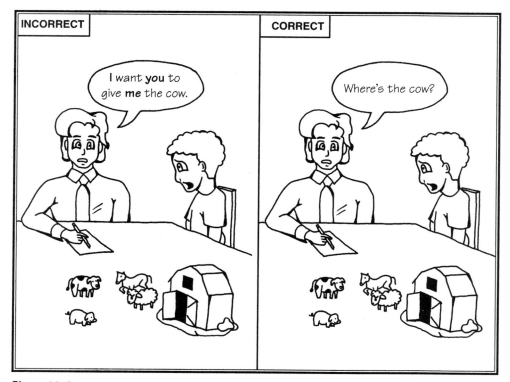

Figure 10.5. Fostering dependency (left side) and fostering independence (right side).

to get the ball and the car," and "I want you to get the baby." The intent of these utterances needs to be conveyed without indirect reference to the power structure as indicated in these examples through usage of *I, you,* and *me*. Revised examples without reference to power structure are as follows: "Listen!" "Get the ball and the car!" and "Get the baby!" Furthermore, instructions given in this fashion are simpler and thus easier for clients to process and understand (see Figure 10.5).

A problem with fostering dependency surfaces when the client is assigned to another speech–language clinician. This change could happen for a variety of reasons, such as the client or clinician moving out of the area, the client leaving preschool services and beginning services for school-age children, the client advancing to a different school within the district, or the clinician taking a leave of absence. If the initial clinician fostered dependency, the client or the client's parents (depending on the client's age) may believe that no other clinician can help. This is not a good beginning for the new clinician. It is extremely difficult to establish a positive relationship in this situation. The new clinician has to struggle to be viewed in the same light as the previous clinician and must prove herself every step of the way. Usually clinicians are viewed as being confident from the start because of their professional role. Therefore, if a clinician encourages clients to take responsibility for both their problem and therapeutic program, switching to a new clinician should not be problematic for either the clinician or the client.

| | Analyze your interaction with your clients. Are you encouraging independence or dependency? |

Problem and Solution 7: Choice Constancy

When a receptive language task involving pictures or objects is presented, it is extremely important to keep the number of choices (the field) constant. The following scenario occurred while a beginning clinician was working on increasing receptive vocabulary with a client. The clinician placed four pictures on the table (cookie, milk, car, and ball). In this example, the child always responded correctly and the schedule of reinforcement was intermittent.

CLINICIAN: Car. Where's the car?
CLIENT: (points to the car)
CLINICIAN: (removes car picture) Cookie. Where's the cookie?
CLIENT: (points to the cookie)
CLINICIAN: (removes cookie picture) Milk. Where's the milk?
CLIENT: (points to the milk)
CLINICIAN: Nice work!

Here is what should have been done:

CLINICIAN: Car. Where's the car?
CLIENT: (points to the car)
CLINICIAN: (removes the picture of the car and adds another picture, perhaps dog) Cookie. Where's the cookie?
CLIENT: (points to the cookie)
CLINICIAN: (removes the picture of the cookie and adds another picture, perhaps juice) Dog. Where's the dog?
CLIENT: (points to dog)
CLINICIAN: Great job! (removes the picture of the dog and adds another appropriate picture)

In the first example, the probability of obtaining correct responses increased. When the client was asked to identify the first picture, a 25% probability existed that he could respond correctly by chance (choose 1 of 4 pictures). The probability increased to 33% when he was asked to identify the second picture (1 of 3), and then to 50% when only two pictures remained (1 of 2). Therefore, each successive identification became easier for the client as the number of choices decreased.

The chance of randomly responding correctly remained the same for each selection throughout the second example. The client was always presented with a field of four pictures and four novel choices. Thus, the probability of responding correctly remained 25% (1 of 4) throughout the task. It is extremely important to replace each selected item with a new item so the difficulty level remains constant.

The same problem exists when the clinician does not remove each previously selected item. Although the number of pictures remains constant, the number of choices available to the client does not. If a client correctly identified one picture, he will not point to that picture again. Thus, the field has decreased as demonstrated in the first example and the chance factor does not remain constant.

QUICK CHECK

When presenting receptive language tasks to a client, answer this question: Am I keeping the number of choices constant?

Problem and Solution 8: Reading Sequence

Because it is important to teach a young child skills necessary for the future, the clinician needs to take into account a young child's native language. The clinician needs to consider the language that the child will learn to read. For example, young clients who will be reading English must learn the left-to-right, top-to-bottom sequence. Therefore, clinicians should not present stimuli in an opposing sequence for these future readers of English.

Beginning clinicians have been observed placing stimulus pictures in a bottom-to-top, right-to-left sequence when sitting opposite the young client. There is a tendency to place the material in correct sequence from one's own perspective, but it is important to remember that the client's perspective is reversed. For the English-speaking child, materials should be placed from the child's left to right and from top to bottom.

When placing stimulus materials in front of an English-speaking child, place them from his left to right and from top to bottom based on his perspective.

Problem and Solution 9: Elicitation Techniques

Language

Because it is important to use techniques that will elicit the desired or target structure, the clinician must strategically design or structure tasks so the desired response is likely to be obtained. In the following example, the beginning clinician is trying to elicit production of the pronoun "he" from a child whose goal is to use the pronouns *he* and *she* correctly.

> CLINICIAN: (shows a picture) What did the boy drop?
> CLIENT: a cookie
> CLINICIAN: Oh, use your special word.

Although the client's response was perfectly normal and appropriate to this situation, this response was not reinforced because it was not what the clinician wanted to hear. She wanted the client to say, "He dropped a cookie," which would be reinforced because of use of the pronoun *he*. In reality, this response is extremely abnormal. First, typical speakers would not answer this question using a complete sentence. Second, a pronoun is a word that takes the place of a noun or any word used as a noun. Typical speakers do not use pronouns until the noun referent is established, and this clinician is requiring the client to use pronouns without first establishing the noun referent.

If a client does not respond with the target or expected response, the clinician should critically evaluate the task. The clinician should restructure the task rather than "teach" the client to be an abnormal communicator, which, in essence, is what happened in the last excerpt. Several tasks are more conducive to eliciting production of "he" or "she." The clinician can ask the client to tell about his best friend (named Billy). The client will use the proper noun "Billy" once or twice, but should also substitute the proper noun with "he." If he does not do this spontaneously, the clinician should provide a model. Another possible task is for the clinician to give the client two puppets, Tony and

Annie. The client is supposed to use the puppets to build a structure (bridge, house, etc.) with blocks behind a screen while explaining how Tony and Annie are building their structure. The screen is essential because the client will have to be more verbal and descriptive to explain what the clinician cannot see. If the client does not spontaneously start using the appropriate pronouns after a few references to the nouns, the clinician should start modeling. Also, if the client confuses the pronouns *he* and *she*, the clinician needs to consider modifications to the task. Two main points are important regarding elicitation techniques: The clinician should (a) carefully design the task so that the target behavior is elicited and (b) be certain that normal communication is emphasized.

In the following two examples, the target response is usage of the regular past tense and usage of the present progressive tense, respectively. Although the target structure differs in the two examples, the same points are evident.

> CLINICIAN: (rolls a ball across the room) What rolled?
> CLIENT: the ball
> CLINICIAN: Say the whole thing.

> CLINICIAN: (shows a picture) What is the girl doing?
> CLIENT: jumping
> CLINICIAN: Say the whole thing.

In both examples, the client's responses are correct and appropriate. The reason that the target responses were not produced is because the clinician did not properly design the tasks. The tasks as designed are conducive to eliciting either a Noun or an Article + Noun response in the first example and a Verb + ing response in the second example. The responses are not conducive to usage of the regular past or present progressive tenses. Therefore, the client should not be penalized when, in fact, he is performing in a correct and appropriate manner. If the clinician has to give the client instructions such as "use your special word" or "say the whole thing," the task needs to be redesigned. In most cases, the stimulus is problematic, not the client's response.

Articulation

Beginning clinicians frequently must try to elicit correct production of errored phonemes even though they are not adept at using cueing and prompting or presenting cues and prompts in any logical order. Therefore, Bain's (1994) hierarchy of cues and prompts to help a client produce an errored sound correctly is presented, starting with those cues that provide the maximum amount of support.

1. Manipulation of Articulators

When a child has difficulty producing a phoneme, the clinician may have to manipulate the child's articulators. For example, when attempting production of an /s/ phoneme with a client who constantly produces /θ/, the clinician may need to use a tongue depressor to push the client's tongue behind his or her teeth so an acceptable production is possible. When the client produces /p/ labiodentally, the clinician may need to place her thumb on the client's lower lip and her index finger of the same hand on the upper lip to get the client's lips to come together while also preventing the upper teeth from getting involved in the production.

2. Placement Cues

Placement cues are frequently referred to as "phonetic placements." The clinician describes or demonstrates the position of the articulators for production of a particular phoneme. For example, if a client frequently produces /θ/ for /s/, the clinician can provide the following phonetic placement cue: "Put your teeth together."

3. Visual and Tactile Imagery

Bain's example of visual and tactile imagery involves a child who stops fricatives. If the client says /t/ for /s/, "the clinician could talk about dripping versus flowing sounds, or run a finger down the child's arm to represent frication and tap the child's arm to represent stops in order to facilitate correct production" (p. 18).

4. Prosodic Emphasis

For prosodic emphasis, the clinician should vary the amount of emphasis placed on the target sound by increasing the intensity and duration. For example, if the error sound is /s/ in the word /sʌn/, the clinician could emphasize the sound to the child by saying, "Say /sssssssʌn/." However, this unnatural emphasis should be eliminated as soon as the client is capable of correct production.

5. Frequency of Stimulus Presentation

The clinician should determine the number of times a stimulus will be presented prior to requesting the client to respond. For example, the clinician may choose to produce the target phoneme five times slowly and distinctly prior to expecting the client to respond. To maximize concentration, there should be silence between the clinician's productions and the client's response.

6. Model of Presentation

The clinician may choose to present a model that is auditory, visual, or both. If the clinician cues, "Listen. Say /s/," the client should be listening but not watching. However, if the clinician presents an auditory and visual model, such as "Watch. Listen. Say /s/," the client should be watching as well as listening. Using both modalities (visual and auditory) gives the client more support than using either modality alone.

7. Phonetic Context

The context in which a phoneme occurs influences production. Some phonemes surrounding an errored phoneme may serve to facilitate production. For example, /t/ preceding /s/ helps many clients achieve correct production of /s/ (*cats*, *boats*, *boots*, etc.). According to Bain, "the *Deep Test of Articulation* (McDonald, 1964) is a useful tool for identifying the influence of surrounding sounds on an errored sound" (p. 17).

8. Contrasts–Minimal Pairs

A client's productions of sounds seem to be positively influenced when the clinician presents stimulus materials that contrast the errored phoneme with the target phoneme. The clinician should present two pictures, each depicting one word of the minimal pair (i.e., one picture containing the target phoneme and the other picture containing the client's usual misarticulated phoneme). For example, a minimal pair that can be used for the process of stopping is *toe* and *sew*. If the process stopping is used, both words will be pronounced as *toe*.

QUICK CHECK

> The type of cue or prompt that should be used depends on the client's errors. Start where the client is likely to have success. If the client never produces the phoneme correctly, begin with the prompt or cue that will give the maximum amount of help or provide the most support. In this case, manipulation of articulators would be a logical starting point if the target phoneme can be approached in this manner. If manipulation of articulators cannot be used for a particular target phoneme, try another prompt or cue, such as a placement cue, which still provides a lot of support. Once the child is able to correctly produce the target phoneme using cues or prompts providing maximum success, continue decreasing the amount of support. Gradually decrease the amount of support provided by prompts or cues to enable the client to correctly produce the target phoneme spontaneously.

Problem and Solution 10: Risky Questions

A clinician should never ask a client a question if she will not accept the response. Beginning clinicians have a tendency to start sessions on the wrong foot, as in this example:

CLINICIAN: Do you want to look at these pictures?
CLIENT: No!

Now what does the clinician do? Typically, the clinician ends up giving the client 10 different reasons why he has to look at the pictures while the client argues that he doesn't want to. This situation can be avoided if the clinician starts the session differently, as in the following example:

CLINICIAN: Pick a card. Remember to use a good sound.

This opening does not give the client an opportunity to say "no." As a result, the clinician does not use valuable time providing a lengthy explanation or arguing. Although clients may still refuse to perform a task, the opportunity to do so should not be initiated by the clinician.

The client, however, should have some control over the session. He should be allowed to make some decisions and choices regarding his therapy sessions, but only when there is no interference with accomplishing goals. Two examples follow:

CLINICIAN: Should we sit on the floor or at the table?

CLINICIAN: Which do you want to do first, the book or the cards?

In the first example, where one sits for therapy has nothing to do with accomplishing goals, so there will be no negative consequences. (Keep in mind the discussions of record keeping with young and active children in Chapter 6 and of seating arrangements in Problem and Solution 1 earlier in this chapter.) In the second example, although the client will "do" both the book and the cards, his decision solely determines the order.

These latter examples differ from the initial one in that the client's responses do not interfere or prevent goal attainment. Other than the actual focus of the therapy session, most clients are capable of making decisions similar to these.

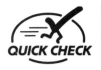

Analyze your use of questions during a session. Never ask a question if you might reject or argue with the client's response.

Problem and Solution 11: Appearing Foolish

Miller (1981) suggested that the clinician not ask questions that the child knows the clinician can answer, because this makes the clinician look foolish. If a question is obvious or simple, as most questions asked during a therapy session are, the client also feels foolish. Some examples follow:

CLINICIAN: What color is this?
CLIENT: red

CLINICIAN: What is the boy doing?
CLIENT: running

CLINICIAN: What is this?
CLIENT: soap

In these examples, the client knows that the clinician knows the answers. Therefore, because the clinician bothers to ask the questions, it appears that the clinician thinks the client does not know this simple, obvious information. The client perceives the clinician as playing the part of a fool and does not appreciate that behavior. Although these types of questions are plentiful in formal tests, they can be prevented, with conscious effort, in therapeutic sessions by abandoning simplistic ways of obtaining responses and being more imaginative in eliciting target responses.

As an alternative to the first example, the clinician can get the child to say a color word in the context of an activity that the client enjoys. This particular client enjoys building with blocks.

CLINICIAN: (places a container of blocks on her lap) What block do you want?
CLIENT: red
CLINICIAN: (holds up a red block) This one?
CLIENT: yes
CLINICIAN: (presents red block to client)

The second example can be restructured similarly. For example, the clinician can use pairs of action cards with pictures of a boy running, a baby crying, a man reading, a lady sitting, a boy playing, a baby crawling, a man sawing, a lady reading, and so on. The client and clinician can play "Go Fish." Neither can see the other's cards. The clinician begins in order to establish the verbal pattern.

CLINICIAN:	Find "the baby is crying."
CLIENT:	I can't. Go fish! Find "the boy is playing."
CLINICIAN:	I can't. Go fish! Find "the man is sawing."
CLIENT:	I can't. Go fish! Find "the boy is running."
CLINICIAN:	Here it is.
CLIENT:	I have a match. I get another turn. Find "the man is reading."

The third example can also be restructured. If the goal is to increase the child's expressive vocabulary, the clinician can fill a "mystery" or "surprise" box with specific objects. She shakes it to evoke interest. Again, the clinician begins in order to establish the verbal pattern.

CLINICIAN:	I close my eyes, reach in, and find money.
CLIENT:	I close my eyes, reach in, and find soap.

The wording of this example can be modified if the wording is too long or complex for a client.

In the two sets of examples, the same responses are being elicited. However, the manner of elicitation makes a difference. Most clients will not feel that anyone is playing the part of a fool in the second set of examples.

Sometimes the initial examples presented earlier in this section *are* appropriate for a client, based on the client's age, the goals of the session, or the client's level of performance. However, if a task makes the clinician or the client feel or appear foolish, then change is necessary.

QUICK CHECK

If your questions can be perceived as *simple* or *obvious* by the client, restructuring is necessary. Change the manner of your elicitation.

Problem and Solution 12: Being Overpowering

To help make clients feel comfortable in the therapeutic setting, the clinician needs to avoid overpowering clients, especially children, without being aware of doing so. For example, a form of overpowering occurs when the clinician sits in a big chair and the client sits in a little chair, or when a child sits on the floor and the clinician sits on a chair or kneels. In these examples, the clinician "towers" over the client, which magnifies the clinician's superiority or authority. Establishing authority of this sort is not conducive to creating a comfortable, positive clinical relationship. Although overpowering may be needed with some clients, for most clients, it is not.

Eye-to-eye contact is best for all relationships, and a clinical relationship is no different. Being at eye level with the client minimizes a sense of superiority or authority. When the client is a child, minor modifications are necessary. For example, the clinician can sit on a little chair and let the child sit on a big chair. When the child is on the floor, the clinician can get as low as possible, even if it means conducting therapy in a prone position. Alternatively, the child can sit in a child-sized chair while the clinician sits on the floor in front of the child. In each of these scenarios, the client and the clinician are at eye level. In this manner, no one towers over the other, and the child should not feel intimidated or overpowered.

QUICK CHECK

> Think about whether you have overpowered a client.

Problem and Solution 13: Directions

Beginning clinicians tend to use lengthy directions, which often confuse the client and are time-consuming. An example follows:

CLINICIAN: If I would say "cat," which one would you point to?

It makes more sense to use clear, precise, and concise directions. The following are examples of how to reword the previous direction:

CLINICIAN: Point to cat!

CLINICIAN: Show me cat!

If the client is working at such a basic receptive level, it is possible that the client has an auditory comprehension problem. Therefore, the client may experience more success if all stimuli are presented in a less complex fashion.

Another problem with directions is that many beginning clinicians have a tendency to overexplain, as in this example:

CLINICIAN: Let's look at these pictures. Look at each picture carefully. Pick out the other member of the pair presented. For example, if I say "cat," point to "dog." If I say "salt," point to "pepper." These types of words are called opposites.

The clinician is overexplaining. She must learn to "get to the point." A revision of the previous example follows:

CLINICIAN: Look at these pictures of opposites. The opposite of "cat" is "dog." Point to "dog." Let's try one. "Up."

QUICK CHECK

> Audiotape a session after obtaining permission on an appropriate release form. Analyze your directions. Are they clear, precise, and concise?

Problem and Solution 14: Receptive Tasks

Receptive tasks must measure exactly what they were designed to measure. In other words, if the client responds correctly, it should be because he understands the language that the clinician is trying to assess. In the following clinician-devised task, the goal was receptive identification of verbs:

CLINICIAN: (shows the client pictures of a boy playing and of a girl cooking) Show me "The boy is playing."
CLIENT: (points to the correct picture)
CLINICIAN: Good work!

Although the client responded correctly, he cannot be credited with understanding the verb *play*. The client might actually have responded to the noun *boy*. Because one picture depicts a boy and the other a girl, the verb does not even have to be considered when making the choice.

This task must be changed to be effective. One suggestion follows:

CLINICIAN: (shows the client pictures of a boy playing and of a boy cooking) Show me "the boy is playing."

CLIENT: (points to the correct picture)

With the task designed in this fashion, there is more evidence that the client understands the verb *play*, or at least can differentiate it from the verb *cook*. The clinician needs to assess many different verbs and assess them in different combinations to be certain. As stated earlier in this chapter, there is a high level of success from random selection when the field consists of only two choices.

Another way the original task can be altered is as follows:

CLINICIAN: (shows the client pictures of a boy playing and of a girl cooking). Show me "play."

CLIENT: (points to the correct picture)

This presentation does not reflect much alteration of the original task; however, minor modification has resulted in an effective task that assesses what it was designed to do. Again, the clinician must give adequate thought to tasks prior to presentation. In this manner, many invalid responses can be anticipated and thus avoided.

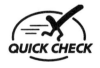

QUICK CHECK

> Make certain that your receptive tasks measure precisely what they were designed to measure. If the client responds correctly, it should be because he understands the language that the clinician is trying to assess.

Problem and Solution 15: Head Nodding and Forward Upper Body Movement

The clinician needs to avoid head nodding and upper body movement when presenting articulatory models to a client. For example, when one clinician modeled /d/, /d/, /d/, she nodded her head and moved her upper body forward (and then backward) three times. She did not intend to convey to the client that these extraneous movements will help him to make a correct production or that these movements are part of what he is to imitate. However, the client incorporated these extraneous movements (head nodding and upper body movements)

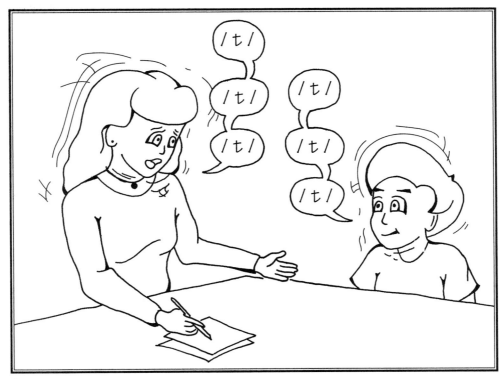

Figure 10.6. Unconsciously exhibiting extraneous movements.

into his production. A clinician who makes such movements may become aware of the client's movements, but may not realize that the client is imitating her movements. If the client presents with unusual behaviors, the clinician needs to become more aware of what she is doing that may cause these behaviors (see Figure 10.6).

QUICK CHECK

Videotape a session after obtaining permission on an appropriate release form. Watch and analyze the tape. See if you are making extraneous movements. If so, observe the effect they have on the client.

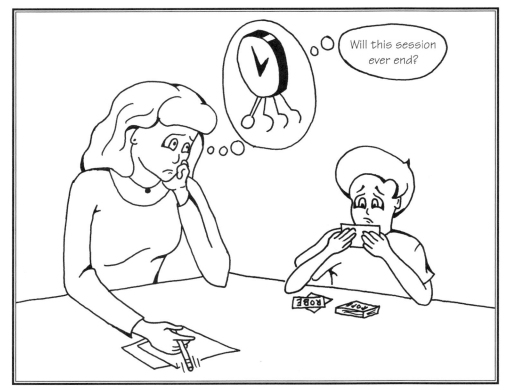

Figure 10.7. Conveying boredom.

Problem and Solution 16: Habits That May Be Misinterpreted

The clinician needs to avoid habits that can be misinterpreted. For example, constantly swinging a leg under the table or twisting hair may be perceived by others as nervousness. The clinician who tends to rest her head or chin on her hand looks bored to others. These habits do not give favorable impressions to clients, families of clients, or other observers. Because observations will continue throughout the clinician's professional career, the clinician needs to eliminate negative behaviors to help make a favorable and professional impression (see Figure 10.7).

Problem and Solution 17: The Game "Mirage"

To avoid having the client respond, "We played games," when his classroom teacher inquires, the clinician must be careful where the emphasis of the session is placed. Games and activities are frequently used to facilitate speech and language goals. Because the games and activities are a means to an end, the clinician should place the emphasis on the speech and language–related goals, not on the games and activities. The following comments should be avoided because they reflect a misplaced emphasis: "Neither of you won because no one got to the end," "We don't have a winner again," "The first one to finish the game gets a prize," and "You both got to the witch's broom. Good job!" A client who "wins" should do so because he reached criterion on a particular objective and not solely because he rolled the higher numbers on the die. The goal in the following excerpt was correct production of the /r/ phoneme in the initial position of words.

CLINICIAN:	Roll the die!
CLIENT 1:	(rolls die) Five.
CLINICIAN:	(shows picture) What's this?
CLIENT 1:	rat
CLINICIAN:	Good. Move five spaces. Your turn.
CLIENT 2:	(rolls die) Three.
CLINICIAN:	(shows picture)
CLIENT 2:	radio
CLINICIAN:	Nice! Move three spaces.

More emphasis can be placed on the actual goal of the session by making a slight modification.

CLINICIAN:	Roll the die!
CLIENT 1:	(rolls die) Five.
CLINICIAN:	(shows pictures) What are these?
CLIENT 1:	rat, razor
CLINICIAN:	Good! These?
CLIENT 1:	rug, rain, rabbit

CLINICIAN:	Good. You said five good /r/ sounds. Move five spaces. (passes die to Client 2)
CLIENT 2:	(rolls die) Three
CLINICIAN:	(shows pictures)
CLIENT 1:	rainbow, ribbon (distorted)
CLINICIAN:	Where's your good sound? Try that one again.
CLIENT 2:	ribbon
CLINICIAN:	That's better.
CLIENT 2:	robot
CLINICIAN:	You had two good /r/ sounds. Move two spaces.

In this example, the clients were told that moving spaces was contingent on correct production of the /r/ phoneme in words. In the first example, the client moved five spaces (the roll of the die) for saying one /r/ word correctly. In the second example, the client moved five spaces only after saying /r/ correctly in five words. A big difference between the first and second example is that in the latter example the client was reminded of the goal (correct production of the /r/ phoneme in the initial position of words) throughout the activity. The clinician made no reference to the goal in the first example. The client's perception of the session, including the goal(s), is a reflection of the manner in which the clinician conducts the session.

QUICK CHECK

> Make certain that your emphasis is on the goals of the session, not on the games or activities.

Problem and Solution 18: Carry-Over

Speech–language pathologists frequently comment that obtaining carry-over (generalization) is problematic. Carry-over is the process in which the client exhibits newly learned techniques (e.g., correct production of a particular sound, use of present progressive tense) in all situations regardless of the environment or the people present. Many clinicians complain that the client simply does not use a technique outside of the environment in which it was initially performed. Carry-over, or generalization, is more likely to be attained when steps are taken to make the client more independent. A client is more likely to become involved and independent if the clinician emphasizes monitoring and performing specific assignments as early as possible in the therapeutic program. In this way, the client becomes responsible for his own performance.

Monitoring

The clinician should emphasize monitoring to help the client move toward becoming independent. When a client begins working on a new goal, he should know the expectations. He should know when responses are correct and when they are not. Although the clinician has to perform the monitoring function initially, if the clinician continues to monitor, dependence can be perpetuated. Change can take place only when a client becomes aware that his behavior is correct or incorrect. If the client perceives that his production is not correct, he will try to correct it by making a change. If the client perceives his production as correct, he will try to stabilize it. Self-listening or self-monitoring should be emphasized as soon as therapy is started. The following example is included as a demonstration of working on monitoring.

CLINICIAN:	Johnny, say /s/.
JOHNNY:	/θ/ (produces a frontal lisp)
CLINICIAN:	Close your teeth. Try again.
JOHNNY:	(produces a distorted /s/)
CLINICIAN:	You're getting closer! Where should your tongue tip be?
JOHNNY:	Here. (points)
CLINICIAN:	Yes. Try again. /s/
JOHNNY:	/s/
CLINICIAN:	Super! /s/
JOHNNY:	/θ/ (produces a frontal lisp)
CLINICIAN:	How were your front teeth?
JOHNNY:	Apart.
CLINICIAN:	How should they be?
JOHNNY:	Together.
CLINICIAN:	Yes. Try again. /s/
JOHNNY:	/s/
CLINICIAN:	Did it sound right?
JOHNNY:	Yes.
CLINICIAN:	Good. Say /s/.
JOHNNY:	/θ/ (produces a frontal lisp)
CLINICIAN:	How was it?
JOHNNY:	Not so hot.
CLINICIAN:	Why?
JOHNNY:	My teeth weren't closed.
CLINICIAN:	Right you are!

The clinician is preparing the client to monitor his productions and take responsibility for his therapeutic program right from the start. The client knows the characteristics of the target phoneme. When monitoring is first introduced, it may be somewhat time-consuming; however, if the groundwork is done properly, monitoring will soon become automatic. An example follows:

CLINICIAN: Let's hear your sound.
CLIENT: /s/. It sounded good.
CLINICIAN: Right. Keep going.
CLIENT: /s/ Good; /s/ Yes; /s/ Good.
CLINICIAN: Right you are!

Monitoring does not have to occur verbally. For example, place two faces (a smiling face and a frowning face) in front of the client. The client points to the smiling face to indicate that his production was correct or to the frowning face to indicate that his production was not correct. Less time is consumed in this manner. Another example of a nonverbal monitoring system is to have a picture of a traffic light. The client points to "green" for a correct response and "red" for an incorrect response. Counters operating red and green lights can also be used. The client can press the lever on the counter with the green light for a correct response and the lever with the red light for an incorrect response. In choosing one of the many ways to monitor responses, the clinician needs to consider what is appropriate for the client's level.

Whatever type of monitoring system is established, the clinician must be certain that the client is actively listening and evaluating each production rather that simply saying "good" or pointing to the smiling face in an automatic fashion. The extra time taken to establish a monitoring system in the early sessions of the therapy program is definitely worthwhile because the client will become more independent, and as a result, progress will be more rapid.

Assignments

To ensure carry-over, the clinician should begin instructing the client to practice the new behavior in other environments and with other people as soon as appropriate. For example, if a client is working on correct production of the /s/ phoneme in isolation, the clinician does not have to wait until /s/ is produced correctly in conversation before attempting to obtain carry-over. Various substeps, as small or insignificant as they may seem, can be made into worthwhile assignments. For example, if the client is having difficulty producing /s/ in isolation, practicing production would not be realistic or helpful at this point. However, the clinician could give an assignment leading up to the accomplishment of the objective as long as it was related to the objective, it was preliminary in nature, and the client had the necessary capabilities.

ASSIGNMENT:
Practice putting front teeth together lightly without tension.

	Tuesday	**Wednesday**
Breakfast	X X ③ X ⑤	① ② X X X
Dinner	① X X ④ X	① X X X X
Bedtime	① X X X X	X X X X X

Key: X = correct; O = incorrect.

Tuesday results: $^{10}/_{15}$ = 67%

Wednesday results: $^{12}/_{15}$ = 80%

Overall results: $^{22}/_{30}$ = 73%

Figure 10.8. Check sheet for carry-over.

For a client who substitutes /θ/ for /s/, focusing on keeping his front teeth together is a definite step toward accomplishment of the objective. Therefore, a possible assignment is to have the client look in a mirror and make certain that his front teeth are together.

I have found that clients are more likely to complete or at least attempt assignments if two conditions exist. First, an assignment must be specific. Second, there must be a way to check the client's performance.

The following example meets the first condition of being a specific assignment: "Every day until our next session, look in the mirror three times a day—around breakfast, dinner, and bedtime. Put your front teeth together lightly and without tension five times." To meet the second condition, there has to be a way to check the client's performance. This can be met by designing a record sheet, such as the completed sheet shown in Figure 10.8. By glancing at the completed record sheet, the clinician can determine how the client performed. The client is much more likely to attempt, and complete, an assignment of this nature when he has a record sheet, an actual piece of paper, that serves as a reminder; he has to put an "X" on the number of the attempt if it was performed correctly or an "O" if performed incorrectly; and he has to return the assignment to the clinician the very next session.

Because the clinician gave the client an assignment, it is the clinician's responsibility to review it at the beginning of the next session. If the client does not automatically present the check sheet, the clinician should ask for it, quickly scan and calculate the client's performance, and ask whether the client had any difficulty. The clinician should reinforce the client in an age-appropriate manner for completion of the assignment.

Beginning clinicians have numerous problems with assignments. One of the most common is designing assignments that are not specific. The following is an example of a nonspecific assignment for a client starting to correctly produce /s/ in conversation:

CLINICIAN: Remember to work on /s/.

This assignment is vague. What exactly is the client to do? How often should the client do it? With whom should it be done? In what environment? Another problem is that this beginning clinician had no way to determine if the client had success.

Another typical problem is a lack of follow-through on the clinician's part. This occurs when the clinician gives an assignment but does not check whether the client completed it or determine how the client performed. Because of this lack of follow-through, the client may get the idea that assignments are not important and conclude that there is no reason to do them.

In planning assignments, the clinician should incorporate situations and materials from the client's life, because these will be more functional and promote carry-over. The clinician should also vary the setting as well as the listeners and speakers as appropriate.

QUICK CHECK

Have immediate success with carry-over. Be certain to implement self-monitoring and the use of specific assignments as early as appropriate in the therapeutic process.

Problem and Solution 19: Too Much Work

Most beginning clinicians probably think, "I have too much work," from the first day of clinical practicum. There are ways, however, that some of the work can be eliminated. One day, I went into the clinic room where student clinicians gather. One student was frantically looking through a dictionary and making a list of words. I asked what she was doing. She said she was preparing for her next therapy session with a university student who had a frontal lisp. There was no reason why this beginning clinician had to construct a word list. Some of this responsibility should have been placed on the client through an assignment, as in the following example:

CLINICIAN: Your next session is Thursday. Make a list of 25 new words beginning with /s/. Bring it with you. You'll practice them next time.

Similarly, a clinician working with a 5-year-old client on the production of /p/ in the initial position of words can help make the client responsible for his therapy and get the family involved by giving an assignment of this nature:

CLINICIAN: (hands the client a paper bag from the supermarket) Look around your house. Find 12 objects that begin with your /p/ sound. Put them in this bag and bring it next time.

In this manner, some of the responsibility for stimulus materials for the next session has been shifted from the clinician to the client and his family.

QUICK CHECK

Make your clients responsible for their stimulus words and materials when appropriate.

Problem and Solution 20: Sign Language

Beginning clinicians frequently approach the teaching of sign language as a totally new and unique experience. Most beginning clinicians, however, are well prepared and can approach this teaching with confidence. Indeed, more and more students are taking sign language instead of a foreign language. They are familiar with language theory and language therapy, which forms the basis for teaching sign language.

The following portion of a therapy session is useful for elaborating on this topic. (Single quotation marks indicate that the words were signed.)

CLINICIAN: (shows a picture) What is the dog doing?
CLIENT: (makes inappropriate sign)
CLINICIAN: No, here's 'sleep.' You try.
CLIENT: 'sleep' (imitates sign correctly)

CLINICIAN: That's right! What is the girl doing?
CLIENT: 'swim'
CLINICIAN: Good! What is the man doing?
CLIENT: 'eat'
CLINICIAN: Good job!

A few changes are necessary to make this session and the clinician's approach productive and effective. First, it is important to remember that language is divided into receptive and expressive modalities. The receptive modality is frequently overlooked when teaching sign language. Clinicians must remember that if a client is going to use sign language to communicate (the ultimate goal), he must also be able to understand or "read" the signs of others when they communicate. Because it is more difficult to "read" the signs of others than to use them for communication, the client should be exposed to the receptive modality first. In the example above, the clinician should place pictures depicting the various actions in front of the client. The clinician should sign one of the verbs and then have the client identify the appropriate picture.

Another change is that this clinician should simultaneously sign everything she says to the client because this client is learning to communicate through signs. Expanding and modeling should be done in the same manner as with hearing clients and those with specific language impairments. Expanding and modeling must always be appropriate to the level at which the client is functioning. These changes are reflected in the following excerpt:

CLINICIAN: (places three pictures in front of the client) 'swim.
              Point to swim.'
CLIENT: (points to the correct picture)
CLINICIAN: 'Good! Girl swim.' (removes and replaces picture)
              'Sleep. Where's sleep?'
CLIENT: (points to the correct picture)
CLINICIAN: 'Yes. Dog sleep.'

QUICK CHECK

> Teach sign language as you would teach spoken language. Remember to begin with the receptive modality. It is important for the client to be able to "read" signs.

Problem and Solution 21: Session Opening

Beginning clinicians tend to forget to "open" their sessions. Sessions should begin with a statement of the goal(s) by either the clinician or the client, depending on the circumstances. If the client has been involved with the therapeutic process for a while and if the client is capable, the client should take an active role in the opening. He can state what he is working on. Examples follow:

> CLINICIAN: What are you working on?
> CLIENT: is Verb + ing
>
> CLINICIAN: What is your sound?
> CLIENT: /s/

If the client is just beginning the therapeutic process or if the goal(s) of the session are changing, then the clinician should specify the goal(s) of the session, using terminology the client can understand. Ideally, however, the client should state the session's goal(s).

QUICK CHECK

Ask yourself, "Do I have a session opening? Am I encouraging the client to take an active role in it?"

Problem and Solution 22: Session Closing

Warning

Although part of closing a session should include providing the client with notice that the session is almost over, beginning clinicians tend to abruptly end their therapy sessions. An example follows:

> CLINICIAN: Make a sentence.
> CLIENT: The dog ran after the cat.
> CLINICIAN: Time is up. See you next week. (hands client his notebook and stands up)

This ending needs to be improved for many reasons. Clinicians typically try very hard to get clients to enjoy therapy, and many clients do like therapy, look forward to their sessions, and do not like to see them end. Therefore, if a warning that the session is going to end is given in advance, it makes the ending easier for the client to accept. Several examples of warnings are provided:

CLINICIAN: Five more sentences. Then it will be time to go.

CLINICIAN: Make a sentence for each of these pictures. (shows the client how many pictures) Then we're done.

CLINICIAN: Two more minutes and then it's time to go.

The warning given must be appropriate to the client's level of functioning. For example, if the client does not understand numbers, telling him "five more sentences" would not be appropriate. If the client does not understand the concept of time, then saying "two more minutes" would not be appropriate. Showing the client how many more he has to complete would be appropriate if he does not understand the concept of time or numbers. These are only a few suggestions. The possibilities of informing the client that the session is ending are numerous.

Wrap-Up

The clinician needs to end the session on a positive note so that the client feels good about himself as well as his accomplishment. If the client did not have much success during the session, the clinician may need to end with an easier task, one on which the client can succeed. In this manner, the client will have something positive to feel good about.

It is also important that the client has a good understanding of his therapeutic program. To make certain the client knows the goal(s) of the session, the goal(s) should be reviewed at the end of the session. This review should ideally be done by the client; however, if this is not possible (for reasons already provided in the section on session opening), then the clinician should provide the review. The following examples are closings by the clinician and the client, respectively.

CLINICIAN: Today you worked on /s/ at the end of words.

CLINICIAN: What did you work on today?
CLIENT: My /s/ sound.

Make certain you have adequate session closure. Provide a specific warning that the session is about to end. The goals should be reviewed. Be certain the client takes an active role in this review when applicable.

Problem and Solution 23: Pause Time

Beginning clinicians frequently do not feel comfortable with or know what to do during moments of silence. Therefore, whenever silence occurs, beginning clinicians tend to fill the silence by talking. They might take this time to explain the task again, repeat the stimulus, rephrase the stimulus, redirect the client, or cue the client. Although the clinician's intent is positive, these verbalizations may disrupt the client's processing, formulation, or production and affect his ability to respond. Some clients require more time to process what a clinician has said or to formulate and produce a response. Some of the more severely involved clients may need as long as 30 seconds to respond. Clinicians need to know their clients and provide adequate response time.

Audiotape or videotape a therapy session after receiving permission on an appropriate release form. Time how long it takes the client to respond. Learn to be quiet and patient while you are waiting for a response. Learn to feel comfortable with silence.

Problem and Solution 24: Mirror Usage

Beginning clinicians know that it is advantageous to experiment using different modalities when helping clients to produce sounds correctly. If a client does not correctly produce a sound when input is presented through the auditory modality, the clinician adds the visual modality, typically through use of a mirror. Two problems frequently occur. The first results when the clinician has not planned ahead to have a suitable mirror available. Because beginning clinicians are taught to be flexible and think on their feet, a clinician might retrieve from her purse a compact used for applying makeup. The clinician opens it, displays a mirror, and has the client listen and watch while she again models the phoneme.

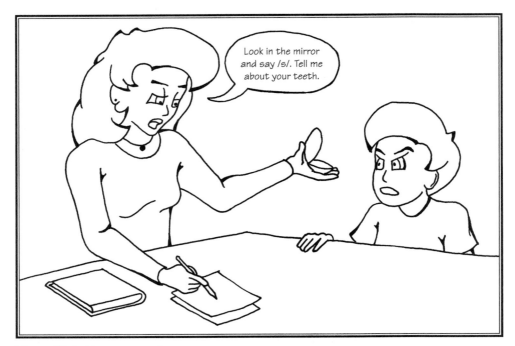

Figure 10.9. Viewing articulaters in a compact.

The client is told to look in the mirror while attempting his production; however, a mirror housed in a compact is extremely small, so the client has difficulty seeing what his articulators are doing (see Figure 10.9). Unless the mirror is an appropriate size and is used correctly, it will not aid the client in correctly producing the phoneme.

A second problem related to use of a mirror, regardless of its size, is having the client be the only one who looks into the mirror. Both the clinician and the client should look into the mirror together. The client should look at the clinician in the mirror as the clinician models the phoneme and watch her articulatory positioning and movements. The client then attempts to match his articulatory positioning and movements to hers by focusing on these aspects in the mirror. For example, the clinician can demonstrate the correct tongue position prior to producing the sound. The client can achieve this correct position. Once he sees that his position matches the model, he is ready for the next step, which is production.

A mirror can be advantageous in therapy if used in the proper manner. Make certain that the mirror is large enough for the client to see your face and his face simultaneously. Be certain the client can see your articulators in the mirror so he can more easily match his to yours.

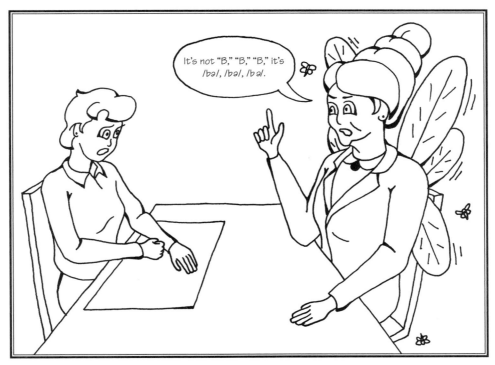

Figure 10.10. Modeling the sound.

Problem and Solution 25:
Differentiating Sound from Letter

When speech–language pathologists work with clients on articulation or phonological problems, they frequently ask the client, "What sound are you working on?" or "What is your special sound?" Notice that the clinician does not ask, "What letter are you working on?" although that is frequently the manner in which the question is answered. If a child responds "T," the clinician should redirect and say, "That is the letter you're working on, but what sound does it make?" Frequently, however, the beginning clinician does not remember to differentiate between the letter and sound. She frequently slips and gives an instruction similar to "Make your 'T' sound," "Say 'T,'" or "Good 'T'" instead of saying to the client, "Make your /t/ sound," "Say /t/," or "Good /t/." It is important to refer to the sound that a phoneme makes and not refer to it by its alphabet name as this does not accurately reflect the focus of therapy (see Figure 10.10).

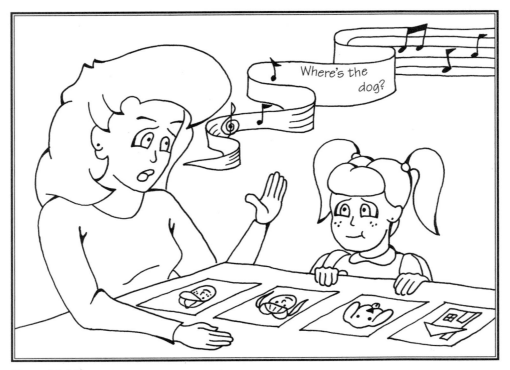

Figure 10.11. Speaking in a singsong voice.

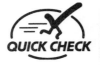

If you want the client to say the sound that the phoneme makes, model this consistently. Do not refer to it sometimes as the alphabet letter and other times by the sound it makes. Refer to the phoneme in accordance with your expectations of the client.

Problem and Solution 26: Singsong Voice

Beginning clinicians frequently adopt a strange way of speaking to young children. This unique pattern is easy to recognize but difficult to describe. The best description is that the voice has a singsong pattern so that the clinician appears to be singing rather than speaking (see Figure 10.11). The easiest and best solution to this problem is for the clinician to be aware of its existence and to avoid lapsing into that pattern.

When working with a young child for the first time, frequently audiotape or videotape your sessions. Become aware of usage of a singsong pattern. If you catch it early on, you can more easily eliminate it.

This chapter contains many suggestions to improve or enhance performance during the therapeutic process. Consider this information as you observe or conduct sessions. This chapter provides an opportunity to learn from the errors of your predecessors. Take advantage of this opportunity and strive to develop to your fullest potential.

After reading this chapter, you should be able to

1. demonstrate an optimal seating arrangement while conducting therapy.
2. demonstrate appropriate usage of reinforcement techniques in 90% of the obligatory contexts, as determined by your supervisor.
3. state three problems that frequently occur with verbal models.
4. demonstrate correct modeling behavior in 90% of the obligatory contexts, as determined by your supervisor.
5. state and explain without error eight cues or prompts used to elicit correct production of errored phonemes, starting with those that provide the maximum amount of support.
6. demonstrate techniques to get the client to monitor his responses in 90% of the obligatory contexts.
7. state two ways to ensure carry-over.
8. present clear, precise, and concise directions in 90% of your attempts, as determined by your supervisor.
9. use your imagination to mentally role-play situations before you are in them.

References

Bain, B. (1994). A framework for dynamic assessment in phonology: Stimulability revisited. *Clinics in Communication Disorders, 4*(1), 12–22.

Carrow-Woolfolk, E. (1999). *Test for Auditory Comprehension of Language–Third Edition.* Austin, TX: PRO-ED.

Dunn, L., & Dunn, L. (1997). *Peabody Picture Vocabulary Test–Third Edition.* Circle Pines, MN: American Guidance Service.

Leahy, M. (1995). *Disorders of communication: The science of intervention.* London: Whurr.

McDonald, E. T. (1964). *A Deep Test of Articulation.* Pittsburgh, PA: Stanwix House.

Miller, J. F. (1981). *Assessing language production in children.* Baltimore: University Park Press.

Reed, V. (1994). *An introduction to children with language disorders* (2nd ed.). New York: Macmillan.

Chapter 11

Self-Evaluation

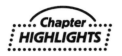

- Importance of self-evaluation
- Techniques used to assist with self-evaluation
- Basic clinical behaviors to include in a self-evaluation
- Complex clinical behaviors to include in a self-evaluation

nderson (1988a) brilliantly conveyed the importance of self-evaluation:

> Supervision must be more than just waiting for someone else to decide what is right and what is wrong. It requires the highest levels of insight about oneself and the other participants. It means action based on that insight. It requires study of the process and, most of all, ... study of self. (p. viii)

It is important for you to continually evaluate all aspects of your professional performance. This self-evaluation, or, as it is sometimes called, self-assessment, self-supervision, or self-observation, should begin as early as possible during the clinical experience and, according to Anderson (1988b), is the most advanced stage of supervision. According to the American Speech-Language-Hearing Association (ASHA, 1989), "Knowledge of the supervisory process helps [supervisees] understand their role as supervisee during their clinical preparation, and prepares them for supervision they most likely will provide later in their careers" (p. 97). At the beginning of your clinical experience, however, you will rely on your supervisor to provide most of the feedback as well as a great deal of direction. How much supervision is required at the beginning and how quickly independence is acquired are determined by hours of experience, number of clients served, experience with the disorder area, experience with the therapeutic approach, the practicum site, the clinician's academic performance, and the clinician's progress in clinical performance.

ASHA's (1985) position statement on the role of clinical supervision in speech–language pathology and audiology reads:

A central premise of supervision is that effective clinical teaching involves, in a fundamental way, the development of self-analysis, self-evaluation, and problem-solving skills on the part of the individual being supervised. The success of clinical teaching rests largely on the achievement of this goal. (p. 57)

Casey, Smith, and Ulrich (1988, p. 27) stated,

Self-supervision is a life-long professional goal and not something that ends with a semester or when a particular supervisory interaction concludes. It is a behavior that will continue and evolve across supervisors, work settings, and clients throughout professional careers. There are many purposes for engaging in self-supervision. The most important include:

1. to assess strengths and needs
2. to facilitate development of clinical and supervisory skills
3. to understand clinical interactions (i.e., clinician effect on client behavior and client effect on clinician behavior)
4. to understand intraprofessional (within the profession) interactions (i.e., clinician effects on supervisor and/or colleagues, supervisor effect on clinician or others)
5. to understand interprofessional (outside the profession) interactions (e.g., non–speech-language pathology or audiology supervisor or administrator, or other health care or education professionals)
6. to assure accountability in both the clinical and supervisory processes
7. to understand issues and be aware of resources related to self-supervision

Being able to accurately and realistically evaluate or analyze your own performance and make indicated changes is a giant step toward achieving independent clinical functioning because you will often provide services without supervision. Early development of the necessary skills to take on the role of being your own supervisor is, therefore, very important. Equally important is the commitment to improving and upgrading your skills for the duration of your professional career. Casey et al. (1988) stated, "Each [speech–language pathologist] continues to engage in some form of supervision as a career-long activity" (p. xii). Therefore, it is extremely important to develop good self-evaluation skills early in your career.

Initial Self-Evaluations

Brasseur and Jimenez (1994) observed that "beginning clinicians are more often concerned about what 'to do' next time and not [with] the how or why procedures" of the current session (p. 113). If your focus remains on the next session, you will not develop good self-evaluation skills. It is necessary to learn to analyze all aspects of the session as well as your performance critically and in depth.

Your initial evaluations of your clinical performance will most likely be shallow and uninteresting. When requested to assess a therapy session, clinicians frequently respond with comments such as "It was a good session," "I feel good about the session," "It was an OK session," "It could have been better," or "It wasn't very good." These evaluations lack rationales to explain why the session was "good," "OK," or "not very good."

When examined further, these session evaluations appear to be based on whether the client was interested in the task or materials, or whether the client changed his speech or language behavior. These "evaluations" rarely contain information about the clinicians' behaviors. Ironically, self-reporting or disclosure may be most valuable when a client does not make progress or when a session does not go well. In these cases, the clinician needs to thoroughly examine her own behavior before placing blame elsewhere because the clinician may sometimes act in a manner that blocks expected progress or prevents the session from being "good." Careful evaluations can determine what went wrong and what changes need to be implemented to improve the next session; however, to do this, the clinician needs good self-evaluation skills. The idea of mental role playing as a means of anticipatory entrance into the speech–language pathology field was introduced in Chapter 1. Once in the field, however, the clinician needs to add other modalities to her self-assessment repertoire.

Six General Strategies

Markel (1981, pp. 166–170) summarized six strategies of self-supervision. Although not designed specifically for speech–language pathology, they are certainly relevant. These strategies are as follows:

1. Self-instruction: Learners tell themselves what to do and when and how to change behavior, gain information, or develop competencies.

2. Problem solving: Learners work through a systematic sequence of activities including problem definition, identification of barriers to productive management, generating and evaluating alternatives, selecting an outcome or outcomes, trying it (or them), observing and evaluating the consequences, selecting other outcomes, or redefining the problem.

3. Modeling: Learners receive direct or mediated presentation of appropriate behavior by a peer or role model.

4. Rehearsal: Learners practice desired behavior, first with assistance and support, then more and more independently.

5. Self-determination of criteria: Learners set their own criterion-referenced objectives and then observe themselves and record the degree to which they are meeting their objectives.

6. Self-contracting: Learners set their own objectives, methods of assessment, time-lines, and consequences or reinforcers.

Actions that flow from these strategies should be self-evident and can provide direction and focus for commencing self-evaluation. Specifying the parameters of competent performance must go beyond these strategies. In a sense, self-evaluation is a form of research in which there is only one subject (you, the clinician). Complicating the research methodology is how the data can be collected on oneself.

Self-Observation Techniques

To be able to evaluate behavior, it is first necessary to observe behavior. Bernthal and Beukelman (1975) defined observation as the "recording of clinical behaviors" (p. 40). They further stated that there are three observation techniques that can be used for evaluating performance: audio recording, video recording, or recording by an observer. If possible, you should use audio or video devices (after obtaining permission on an appropriate consent form) as early as practical in the progression toward becoming your own supervisor. These tapes should be reviewed with Chapter 10 in mind and in light of any existing supervisory comments. Dowling (1992) agrees that videotaping is valuable. Observing videotapes of your sessions enables you to step outside yourself and learn not only about yourself but also the impact you have on the client's performance. You will be able to determine aspects of the session that went well and identify aspects that need to be improved. You may be able to further develop your evaluation skills if you occasionally invite your supervisor or a peer to observe a portion of the videotape to give you feedback. Oldenburg (2000) recommended addressing the areas listed in Figure 11.1 when critiquing a videotape.

VIDEO CRITIQUE

Clinician's Name: _____

Client's Initials: _____ Date of Critique: _____

Objective/Activity: _____

Rating Scale: 1 = rarely; 5 = consistently; NA = not applicable

1. Selected goals were appropriate for this session.	1 2 3 4 5 NA
2. The task difficulty level for this session was appropriate.	1 2 3 4 5 NA
3. Instructions to your client were clear and simple.	1 2 3 4 5 NA
4. The client understood what was expected of him/her.	1 2 3 4 5 NA
5. The client attended to you and your instructions.	1 2 3 4 5 NA
6. The client interrupted therapy inappropriately.	1 2 3 4 5 NA
7. You maintained your focus on your treatment plan.	1 2 3 4 5 NA
8. Stimuli were paced appropriately.	1 2 3 4 5 NA
9. The client was given sufficient processing time.	1 2 3 4 5 NA
10. Positive reinforcement was given for correct responses.	1 2 3 4 5 NA
11. Evaluative feedback was provided in a timely manner.	1 2 3 4 5 NA
12. A sufficient number of correct responses were obtained.	1 2 3 4 5 NA
13. All responses were charted.	1 2 3 4 5 NA
14. The clinician talked more than necessary.	1 2 3 4 5 NA
15. The clinician's language level was appropriate for the age and ability of the client.	1 2 3 4 5 NA
16. The client displayed a significant amount of frustration.	1 2 3 4 5 NA
17. Sufficient time was allotted to each therapy activity/goal.	1 2 3 4 5 NA
18. Therapy and materials appeared to be disorganized.	1 2 3 4 5 NA
19. Materials were available, but not distracting to the client.	1 2 3 4 5 NA
20. Error responses were accurately identified.	1 2 3 4 5 NA
21. The learning steps were sequenced appropriately.	1 2 3 4 5 NA
22. Modified task difficulty (branching) was appropriate.	1 2 3 4 5 NA
23. Behavioral limits were set and followed.	1 2 3 4 5 NA
24. The lesson plan reflected the therapy conducted.	1 2 3 4 5 NA

State one thing you liked about this session: _____
_____
_____

State one thing you need to change before the next session: _____
_____
_____

Comments: _____
_____
_____

Figure 11.1. Worksheet for evaluating a videotape of a speech–language pathology therapy session. *Note.* Adapted with permission from L. Oldenburg, Speech Disorders III Course Practicum Syllabus (Fall 2000), California State University, Sacramento, CA.

Although introspective self-observation—looking at oneself with objective detachment—is not easy for most beginning clinicians, it can help tremendously. The remainder of this chapter has information to help you learn to observe and evaluate yourself and your sessions.

Initial Focus: Benchmark Measurements

You will be better able to evaluate your therapy sessions and your own performance when you have some guidelines. Bernthal and Beukelman (1975, pp. 40–43) described six aspects of clinical behavior that can be used to evaluate a session. Each is stated, summarized, and discussed here.

1. Determining Participation Percentages and Patterns

Because a therapy session is limited in time, every minute must focus on remediation of the client's problem. Time must be used efficiently and effectively. It is not in the client's best interest for the session to be dominated by irrelevant interchanges, socializing, or other behaviors that are not geared toward direct remediation. Extraneous interchange limits available time for the client to work on the therapeutic objectives and to make necessary changes.

Participation percentages may be calculated in one of two ways: by counting the number of words spoken by you and by the client or by determining the amount of time you and the client each spoke. In either case, make an audio or video recording of a session. If the number of words spoken is the focus, count the words during a segment of therapy that is representative of the session. Count your words and the client's words. The participation percentage for each speaker is calculated as follows:

$$\frac{\text{Number of words spoken by client (or clinician)}}{\text{Total number of words produced}} \times 100 = \text{Participation percentage.}$$

If the focus is the amount of time you and the client each spoke, select a representative segment of the session. Play the tape and determine the amount of time you talk as well as the amount of time the client talks. Also determine the total time of the segment. The participation percentage is calculated as follows:

$$\frac{\text{Amount of time client (or clinician) talks}}{\text{Total amount of all talking time}} \times 100 = \text{Participation percentage.}$$

This information, calculated in words or time, will show whether you are monopolizing the session. When you are talking, the client's therapeutic objectives are not being met.

2. Determining Response Rate of Target Behaviors

It also is useful to determine whether a particular therapeutic technique results in obtaining a desired number of responses per minute. "Mowrer (1973) recommends that response rates should average between 15 and 25 responses per minute during the initial phases of articulation instruction and between 6 and 10 responses per minute during connected speech or carry-over activities" (Bernthal & Beukelman, 1975, p. 41). Usually, a professional half-hour therapy session is actually 25 minutes in length. Therefore, based on Mowrer's numbers given above, between 375 and 625 responses per session should be obtained during the initial phases of articulation instruction and between 150 and 250 responses per session should be obtained during connected speech or carry-over activities (assuming the entire session is devoted to these tasks). The response rate is determined as follows:

$$\frac{\text{Number of client responses}}{\text{Number of minutes in session}} = \text{Response rate.}$$

If, however, different tasks are performed in a session, individual response rates should be obtained for each. It is best to calculate an overall response rate as well as individual response rates for each task.

In a later study, Mowrer (1988) identified both clinician and client behaviors associated with low- and high-target response rates. Clinicians' behaviors associated with low response rates were "talking about subjects which were unrelated to evoking the target response (social interchanges, homework assignments, game instructions, etc.), reinstructing children who failed to repeat all the words of [the] sentence model, [and] ignoring children who were silent" (p. 107). Children's behaviors associated with low response rates were

> talking about subjects unrelated to the target response (social interchange), watching others perform motor tasks such as those performed in game and playing activities, listening to various auditory stimuli (others responding, word discrimination), [and] performing motor tasks which were unrelated to producing the target response (drawing cards, opening Easter eggs, cutting and pasting, etc.). (p. 107)

On the other hand, clinicians' behaviors that were related to high response rates were "presenting picture cues containing the target sound,

[and] presenting auditory cues containing the target sound" (p. 107). The only children's behavior identified that was associated with a high response rate was "replying to the teacher's instructions to name or repeat a word or phrase containing the target sound" (p. 107).

3. Determining Percentage of Correct Responses

One way of measuring a client's success on a task is to determine the percentage of correct responses:

$$\frac{\text{Number of correct responses}}{\text{Number of responses}} \times 100 = \text{Percentage of correct responses.}$$

Mowrer (1988) analyzed behaviors of clinicians who had students with (a) low accuracy rates and (b) high accuracy rates. The only clinician behavior that related to a high accuracy rate was "recognition of a correct response when that response was correct" (p. 108). Clinician behaviors related to a low accuracy rate were "providing verbal praise ('Good') following an incorrect response, presenting tasks beyond the child's skill level, [and] ignoring a correct response" (p. 108).

4. Determining Accuracy of Reinforcement

Reinforcement is an extremely powerful tool in modifying speech or language behavior. Therefore, it is extremely important that the clinician reinforce a client's behavior promptly and accurately. A continuous reinforcement schedule is one in which all correct responses are reinforced. This type of schedule is most effective for establishing new behaviors. Once a behavior is established, a change to an intermittent schedule is necessary to help maintain behaviors. Intermittent reinforcement schedules provide "greater resistance to extinction" (Mowrer, 1988, p. 209).

You should evaluate your behavior to determine (a) the number of accurate reinforcement sequences (i.e., how often the target behavior is promptly followed by a reinforcer) and (b) the number of inaccurate reinforcement sequences (i.e., how often the target behavior is followed by no reinforcement or the reinforcer is given when no correct response occurs). Because of the importance of reinforcement, all clinicians should strive for perfection in administering reinforcement.

5. Comparing the Instructional Plan to the Behavioral Record

Prior to a session, you need to develop a lesson (instructional) plan (see Chapter 2). Following the session, you should review what was done in the session (behavioral record) to determine whether the instructional plan was followed or whether activities other than those specified were implemented. If deviation from the plan occurred, you must be able to justify all changes. If you find that there are frequent deviations from your plans, your method of developing plans should be examined. Flexibility is desirable but must be explained.

6. Systematic Recording of Client Behavior

For you to know if the client's behavior is changing, you need to keep accurate records on the client's behavior. (To review record keeping, consult Chapter 6.) Records on the number of correct and incorrect responses on each target behavior must be carefully and regularly kept and reviewed. According to Bernthal and Beukelman (1975), these records make it possible to "determine the time frame in which the client changes his behavior, determine the behavioral change patterns associated with specific instructional procedures, and determine the learning curves associated with several procedures designed to teach the same target behavior" (p. 43).

Summary of Initial Focus

To adequately perform a self-evaluation, you need to calculate and review the indices just described. These six suggestions, however, are not ends in themselves but are an attempt to present you with concrete ways to start evaluating your performance. Use of these suggestions will help to avoid shallow and nondirective self-reviews. This is just the beginning of the path to developing accurate self-evaluation skills—a path that should never end.

Later Focus: Fine-Tuning Clinical Competence

When you can accurately evaluate your performance using Bernthal and Beukelman's (1975) benchmark measurements and make positive changes when warranted, it is time to focus on evaluating more complex clinical behaviors that are expected by supervisors. Because these behaviors are more abstract, they will not be as easy to evaluate as those included in the initial focus.

The *Wisconsin Procedure for Appraisal of Clinical Competence* (W-PACC), designed by Shriberg et al. (1975), is a comprehensive instrument created to appraise "the extent to which effectiveness is dependent upon continued supervisory input" (p. 160). This instrument focuses on three categories: interpersonal skills, professional–technical skills, and personal qualities. Although different terms may be used by others to describe these three categories, these are the behaviors that supervisors deem important to develop and later evaluate in beginning clinicians. All categories are equally important, but more behaviors are addressed under the professional–technical skills domain because four major subdomains (developing and planning, teaching, assessment, and reporting) are included in this domain.

The Clinician Appraisal Form, a part of the W-PACC, is thorough in terms of the behaviors on which beginning clinicians should be evaluated. Because these are the behaviors that clinical supervisors assess, you also should be evaluating these behaviors to improve your performance. The interpersonal skills scale has 10 items. According to Anderson (1988b), these items "appraise the clinician's ability to relate to and interact with the client, the client's family, and other professionals in a manner which is conducive to effective management" (p. 340). The following items (Shriberg et al., 1975) describe the clinician's interpersonal skills:

1. Accepts, empathizes, shows genuine concern for the client as a person and understands the client's problems, needs, and stresses.

2. Perceives verbal and non-verbal cues which indicate the client is not understanding the task; is unable to perform all or part of the task; or emotional stress interferes with performance of the task.

3. Creates an atmosphere based on honesty and trust; enables client to express his/her feelings and concerns.

4. Conveys to the client in a nonthreatening manner what the standards of behavior and performance are.

5. Develops understanding of teaching goals and procedures with clients.

6. Listens, asks questions, participates *with* supervisor in therapy and/or client related discussions; is not defensive.

7. Requests assistance from supervisor and/or other professionals when appropriate.

8. Creates an atmosphere based on honesty and trust; enabling family members to express their feelings and concerns.

9. Develops understanding of teaching goals and procedures with family members.
10. Communicates with other disciplines on a professional level.

The professional–technical skills scale has 28 items in four subdomains. The developing and planning subdomain comprises eight items (Shriberg et al., 1975):

1. Applies academic information to the clinical process.
2. Researches problems and obtains pertinent information from supplemental reading and/or observing other clients with similar problems.
3. Develops a semester management program (conceptualized or written) appropriate to the client's needs.
4. On the basis of assessment and measurement can appropriately determine measurable teaching objectives.
5. Plans appropriate teaching procedures.
6. Selects appropriate stimulus materials (age and ability level of client).
7. Sequences teaching tasks to implement designated program objectives.
8. Plans strategies for maintaining on-task behavior (including structuring the teaching environment and setting behavioral limits).

The teaching subdomain consists of nine items that are geared toward the clinician's ability to modify behavior (Shriberg et al., 1975):

9. Gives clear, concise instructions in presenting materials and/or techniques in management and assessments.
10. Modifies level of language according to the needs of the client.
11. Utilizes planned teaching procedures.
12. Adaptability—makes modifications in the teaching strategy such as shifting materials and/or techniques when the client is not understanding or performing the task.
13. Uses feedback and/or reinforcement which is consistent, discriminating, and meaningful to the client.
14. Selects pertinent information to convey to the client.
15. Maintains on-task behavior.
16. Prepares clinical setting to meet individual client and observer needs.
17. If mistakes are made in the therapy situation, is able to generate ideas of what might have improved the situation.

The assessment subdomain comprises seven items that focus on the clinician's ability to assess behavior and make recommendations (Shriberg et al., 1975):

18. Continues to assess client throughout the course of therapy using observational recording, standardized and nonstandardized measurement procedures and techniques.
19. Administers diagnostic tests according to standardization criterion.
20. Prepares prior to administering diagnostic tests by: (a) having appropriate materials available [and] (b) familiarity with testing procedures.
21. Scores diagnostic tests accurately.
22. Interprets results of diagnostic testing accurately.
23. Interprets accurately results of diagnostic testing in light of other available information to form an impression.
24. Makes appropriate recommendations and/or referrals based on information obtained from the assessment or teaching process.

The reporting subdomain consists of four items dealing with the clinician's ability to formulate oral and written reports (Shriberg et al., 1975):

25. Reports information in written form that is pertinent and accurate.
26. Writes in an organized, concise, clear, and grammatically correct style.
27. Selects pertinent information to convey to family members.
28. Selects pertinent information to convey to other professionals (including all nonwritten communication such as phone calls and conferences).

The last 10 items of the Clinical Appraisal Form pertain to the personal qualities domain and "provide additional information about the clinicians' general responsibility in clinical tasks" (Anderson, 1988b, p. 340). The following are those final 10 items (Shriberg et al., 1975):

1. Is punctual for client appointments.
2. Cancels client appointments when necessary.
3. Keeps appointments with supervisor or cancels appointments when necessary.
4. Turns in lesson plans on time.
5. Meets deadlines for reports.
6. Turns in attendance sheets on time.

7. Respects confidentiality of all professional activities.
8. Uses socially acceptable voice, speech, and language.
9. Personal appearance is appropriate for clinical setting and maintaining credibility.
10. Appears to recognize own professional limitations and stays within boundaries of training.

Clinicians receive a numerical rating, when applicable, on each item on the interpersonal skills and professional–technical skills scales. A rating of 1 is given to the clinician if "specific direction from supervisor does not alter unsatisfactory performance and inability to make changes" (Anderson, 1988b, p. 356). If the clinician "needs specific direction and/or demonstration from supervisor to perform effectively," she is rated 2, 3, or 4 depending on performance (p. 356). A rating of 5, 6, or 7 is earned if a clinician "needs general direction from supervisor to perform effectively," whereas a rating of 8, 9, or 10 is earned if the clinician "demonstrates independence by taking initiative; makes changes when appropriate; and is effective" (p. 356). Items in the personal qualities domain are not numerically rated but are scaled in five categories: "does not apply," "lack information," "unsatisfactory," "inconsistent," and "satisfactory." For clarification on any of the above items, see Shriberg et al. (1975) or Anderson (1988b).

Another instrument, the *Indiana University Evaluation of Speech–Language Pathology Student Practicum* (IUESP), was developed to evaluate students' progress in practicum (McCrea & Brasseur, 2003, pp. 147–153). Twelve areas of performance are evaluated: beginning program preparation; initial documentation; program development; documentation/lesson plan; documentation/SOAP (Subjective-Objective-Assessment-Plan); program implementation; treatment process–feedback/reinforcement; treatment process–data; treatment process–interaction skills; documentation/report writing; response to supervision; and professional behavior. Focusing on the items on this form will provide the beginning clinician with direction. McCrea and Brasseur (2003) state that an instrument like this "could help both supervisors and supervisees focus on the general goal of clinician/supervisee independence and professional maturity rather than on individual client behavior" (p. 112).

Additional Strategies
To Facilitate Self-Evaluation

Dowling (1992) addressed additional strategies that you can use, independent of your supervisor, to gain control over your growth in the area of self-evaluation. These are being familiar with the clinical evaluation form used, observing more experienced clinicians, and seeking assistance from peers.

Familiarity with the Clinical Evaluation Form

Become thoroughly familiar with the behaviors listed on the clinical evaluation form used at your university. Use this form as a checklist to plan your therapy session, making certain to address all the necessary areas. After your therapy session, complete the clinical evaluation form with regard to your behavior. This will help you "focus on the specific subcomponents of therapy and stimulate thought in regard to the clinical process" (Dowling, 1992, p. 254). On the basis of your evaluation, either continue your therapy in the same manner or make modifications for the next session. If your supervisor has observed and evaluated your session by completing the clinical evaluation form, you can further develop your evaluation skills by comparing the two sets of results prior to receiving additional supervisory feedback. This comparison provides valuable insight into the accuracy of your perceptions. As you become better able to accurately analyze your performance, more agreement will be found between your results and your supervisor's.

Observation of More Experienced Clinicians

To further your clinical growth, observe therapy sessions conducted by clinicians who have more experience than you or who excel in an area in which you are having difficulty. Dowling (1992) suggested that you may "learn clinical flexibility, in discovering that a variety of options exist for achieving a specific goal" (p. 254). These observations will also help you "build an internal concept of what constitutes successful therapy" (Dowling, 1992, p. 255) and will help build a knowledge base on which to evaluate your own performance.

Utilization of Peers

Peers can help you develop your evaluation skills in several ways. By discussing various issues with colleagues, you may be able to extract some information and apply it to your functioning in the clinical setting. You can also learn from observing a peer's therapy session or a videotape of a peer's session. Together you and a peer can identify each other's strengths as well as areas that need to be developed, and you can brainstorm strategies for future sessions. Getting insight from another person knowledgeable in speech–language pathology can increase your knowledge base and consequently give you additional ways to evaluate your own clinical performance.

Student Self-Appraisal

According to McLeod (1994, p. 98), "Student Self-Appraisal is a formalised procedure which enables students to self-evaluate and reflect on their clinical experience." It encourages students to evaluate their own performance and identify both their strengths and any areas that they need to change. "It provides a forum for students to take control of their own learning and to develop their own learning goals" (McLeod, 1994, p. 99). The Student Self-Appraisal focuses on a structured discussion between you and your supervisor. These discussions deal with your clinical placement and experience in a broad sense and do not focus predominantly on performance during the most recent clinical interaction, as most meetings with supervisors do. As a result of these discussions, make a list of goals you want to achieve and a list of accomplishments you have already achieved. A series of questions and probes are used to assist you with reflecting on your clinical placement. The first questions deal with the positive aspects of your clinical experience: "What have been the most satisfying aspects of your placement over this review period? What have been the high points?" and "What do you consider are the most important activities you have performed over this review period?" (p. 101). You then comment on the quantity and variety of your present caseload, other tasks and roles you would like to try, negative aspects of your current clinical experience and what you have done or can do to improve them, the supervision you have received, opportunities for self-development, and any other aspects about which you have concerns.

These discussions run from 30 minutes to 1 hour. You are to consider the questions and answer them in writing prior to your scheduled appointment with your supervisor. Your written responses are not given to your supervisor but serve as a way of preparing yourself for the meeting. These Student Self-Appraisal meetings should be conducted twice during each clinical experience, once at the midpoint and again at the end. The outcome of these Student Self-Appraisals are not supposed to be linked to a grade.

In a follow-up survey to determine the effectiveness of this procedure, McLeod (1994) reported positive comments. For example, students said, "Student Self-Appraisal enables an objective examination of my skills," "Student Self-Appraisal forces me to reflect on my clinical experiences," and "Student Self-Appraisal encourages problem solving" (p. 94). Given the positive impact this procedure made on the students involved, it would be in your best interest to continue to reflect on your experience in this manner.

Self-evaluation is an extremely important part of the clinical process. It is necessary for you to become cognizant of everything that occurs during client interactions. If you know what behaviors and skills are important in the role of a speech–language pathologist, you can strive to become competent in those areas. The behaviors discussed in this chapter are those deemed important by supervisors and, therefore, are those that are important for you to master as early in your career as possible. Knowing how to perform in clinical encounters is the first step because this is where being able to accurately and realistically evaluate your own performance is vital. Only when you are aware of your own behavior can you improve performance. When good self-evaluation skills have been developed, it is then possible to become independent.

After reading this chapter, you should be able to

1. state at least five reasons for engaging in self-evaluation.
2. state at least five techniques you can use to help self-evaluate your performance.
3. list at least six basic clinical behaviors you will include in your initial self-evaluations.
4. state at least 30 higher level clinical behaviors you will eventually incorporate into your self-evaluations.

References

American Speech-Language-Hearing Association. (1985). Clinical supervision in speech–language pathology and audiology. *Asha, 27,* 57–60.

American Speech-Language-Hearing Association. (1989). Preparation models for the supervisory process in speech–language pathology and audiology. *Asha, 31,* 97–106.

Anderson, J. L. (1988a). Foreword. In P. L. Casey, K. J. Smith, & S. R. Ulrich, *Self-supervision: A career tool for audiologists and speech–language pathologists* (pp. vii–viii). Rockville, MD: National Student Speech-Language-Hearing Association.

Anderson, J. L. (1988b). *The supervisory process in speech–language pathology and audiology.* Boston: College-Hill.

Bernthal, J. E., & Beukelman, D. R. (1975). Self-evaluation by the student clinician. *The Journal of the National Student Speech and Hearing Association, 3,* 39–44.

Brasseur, J., & Jimenez, B. (1994). Supervisee self-analysis and changes in clinical behavior. In M. Bruce (Ed.), *Proceedings of the 1994 International & Interdisciplinary Conference on Clinical Supervision: Toward the 21st century* (pp. 111–125). Houston: University of Houston.

Casey, P. L., Smith, K. J., & Ulrich, S. R. (1988). *Self-supervision: A career tool for audiologists and speech–language pathologists.* Rockville, MD: National Student Speech-Language-Hearing Association.

Dowling, S. (1992). *Implementing the supervisory process.* Englewood Cliffs, NJ: Prentice Hall.

Markel, G. (1981). Self-management in classrooms: Implications for mainstreaming. In P. Bates (Ed.), *Mainstreaming: Our current knowledge base* (pp. 161–183). Minneapolis: University of Minnesota.

McCrea, E., & Brasseur, J. (2003). *The supervisory process in speech–language pathology and audiology.* Boston: Allyn & Bacon.

McLeod, S. (1994). Student self-appraisal: Facilitating mutual planning in clinical education. *The Clinical Supervisor, 15*(1), 87–101.

Mowrer, D. (1973). A behavioristic approach to modification of articulation. In W. Wolfe & D. Goulding (Eds.), *Articulation and learning.* Springfield, IL: Charles C. Thomas.

Mowrer, D. (1988). *Methods of modifying speech behaviors* (2nd ed.). Prospect Heights, IL: Waveland Press.

Oldenburg, L. (2000). Video critique [Course syllabus for Speech Disorders III]. Sacramento: California State University.

Shriberg, L., Filley, F., Hayes, D., Kwiatkowski, J., Schatz, J., Simmons, K., & Smith, M. (1975). The Wisconsin Procedure for Appraisal of Clinical Competence (W-PACC): Model and data. *Asha, 17,* 158–165.

Epilogue:
The Basics
Are Not Enough!

This book has presented a comprehensive overview of how you as a beginning speech–language clinician can be successful in your clinical endeavors. It has identified topical areas in which you must demonstrate competence and it has provided many tools to use in gaining this competence. Because there is so much information to remember, frequent use of this book should help you make an easier, smoother, and more graceful transition from the context of learning (the classroom) to the context of application (the clinical setting) (see Figure E.1).

After reading this book, you will have been introduced to the most troublesome pitfalls, both large and small, that have perplexed many, if not all, former beginning clinicians. I hope the suggestions to prevent you from falling into these traps have been helpful. Please keep in mind, however, that even when you have mastered the basic clinical procedures, the journey is not over. You must proceed to a higher level of competence in which knowledge and application of more complex clinical procedures are necessary. You must proactively continue to obtain, apply, and evaluate new knowledge throughout your professional career.

Most university programs provide you with the basics of the profession in an ideal, but somewhat unrealistic, environment because the first clinical experience is usually performed in the university's in-house clinic. Clients are frequently seen individually. This environment is conducive to learning the basics about the clinical process and applying the information previously learned in lectures and textbooks. Once the basics have been mastered, however, you must learn to work with clients with less common and more complex problems. You must also become comfortable conducting different types of therapy.

Even in the relatively friendly and structured environment of the university program, you must provide all services as competently and as professionally as possible. According to the American Speech-

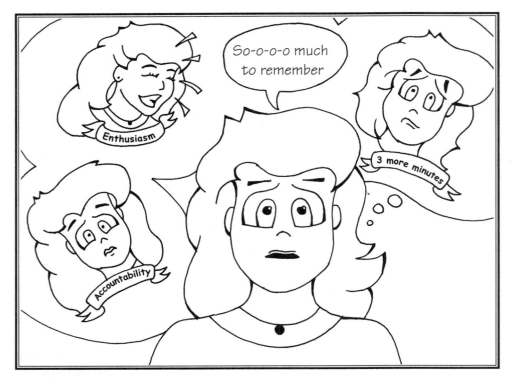

Figure E.1. So much to remember!

Language-Hearing Association's (ASHA, 2001a) code of ethics, "Individuals shall provide all services competently" and "shall engage in only those aspects of the professions that are within the scope of their competence, considering their level of education, training, and experience" (p. 2). Therefore, it is your professional responsibility to be competent in a particular area of service delivery prior to providing services in that area, regardless of the clinical setting.

Speech–language pathology as a profession is constantly changing. Therefore, it is the responsibility of each professional to keep up with and adapt to these changes. Similarly, it is the responsibility of each professional to continually upgrade his or her knowledge base. This can be done by attending workshops presented by the various regional speech–language pathology associations or by other sponsors such as hospitals, universities, and rehabilitation centers; attending conventions held by state associations or by ASHA; reading journals and books in speech–language pathology; and using the Internet to learn new research tactics, get in on professional chats, and look for career openings.

You also have an obligation to get actively involved in the profession. If you have not yet become a member of the National Student

Speech-Language-Hearing Association (NSSLHA), which is the student branch of ASHA, do so immediately. (The address for both NSSLHA and ASHA is 10801 Rockville Pike, Rockville, Md 20852. You may download a membership application from the following site: www.nsslha.org/join) The benefits are numerous, but most important, you will receive journals at a substantially discounted price.

It is important not only to keep up with the trends but also to anticipate them. Because of a change in demographics, the need for services to the elderly is increasing. The U.S. Census Bureau (2000) estimates that approximately 27% of the population will be 55 years of age or older in the years 2011 to 2015. Many of these people may develop speech or language difficulties. For example, some years ago, Cornett and Chabon (1988) stated that, "by the year 2000, 25% of persons over age 65 are expected to have a speech or language impairment, and 46% may have a hearing impairment" (p. 197). It is also necessary for you to keep abreast of the continuing evolution of technology in the profession. You need to keep pace with new developments and learn to use appropriate tools to enhance some or all phases of clinical practice.

In a related vein, it is also important that you prepare for the geographic area in which you will work. Learn as much as possible about the population that you will be serving. Specifically, learn about the cultural and linguistic diversity of the populations you will most likely encounter because it is not possible to effectively evaluate or treat clients without this important background knowledge.

It is your professional responsibility to know and adhere to the regulations governing your performance. All professionals in the field of speech–language pathology must be aware of ASHA's code of ethics (2001a) and scope of practice (2001b), as well as its various position papers. You must also be aware of legislation affecting the profession. If employed in an educational setting, you also need to keep abreast of special education regulations. You also should be familiar with outcome-based education, curriculum-based assessment, inclusion, instructional support teams, collaborative problem solving, collaborative consultation, whole language, classroom-based assessment, classroom-based treatment, as well as many other areas that affect speech–language clinicians.

Regardless of your future employment setting—be it a school, private practice, or some branch of health care (e.g., a hospital, long-term care facility, day hospital, rehabilitation center, adult day-care program, community group home, home care, community clinic, health maintenance organization, preferred provider organization)—it is of utmost importance that you be aware of all the legislation, regulations, and insurances that have an impact on your position. It is important to be on the cutting edge of new developments. You need to keep an open mind and remain flexible—you must recognize, understand, and welcome change. Do not look at changing times or trends with fear, but derive comfort from the fact that you are prepared to meet them.

I conclude this book on a positive note. According to the U.S. Bureau of Labor Statistics (2002), jobs in the field of speech–language pathology and audiology are projected to increase 40% between the years 2000 and 2010, meaning that 40,000 additional positions will be created. "Growth will result from the increased demand for health services as the population ages and as medical advances allow more people to survive strokes and other ailments" (p. 23). The bureau states that another reason for growth of the profession is "rising school enrollments and an increase in services for special education students" (p. 23). The obvious conclusion is that once you earn your graduate degree, a job should be waiting for you in your chosen profession of speech–language pathology or audiology. The next step is yours to take. May you not stumble.

References

American Speech-Language-Hearing Association. (2001a, December 26). Code of ethics (revised). *the ASHA leader, 6*(23), 2.

American Speech-Language-Hearing Association. (2001b). *Scope of practice in speech–language pathology*. Rockville, MD: Author.

Cornett, B. S., & Chabon, S. S. (1988). *The clinical practice of speech–language pathology*. Columbus, OH: Merrill.

U.S. Bureau of Labor Statistics. (2002, Spring). The 2000–10 job outlook in brief. *Occupational Outlook Quarterly*, p. 23. http://www.bls.gov/opub/ooq/2002/spring/art01.pdf

U.S. Census Bureau. (2000). *Population projection program*. Retrieved November 7, 2003, from http://www.census.gov/population/projections/nation/summary/np-t3-d.pdf

Glossary

Academic standards. Standards developed by each state's department of education that define the knowledge and skills students need to learn in each subject area by designated grade levels (3rd, 5th, 8th, and 11th grades); establish a framework of achievement for all students; and serve as a baseline from which school districts develop their own standards that contain the district's goals and objectives.

Accountability (clinical). Having complete, accurate, thorough records on the clients you are servicing; making sure that the required paperwork (e.g., evaluation, reevaluation, progress report, progress notes) is thorough, accurate, and complete; and keeping track of your clinical hours (a) to count toward your Certificate of Clinical Competence and (b) for possible legal entanglements.

Articulation. The distinct production of individual phonemes. Use of the articulators (lips, tongue, teeth, etc.) to produce speech sounds.

ASHA. An acronym for the American Speech-Language-Hearing Association, which is the national organization for speech–language pathologists. It is located at 10801 Rockville Pike, Rockville, MD 20852. The phone number is 800/498-2071.

Assessment. The evaluation of a client's speech, language, and overall communicative ability. Related to accountability.

Attending behavior. The ability of a client to focus on a task.

Augmentative device. A device or physical object used to supplement communication. It may be of high or low technological sophistication.

Background information. Information you obtain about a client. Pertinent background information that appears at the beginning of the written evaluation (e.g., referral source, previous therapy, speech and language milestones, developmental milestones, birth history, medical history, educational history, vocational history) depending on the client's age and the nature of the problem.

Behavioral objectives. Performance or behavior that the client is supposed to exhibit at some point in the therapy process. A behavioral objective should contain three components: performance, condition, and criterion. Behavioral objectives are found in lesson plans, evaluations, reevaluations, and progress reports. They contribute to clinical accountability. Objectives may be revised as clients progress from one level to another. See also *Lesson objectives, Long-range objectives, Objectives, Session objectives, Short-range objectives,*

Short-term instructional objectives, Terminal objectives, Therapeutic objectives, and *Transitional objectives.*

Benchmark. General statements that represent a client's milestones to goals. Statements about reference points along the way to learning a new skill or group of skills.

Branch step. A therapy objective of lesser complexity than the one on which the client did not have success. This is accomplished by breaking the objective down into its component parts so the client will have success.

CAA. An acronym for the Council on Academic Accreditation in Audiology and Speech–Language Pathology, a body of ASHA that defines the standards for the accreditation of graduate educational programs.

Carry-over. Using a newly learned speech, language, or communication technique in everyday situations. See *Generalization.*

Certificate of Clinical Competence (CCC). Granted by ASHA to those persons who qualify by meeting specific requirements with regard to degree, coursework, practicum, supervised professional experience, and the national exam in speech–language pathology.

CCC-A. Certificate of Clinical Competence in audiology.

CCC-SLP. Certificate of Clinical Competence in speech–language pathology.

Client. A person (patient) receiving therapy from a speech–language pathologist.

Clinical strategy outline. A plan for a therapy session that includes objectives (lesson objectives, session objectives, short-range objectives, short-term objectives, subobjectives) and procedures to be used to meet those objectives. Sometimes materials to be used are indicated. Same as a *Lesson plan, Instructional plan,* or *Pretherapy plan.* Related to *Accountability.*

Clinician. A person providing speech and language therapy. A *beginning clinician* is one who is in an educational training program, is enrolled in clinical practicum, and is providing services in speech, language, and/or communication. Frequently, the term *speech–language clinician* is given to those professionals employed in the schools.

Continuous reinforcement. Reinforcement that follows every correct response; useful for establishing a new skill or behavior.

Covert verb. Relevant to the performance component of a behavioral objective. A verb referring to performance or behavior that cannot be directly observed. Examples include *recognize, infer, analyze, recall, identify, solve,* and *know.* See *Overt verb.*

Curriculum-based IEPs (Curriculum-linked IEPs). Individualized Education Programs that are directly connected to the curriculum. Each of the student's needs must be matched with elements of the general education curriculum.

Curriculum-based therapy. Therapy based on the general education curriculum.

Daily log. A record of the client's performance during therapy sessions. Same as *Progress note*. Related to *Accountability*.

Dependency (fostering). When the clinician shares the client's problem and behaviors by encouraging the client to perform tasks for the benefit of the clinician and not for the client's betterment. The clinician often exhibits authoritarian behavior and does not encourage the client to be responsible for his problem or therapy program.

Evaluation. The written assessment of a person's speech, language, or communication abilities. Part of the paperwork process and part of accountability.

Evaluation Report (ER). One of the pieces of paperwork required of speech–language clinicians employed in the public schools. A copy must be presented to the student's parents no later than 60 school days after the written permission is received by the school.

Expressive language. Encoding language. The production of language. Communicating through the spoken or printed word or other forms of language.

Fixed-ratio reinforcement. A type of intermittent reinforcement in which reinforcement occurs after a fixed number of correct responses. It may occur after every three correct responses, or after every five correct responses, and so forth.

Fluency. The smooth, effortless, uninterrupted flow of speech.

General education curriculum. The content taught in regular education. All instruction is from regular courses at the regular grade level. All special education teachers use the same materials as other teachers.

Generalization. Using a newly learned speech, language, or communication technique in everyday situations. See *Carry-over*.

Group therapy. A type of therapy in which all clients in the group are interacting. This interaction may involve non–goal-related activities or goal-related activities. This latter type is the more desirable form, although it takes more planning to achieve. See *Therapy in a group*.

IDEA Amendments of 1997 (IDEA '97) (P.L. 105-17). The federal Public Law that changed the role of school-based speech–language pathologists.

IEP process. Also called *Multidisciplinary evaluation process* (MDE), *Special education process*, and *Procedural safeguards process*. Dictates the paperwork required by school-based speech–language clinicians. It includes *Permission to Evaluate; Evaluation Report (ER); Individualized Education Program (IEP); Procedural Safeguards Letter; Procedural Safeguards Notice; Permission to Reevaluate; Invitation to Participate in the IEP Meeting or Other Meeting;* and *Notice of Recommended Educational Placement (NOREP)*.

Indicator behavior. Used to clarify the performance portion of a behavioral objective when a covert verb is used. The indicator behavior appears in parentheses. For example, "identify (point to) pictures receptively."

Individualized Education Program (IEP). One of the pieces of paperwork required of speech–language clinicians employed in the public schools. The IEP must be developed within 30 calendar days from the date of the *Evaluation Report*.

Individuals with Disabilities Act of 1990 (IDEA) (P.L. 101-336). The federal Public Law that regulates the delivery of services to children with disabilities in public schools.

Informant. The person providing background information on the client. Depending on the situation, it is possible for the client to be his or her own informant.

Initial evaluation. The first time a person's speech, language, or communication abilities are assessed, or the first time the clinician is evaluating the person. Part of *Accountability*.

Instructional plan. See *Clinical strategy outline*.

Intermittent reinforcement. A type of reinforcement schedule that produces greater resistance to extinction; useful for maintaining a behavior. See *Continuous reinforcement*.

Invitation to Participate in the IEP Team Meeting or Other Meeting. One of the pieces of paperwork required of speech–language clinicians employed in the public schools. This invitation invites the parent(s) or guardian(s) to attend and participate in the IEP meeting. If it is not an IEP meeting, the nature of the meeting must be stated.

Language. The relationship between sound and meaning; a socially shared code that represents ideas through arbitrary symbols and rules that govern combinations of these symbols; a systematic set of symbols used in various modes for communication and thought.

Language assessment. Using both formal and informal procedures to determine where the person is functioning with regard to the mastery of language. Both receptive and expressive language is evaluated and included in the initial evaluation and reevaluation. Related to *Accountability*.

Lesson objectives. The goals to be accomplished in one therapy session.

Lesson plan. See *Clinical strategy outline*.

Long-range objectives. The outcome that the clinician is guiding the client to achieve at a distant point in time. The time frame varies with the setting. In a university setting, the time frame is usually defined as a semester. See also *Behavioral objectives, Lesson objectives, Objectives, Session objectives, Short-range objectives, Short-term instructional objectives, Short-term objectives, Subobjectives, Terminal objectives, Therapeutic objectives,* and *Transitional objectives*.

Long-term objectives. See *Long-range objectives*.

Monitor. Determining the correctness or incorrectness of a behavior.

Multidisciplinary evaluation process (MDE). See *IEP process.*

Notice of Recommended Educational Placement (NOREP). One of the pieces of paperwork required of speech–language clinicians employed in the public schools. It summarizes recommendations for the student's educational program. The NOREP should be implemented as soon as possible but no later than 10 days after its completion.

NSSLHA. Acronym for the National Student Speech-Language-Hearing Association, the national organization for students majoring in speech–language pathology and audiology. It is located at 10801 Rockville Pike, Rockville, MD 20852, and the Web site is www.nsslha.org.

Objectives. Goals set for client performance. Usually listed in a specific order but may be altered to suit client progress. See also *Behavioral objectives, Lesson objectives, Long-range objectives, Long-term objectives, Session objectives, Short-range objectives, Short-term instructional objectives, Short-term objectives, Subobjectives, Terminal objectives, Therapeutic objectives,* and *Transitional objectives.*

Overt verb. Relevant to the performance component of a behavioral objective. A verb referring to performance that is directly observable through vision or audition. Examples are *list, name, point, write,* and *repeat.* See *Covert verb.*

Paperwork. That which you must do, cannot avoid, and will never outlive. Documents required vary among service providers. Within university programs, it usually refers to some or all of the following: writing *Behavioral objectives, Evaluations, Reevaluations, Semester plan of treatment, Lesson plans, Session evaluations, Progress notes,* and *Progress reports.* The bedrock of clinical accountability that can have professional or legal implications. See *Accountability.*

Patient. A person (client) receiving therapy from a speech–language pathologist.

Permission to Evaluate. One of the pieces of paperwork required of speech–language clinicians employed in the public schools. This is sent to the parent(s) or guardian(s) to gain consent to proceed. Tests and procedures that will be performed during the evaluation must be indicated.

Permission to Reevaluate. One of the pieces of paperwork required of all speech–language clinicians employed in the public schools. It informs the parent(s) or guardian(s) that the student will be reevaluated and why. Tests and procedures that will be used will be stated. The proposed date for the reevaluation is provided.

Phonology. The study of the sound system of the language. It includes speech sounds (phonemes), speech patterns, and the rules that apply to those sounds.

Play therapy. A type of nondirective therapy that is frequently used with young children or with children who are functioning at a low cognitive level.

Pragmatics. The use of language in social context.

Pretherapy Plan. See *Clinical strategy outline.*

Problem behavior. Behavior that interferes with the client's achievement of the objectives; includes inattentiveness, not following directions, refusing to perform tasks, kicking, shouting, biting, and so forth.

Procedural Safeguards Letter. One of the pieces of paperwork required of speech–language clinicians employed in the public schools. It must be made available to the student's parent(s) or guardian(s) at a minimum of four different times during the process. It includes information for parents about state or local advocacy organizations.

Procedural Safeguards Notice. One of the pieces of paperwork required of speech–language clinicians employed in the public schools. It must be made available to the student's parent(s) or guardian(s) at a minimum of four different times during the process. The parent's rights and the procedures for safeguarding these rights are described.

Procedural safeguards process. See *IEP process.*

Progress Note. See *Daily log.*

Progress report. A report written after the client has received therapy for a period of time. The actual amount of time that lapses varies depending on the setting. In a university setting, this report is usually written at the end of the semester. The purpose is to document any improvement that has been made. Related to *Accountability.*

Receptive language. Decoding language. Understanding or comprehending spoken or written messages as well as other forms of language.

Reevaluation. To evaluate the client again to obtain additional information, to determine whether the previous diagnosis has changed or remains accurate, or to obtain additional information about how to proceed with the client's therapy program. A type of report. Related to *Accountability.*

Reinforcement. The procedure of following a correct response with a reinforcer. See *continuous reinforcement, intermittent reinforcement.*

Self-evaluation. The ability to critically analyze your own professional performance accurately and in depth in order to improve your clinical skills and be the best clinician you can.

Self-monitoring. When the client independently evaluates the correctness and incorrectness of his responses. This is a step toward the client's becoming independent. This procedure assists with the carry-over process. See *Carry-over, Dependency.*

Semantics. The study of the meaning of language. This includes meaning at the word, sentence, and conversational levels.

Semester (or quarter) plan of treatment. This plan is specific to the university setting due to the reference to "semester" or "quarter" and is composed of both long-range goals and short-term objectives. It is based on both formal and informal testing as well as observations formulated during the initial evaluation. Related to *Accountability.*

Session. Refers to the time when the clinician and client are involved in therapy.

Session evaluation. A critique of the session upon completion. Some things to include are whether the objectives were met, whether the procedures were helpful, whether progress was made, what could have been done differently, strengths of the session, weaknesses of the session, and changes to be made for the next session. It may be required that this session evaluation be written on the back of the lesson plan. Sometimes it also needs to be presented verbally while conferencing with your supervisor. Related to *Accountability*.

Session objectives. Objectives to be addressed in a specific session. See also *Short-range objectives*.

Short-range objectives. Those objectives that are attainable in a short period of time. In some settings, this period may be 1 session, 1 week, or 1 month. Also called *Short-term objective*. See also *Behavioral objectives, Lesson objectives, Long-term objectives, Long-range objectives, Session objectives, Short-term instructional objectives, Short-term objectives, Subobjectives, Terminal objectives, Therapeutic objectives,* and *Transitional objectives*.

Short-term instructional objectives. Required by law for Individualized Education Program. See also *Session objective*.

Short-term objectives. See *Short-range objective*.

Smothering (the client). Using language that is beyond the client's expressive language ability.

Special education. Specially designed instruction.

Special education process. See *IEP process*.

Speech–language pathologist. A person holding a degree and certification in speech–language pathology who is qualified to diagnose and treat speech, language, voice, and communication problems. Holds state licensure.

Speech–language pathology assistant. Support personnel in speech–language pathology who can perform tasks as prescribed, directed, and supervised by certified speech–language pathologists following academic or on-the-job training.

Student self-appraisal. A procedure that helps students self-evaluate and reflect on their clinical experiences.

Subobjectives. See *Session objectives*.

Subjective-Objective-Assessment-Plan (SOAP). One format for writing progress notes.

Terminal objectives. Those objectives that need to be accomplished prior to the client's discharge from therapy. See *Behavioral objectives, Lesson objectives, Long-range objectives, Long-term objectives, Objectives, Session objectives, Short-range objectives, Short-term instructional objectives, Short-term objectives, Subobjectives, Therapeutic objectives,* and *Transitional objectives*.

Therapeutic objectives. The objectives that should be the focus of therapy. See *Behavioral objectives, Lesson objectives, Long-range objectives, Long-term objectives, Objectives, Session objectives, Short-range objectives, Short-term instructional objectives, Short-term objectives, Subobjectives, Long-range objectives, Terminal objectives,* and *Transitional objectives.*

Therapy. The process whereby the clinician guides the client in working on and meeting his objectives. The process of guiding the client from his current level of functioning to the level where he or she should be functioning.

Therapy conference. A conference conducted by a speech–language pathologist with the parent or spouse of a client who is receiving services. The purpose is to provide information to and share information with the parent or spouse. The client's current functioning level should be explained and progress related to the client's short-range and long-range objectives should be presented. Any questions the parent or spouse has should be answered. Recommendations should be given.

Therapy conference report. The report that is written following the *Therapy conference* to detail what occurred during the conference. It becomes a part of the client's permanent record.

Therapy in a group. The process whereby the clinician provides individual therapy to each of the clients in a group setting. See *Group therapy.*

Therapy program. The plan through which the speech–language pathologist guides the client in order to remediate or decrease the severity of his or her problem. Related to *Accountability.*

Transitional objectives. Session objectives presented in a specific order subject to alteration based on client performance. See *Session objectives.*

Treatment plan. A plan for a therapy session that includes objectives (*Short-term objectives*) and procedures to be used to meet these objectives. Sometimes materials are included. Same as a *Clinical strategy outline, Instructional plan,* or *Lesson plan.* Related to *Accountability.*

Video critique. Analyzing a videotape of a therapy session. A procedure that helps you self-evaluate and reflect on your clinical performance.

Voice. Sound produced by the vibration of the vocal folds and modified by the resonators (oral cavity, nasal cavity, pharynx, etc.).

Index

Abbreviations, in evaluation reports, 85
Academic standards, 208–209, 219, 272–274, 351
Access to client during therapy, 282, 283
Accountability
    clinical tracking sheets, 180–185
    continuing education requirements and, 187, 190, 191
    definition of, 351
    licensure for speech–language pathologists, 190, 191
    professional accountability, 187–190
    record keeping and, 166–167, 177–192
    record sheet for clinical hours during practicum, 190, 192
    tracking clinical hours (if applying for CCC after Jan. 2005), 185–187, 192
    tracking clinical hours (if applying for CCC before Dec. 2004), 178–185, 192
    worksheet for recording evaluation and diagnostic hours in speech–language pathology, 188
    worksheet for recording therapy hours in speech–language pathology, 189
Accuracy
    in record keeping, 166–167, 169–170, 177–178, 337
    of reinforcement, 336
Action verbs for behavioral objectives, 14
Active children, record keeping with, 173
Active voice in evaluation reports, 85–86
ADD (attention-deficit disorder), 213
Addition of final consonants, 148
Additional Testing section in progress reports, 96
ADHD (attention-deficit/hyperactivity disorder), 213
Age of client in evaluation reports, 88
Alternative communication. See Augmentative and alternative communication
American Speech-Language-Hearing Association (ASHA), 93n, 141, 178–180, 185–186, 187, 190, 192, 208, 210, 329–330, 347–348, 351
Anticipatory socialization, 279–280
Appearing foolish during therapy, 306–307
Arizona Articulation Proficiency Scale: Third Revision, 102–103
Articulation
    behavioral objectives for, 23–24, 38
    condition examples for, 18
    contrasts minimal pairs, 304
    definition of, 351
    elicitation techniques for, 302–304
    evaluation report on, 100, 102–106
    frequency of stimulus presentation, 303
    manipulation of articulators, 303
    model of presentation, 304
    performance examples for, 15
    phonetic context, 304
    placement cues, 303
    progress reports on, 128, 129–134
    prosodic emphasis, 303
    reevaluation report on, 120–124
    visual and tactile imagery, 303
Artificial reinforcement, 288–290
ASHA (American Speech-Language-Hearing Association), 93n, 141, 178–180, 185–186, 187, 190, 192, 208, 210, 329–330, 347–348, 351
Assessment. *See also* headings beginning with Evaluation
    clinician's skills in, 340
    definition of, 351
    IEP indication of student's participation in, 215–216, 252–253
    in progress notes, 158–159
Assignments, 316–317, 318
Attending behavior
    definition of, 351
    progress report on, 128, 135–138
Attention-deficit disorder (ADD), 213
Attention-deficit/hyperactivity disorder (ADHD), 213
Audio and video critiques, 296, 311, 313, 323, 332–334, 343, 358
Audiometry, 93, 93n
Auditory sensitivity
    in evaluation reports, 93, 104, 108, 114, 119
    in reevaluation reports, 123, 126
Augmentative and alternative communication
    behavioral objectives for, 32–33
    condition examples for, 20
    definition of, 351
    performance examples for, 16–17

Background information
    definition of, 351
    in evaluation reports, 80, 82–83, 88–90, 102, 106, 110–111, 117
    in progress reports, 96, 129, 131, 135

in reevaluation reports, 121, 125

Behavioral objectives
components of, 12–22
condition component of, 17–20, 69–71
consistency in, 65
criterion component of, 20–22, 71–74
definition of, 11, 351–352
exercise on, 41–60
in grant writing, 33
in IEPs, 39, 215, 248–250
importance of, 11–12
incorrect format following lead-in, 63–65
lead-in for, 63–65
in lesson plans, 33–39
long-range objectives, 34–39, 354
performance component of, 12–17, 66–69
problems to avoid while writing, 63–77
in progress notes, 143–149
in reports, 39
samples of, 22–33
short-term objectives, 34–38, 215, 248–250, 357
support or harmony between procedures and, 74–77
terminal objectives, 38–39, 357
verbs for, 13, 14

Benchmark, 215, 334–337, 352
Birth history in evaluation reports, 89, 102, 110
Block style for evaluation reports, 87
Body movements of clinician, 309–310
Boredom of clinician, 312–313
Branch step, 352
Breath features, 125–126
Bureau of Labor Statistics, U.S., 350

CAA (Council on Academic Accreditation in Audiology
    and Speech–Language Pathology), 352
Carry-over, 314–318, 352
CCC (Certificate of Clinical Competence)
application for, after Jan. 2005, 185–187, 192, 352
application for, before Dec. 2004, 178–185, 192
Census Bureau, U.S., 349
Certificate of Clinical Competence (CCC)
application for, after Jan. 2005, 185–187, 192
application for, before Dec. 2004, 178–185, 192
definition of, 352
*Certification & Membership Handbook: Speech–Language
    Pathology* (ASHA), 178–180, 185–186, 187, 192
Choice constancy, 299–300
CLEF–3 (*Clinical Evaluation of Language
    Fundamentals–3*), 238
Client, definition of, 352
Clinical assessment. *See* Evaluation section
Clinical Evaluation Form, 342
Clinical Evaluation of Language Fundamentals–3
    (CLEF–3), 238
Clinical hours tracking
for CCC application after Jan. 2005, 185–187, 192
for CCC application before Dec. 2004, 178–185, 192
clinical tracking sheets, 180–185

Clinical strategy outline, 337, 352. *See also* Lesson plans
Clinical supervision, 329–330. *See also* Self-evaluation
Clinical tracking sheets, 180–185
Clinicians. *See* Speech–language clinicians
Closing of therapy session, 321–323
Cluster production, 148–149
Computer software for record keeping, 165–166
Condition component of behavioral objectives, 17–20,
    69–71
Consent for Evaluation Form, 211, 223–224
Consent for Placement in Special Education Servcices,
    235–236
Consistency in behavioral objectives, 65
Consonants, 148
Continuing education requirements, 187, 190, 191
Continuous reinforcement, 285, 352
Contractions in evaluation reports, 85
Contrasts minimal pairs, 304
Correct responses, percentage of, 336
Council on Academic Accreditation in Audiology and
    Speech–Language Pathology (CAA), 352
Counseling process, 197. *See also* Therapy conferences
Covert verbs for behavioral objectives, 14, 352
Criterion
definition of, 20
self-determination of, 332
success on, indicated in progress notes, 143
Criterion component of behavioral objectives, 20–22,
    71–74
CTOPP, 238
Cues. *See* Elicitation techniques
Current status in progress reports, 97
Curriculum-based IEPs, 352
Curriculum-based therapy, 272–276, 352

Daily logs, 141, 353. *See also* Progress notes
Deep Test of Articulation, 133
Dependency, fostering of, 297–299, 353
Developing and planning skills of clinicians, 339
Developmental milestones in evaluation reports, 89,
    102, 110–111
Diagnoses in evaluation reports, 83–84
Directions during therapy, 308–309
Dysphagia
behavioral objectives for, 31–32
condition examples for, 20
performance examples for, 16

Education for All Handicapped Children Act
    (P.L. 94–142), 39
Elicitation techniques, 301–304
Encouragement during testing, 290–291
Ending of therapy session, 321–323
ER. *See* Evaluation Report (ER)
Ethical issues, 93n, 348
Evaluation of clients. *See also* Evaluation reports;
    Reevaluation reports
consent form for, 211, 223–224

definition of, 353
paperwork requirements for, 167–168, 169
permission form for, 211, 220–222
Evaluation of treatment session, 167–168, 169
Evaluation Report (ER), 211–213, 237–243, 353
Evaluation reports. *See also* Progress reports;
    Reevaluation reports
age of client in, 88
analysis of poorly written evaluation report, 80–87
articulation report, 100, 102–106
background information in, 80, 82–83, 88–90
behavioral objectives in, 39
block style for, 87
dates in, 82
diagnoses in, 83–84
Evaluation section in, 83–84, 90–93, 102–104,
    107–108, 111–115, 117–119
fluency report, 101, 117–119
guidelines for, 87–95, 99–100
headings and subheadings in, 87
identifying information in, 88, 102, 106, 110, 117
Impressions section in, 93, 104, 108–109, 115, 119
language report, 100–101, 106–116
length of, 88
paragraph format for, 87
in public schools, 211–213, 237–243
recommendations in, 94, 105, 109, 115–116, 119
samples of, 100–119, 237–243
signatures in, 94, 105, 109, 116, 119
social and developmental history in, 82–83
source of information in, 80, 82
writing style and grammar in, 84–87
Evaluation section
of evaluation reports, 83–84, 90–93, 102–104,
    107–108, 111–115, 117–119
in reevaluation reports, 121–123, 125–126
Expressive language
definition of, 353
in evaluation reports, 92, 104, 107–108, 112–113
in reevaluation report, 123
Expressive One-Word Picture Vocabulary Test–2000,
    107n
Expressive One-Word Picture Vocabulary Test–Revised, 107,
    107n

First-person writing style in evaluation reports, 85–87
Fixed-ratio reinforcement, 353
Fluency
behavioral objectives for, 27–28
condition examples for, 19
definition of, 353
evaluation report on, 101, 117–119
performance examples for, 16
section on, in evaluation report, 91
*Fluharty Preschool Speech and Language Screening
    Test–Second Edition*, 106
Fostering dependency during therapy, 297–299
Frequency of stimulus presentation, 303

Game "mirage," 313–314
General education curriculum, 208, 353
Generalization (carry-over), 314–318, 353
Goals in IEPs, 215, 248–250
Goldman–Fristoe Test of Articulation–2, 113–114,
    121–122
Grammar, 84–87
Grant writing, 33
Group therapy
clinician–client ratio in, 261
definition of, 353
goal-related interaction in, 264
interaction during, 263–267
non–goal-related and goal-related combination in,
    264–266
non–goal-related interaction in, 263–264
record keeping during, 171–172
therapy in a group versus, 171, 262–263, 358

Harmony between behavioral objective and procedures,
    74–77
Head nodding by clinician, 309–310
Headings and subheadings in evaluation reports, 87
Hearing threshold test, 93n
Horizontal example of recording responses, 173–175

IDEA (Individuals with Disabilities Education Act), 208,
    354
IDEA Amendments of 1997 (IDEA '97), 208–210, 214,
    272, 353
Identifying information
in evaluation reports, 88, 102, 106, 110, 117
in IEPs, 244
in progress reports, 95, 129, 131, 135
in reevaluation reports, 121, 125
in therapy conference reports, 199, 200, 202, 204
IEPs. *See also* Public schools
behavioral objectives in, 39, 215, 248–250
curriculum-based IEPs, 352
definition of, 353, 354
Evaluation Report (ER) and, 211–213, 237–243
form for, 214
Invitation to Participate in IEP team meeting or other
    meeting, 213, 232–234, 354
Least Restrictive Environment (LRE) section in, 216,
    253
Measurable Annual Goal in, 215, 248–250
Participation in State and District-Wide Assessments
    section in, 215–216, 252–253
Present Levels of Educational Performance (PLEP)
    section of, 214, 246–247
record keeping for, 210–217
sample of, 244–255
Special Education/Related Services section in, 215,
    251–252
stages of IEP process, 214
state standards and, 208–209, 219, 272–274
Transition Planning section in, 254–255

Impressions section
in evaluation reports, 93, 104, 108–109, 115, 119
in progress reports, 97, 130, 133–134, 137
in reevaluation reports, 123–124, 126–127
Improving Education Results for Children with
Disabilities Act (2003), 210
*Indiana University Evaluation of Speech–Language
Pathology Student Practicum* (IUESP), 341
Indicator behavior, 14, 353
Individual therapy. *See also* Therapy
focus of, 261
record keeping during, 169–171, 280–282
seating arrangement during, 280–282
Individualized Education Programs. *See* IEPs
Individuals with Disabilities Education Act (IDEA), 208,
354. *See also* IDEA Amendments of 1997 (IDEA
'97)
Informants, definition of, 354
Initial evaluation, 354
Initial self-evaluations, 331
Instructional plan, 337, 354
Intermittent reinforcement, 285–286, 354
Interpersonal skills of clinicians, 338–339
Invitation to Participate in IEP team meeting or other
meeting, 213, 232–234, 354
IUESP (*Indiana University Evaluation of Speech–Language
Pathology Student Practicum*), 341

Language
behavioral objectives for, 25–26, 37–39
condition examples for, 18–19
definition of, 354
elicitation techniques for, 301–302
evaluation reports on, 100–101, 106–116
performance examples for, 15
progress report on, 128, 135–138
reevaluation report on, 120–124
section on, in evaluation reports, 91–92, 104, 107,
111–113
section on, in reevaluation reports, 122–123
standards for language arts, 219, 272–274
Language assessment, 354
Lead-in for behavioral objectives, 63–65
Least Restrictive Environment (LRE), 216, 253
Lesson objectives, 354
Lesson plans
behavioral objectives in, 33–39
paperwork requirements for, 167, 169
Letter differentiated from sound, 325–326
Licensure for speech–language pathologists, 190, 191
Long-range objectives, 34–39, 354
Loquaciousness of clinician, 296
Loudness, 125–126
LRE (Least Restrictive Environment), 216, 253

Manipulation of articulators, 303
McRel standards, 208–209
Mean length of utterance (MLU), 113

Measurable Annual Goal in IEPs, 215, 248–250
Medical history in evaluation reports, 89, 102, 106, 110
Mental role playing, 279–280
Mirror usage during therapy, 323–324
MLU (mean length of utterance), 113
Model of presentation, 304
Modeling
self-evaluation by clinician and, 332
verbal models used by clinicians, 292–296
Monitoring
carry-over and, 315–316
definition of, 354
Multidisciplinary evaluation process (MDI). *See* IEPs

National Student Speech-Language-Hearing
Association (NSSLHA), 348–349, 355
Naturalistic reinforcement, 288–290
Nervousness of clinicians and students, 4, 195–196,
279–280, 312–313
NOREP (Notice of Recommended Educational
Placement), 216, 235–236, 256–257, 355
Notes. *See* Progress notes
Notice and Consent for Placement in Special Education
Services, 235–236
Notice of Procedural Safeguards, 211, 217, 225–231,
356
Notice of Recommended Educational Placement
(NOREP), 216, 235–236, 256–257, 355
NSSLHA (National Student Speech-Language-Hearing
Association), 348–349, 355

Objective component of progress notes, 157–158
Objectives. *See also* Behavioral objectives; Therapeutic
objectives
definition of, 355
lesson objectives, 354
session objectives, 357
transitional objectives, 358
Observation
definition of, 332
of more experienced clinicians for self-evaluation, 342
self-observation techniques, 332–334
worksheet on observation and practicum requirements, 182
"OK" syndrome, 292–294
Opening of therapy sessions, 321
Oral function
in evaluation reports, 92, 104, 108, 115
in reevaluation reports, 123, 126
Oral-peripheral examination
in evaluation reports, 92, 104, 108, 114–115, 119
in reevaluation reports, 123, 126
Oral structure
in evaluation reports, 92, 104, 108, 114
in reevaluation reports, 123, 126
Overpowering clients during therapy, 308
Overt verbs for behavioral objectives, 14, 355
Overwork, elimination of, 318–319

P.L. 94-142 (Education for All Handicapped Children Act), 39
P.L. 101-336 (IDEA), 208, 354
P.L. 105-17 (IDEA '97), 208–210, 214, 272, 353
Paperwork. *See* Record keeping
Paragraph format for evaluation reports, 87
Participation in State and District-Wide Assessments section in IEPs, 215–216, 252–253
Participation percentages and patterns, 334–335
Passive voice in evaluation reports, 85–86
Patient, definition of, 355
Pause time during therapy, 323
Peabody Picture Vocabulary Test–Revised, 107, 107n
Peabody Picture Vocabulary Test–Third Edition, 107n, 111, 291
Peers and self-evaluation, 343
Percentage of correct responses, 336
Performance component of behavioral objectives, 12–17, 66–69
Permission to Evaluate Form, 211, 220–222, 355
Permission to Reevaluate Form, 216–217, 220–222, 355
Personal qualities of clinicians, 340–341
Phonetic context, 304
Phonics Screening Survey, 239
Phonological awareness
    behavioral objectives for, 30–31
    condition examples for, 19
    definition of, 355
    performance examples for, 16
Phonology
    behavioral objectives for, 24–25, 36–37
    condition examples for, 18
    performance examples for, 15
Pitch, 125
Placement cues, 303
Plan of treatment, 167, 169
Plan section of progress notes, 159
Play therapy, 261, 267–272, 355
PLEP (Present Levels of Educational Performance) in IEP, 214, 246–247
PLS-3 (*Preschool Language Scale–3*), 111–113, 122–123
Population trends, 349
Practicum record keeping, 182–184, 190, 192
Pragmatics
    behavioral objectives for, 28–29
    condition examples for, 19
    definition of, 355
    performance examples for, 16
Praise during testing, 290–291
Preschool Language Scale–3 (PLS–3), 111–113, 122–123
Present Levels of Educational Performance (PLEP) in IEP, 214, 246–247
Pretherapy plan. *See* Clinical strategy outline; Lesson plans
Prior Notice About Evaluation Form, 223–224
Problem behavior
    behavioral objectives for, 29–30
    condition examples for, 19

definition of, 356
performance examples for, 16
Problem solving and self-evaluation, 332
Procedural Safeguards Letter, 211, 356
Procedural Safeguards Notice, 211, 217, 225–231, 356
Procedural safeguards process. *See* IEPs
Professional accountability. *See* Accountability
Professional technical skills of clinicians, 339–340
Progress notes
    ambiguity in, 153–154
    analysis of, 148–150
    background on, 141–143
    behavioral objectives in, 143–149
    content of, 142
    cumulative progress note entries, 143–156
    data incomplete in, 152–153
    date for, 142
    format of, 143
    function of, 141–143
    no objective stated in, 150–152
    objective nature of, 142
    problematic entries, 150–156
    samples of, 143–148, 159–162
    self-contained nature of, 142
    signature in, 142
    SOAP (subjective-objective-assessment-plan) format for, 156–162, 357
    streamlining system for, 167, 168, 169
    wrong emphasis in, 154–156
Progress Report Form, 218
Progress reports
    Additional Testing section in, 96
    articulation reports, 128, 129–134
    attending behavior report, 128, 135–138
    background information in, 96, 129, 131, 135
    behavioral objectives in, 39
    current status in, 97, 130, 133–134, 137
    definition of, 128, 356
    form for, 218
    frequency of, 128
    guidelines for, 99–100
    identifying information in, 95, 129, 131, 135
    Impressions section in, 97, 130, 133–134, 137
    language report, 128, 135–138
    organization and content of, 95–98
    progress and procedures in, 96–97, 129–130, 132, 135–136
    recommendations in, 97, 130, 134, 138
    results of standardized testing in, 133, 136–137
    samples of, 128–138
    signatures in, 97, 130, 134, 138
    therapeutic objectives in, 96, 129, 131, 135
Prompts. *See* Elicitation techniques
Pronouns in evaluation reports, 84–86
Prosodic emphasis, 303
Public schools. *See also* IEPs
    Consent for Evaluation Form, 211, 223–224
    curriculum-based therapy in, 272–276

Evaluation Report (ER), 211–213, 237–243, 353
IDEA and, 208–210, 214, 272, 353
IEPs and, 39, 208–209, 244–255
Invitation to Participate in IEP team meeting or other meeting, 213, 232–234, 354
Notice and Consent for Placement in Special Education Services, 235–236
Notice of Recommended Educational Placement (NOREP), 216, 235–236, 256–257, 355
paperwork requirements in, 210–217
Permission to Evaluate Form, 211, 220–222, 355
Permission to Reevaluate Form, 216–217, 220–222, 355
preparation for, 207–217
Procedural Safeguards Letter, 211, 356
Procedural Safeguards Notice, 211, 217, 225–231, 356
Pure-tone hearing screening test, 93

Quality of voice, 125–126
Questions during therapy
risky questions, 305–306
simple or obvious questions and appearing foolish, 306–307

Rapid Letter Naming test, 239
Rate of speech
in evaluation report, 91
in reevaluation report, 125–126
Reading sequence, 300–301
Receptive language
definition of, 356
in evaluation reports, 91–92, 104, 107, 111–112
in reevaluation reports, 122–123
during therapy, 309–310
Recommendations
in evaluation reports, 94, 105, 109, 115–116, 119
in progress reports, 97, 130, 134, 138
in reevaluation reports, 124, 127
Record keeping. *See also* IEPs
accountability and, 166–167, 177–192
accuracy of, 166–167, 169–170, 177–178, 337
for clinical hours during practicum, 190, 192
clinical tracking sheets, 180–185
computer software for, 165–166
continuing education requirements and, 187, 190, 191
as continuous process during entire therapy session, 170
definition of paperwork, 355
during group sessions, 171–172
horizontal example of recording responses, 173–175
for IEPs, 210–217
during individual sessions, 169–171, 280–282
problems with paperwork, 5, 165–166
professional accountability and, 187–190
in public schools, 210–217
response sheets, 169, 170–171, 177
sampling approach to, 170, 172

self-evaluation on, 337
steps in therapeutic process and paperwork requirements, 167–169
system for streamlining paperwork process, 167–177
tracking clinical hours (if applying for CCC after Jan. 2005), 185–187, 192
tracking clinical hours (if applying for CCC before Dec. 2004), 178–185, 192
vertical example of recording responses, 175–177
ways to record, 173–177
worksheet for recording evaluation and diagnostic hours in speech–language pathology, 188
worksheet for recording therapy hours in speech–language pathology, 189
with young or very active children, 173
Reevaluation. *See also* Reevaluation reports
definition of, 356
permission form for, 216–217, 220–222
Reevaluation reports
articulation report, 120–124
background information in, 121, 125
compared with evaluation reports, 120
Evaluation section in, 121–123, 125–126
form for, 242–243
guidelines for, 99–100
identifying information in, 121, 125
impressions in, 123–124, 126–127
language report, 120–124
in public schools, 242–243
recommendations in, 124, 127
samples of, 120–127
signatures in, 124, 127
voice report, 120, 125–127
Rehearsal and self-evaluation, 332
Reinforcement
accidental or inappropriate usage of, 283–285
continuous reinforcement, 285, 352
definition of, 356
fixed-ratio reinforcement, 353
intermittent reinforcement, 285–286, 354
naturalistic versus artificial reinforcement, 288–290
self-evaluation on accuracy of, 336
specific and varied reinforcement, 286–287
tangible reinforcement, 287–288
during testing, 290–291
during therapy, 282–290
Reporting skills of clinicians, 340
Reports. *See* Evaluation reports; Progress reports; Reevaluation reports; Therapy conference reports
Response rate of target behaviors, 335–336
Response sheets, 169, 170–171, 177
Risky questions during therapy, 305–306

Schools. *See* Public schools
Screening Deep Test of Articulation, 133
Seating arrangement during therapy, 280–282
Self-contracting, 332

Self-determination of criteria, 332
Self-evaluation
    of accuracy of reinforcement, 336
    of assessment skills, 340
    benchmark measurements for, 334–337
    comparing instructional plan to behavioral record, 337
    definition of, 356
    of developing and planning skills, 339
    familiarity with Clinical Evaluation Form, 342
    fine-tuning clinical competence, 337–341
    importance of, 329
    initial self-evaluations, 331
    instruments for, 338–341
    of interpersonal skills, 338–339
    observation of more experienced clinicians, 342
    participation percentages and patterns, 334–335
    peers and, 343
    percentage of correct responses, 336
    of personal qualities, 340–341
    of professional technical skills, 339–340
    purposes of, 330
    of reporting skills, 340
    response rate of target behaviors, 335–336
    self-observation techniques, 332–334
    strategies for, 331–343
    Student Self-Appraisal, 343–344, 357
    of teaching skills, 339
Self-instruction, 331
Self-monitoring, 315–316, 356
Self-observation techniques, 332–334
Semantics, 356
Semester plan of treatment, 167, 169, 356
Session, 357. *See also* Therapy
Session evaluation, 357. *See also* Evaluation reports
Session objectives, 357
Short-term objectives
    definition of, 357
    in IEPs, 215, 248–250
    in lesson plans, 34–38
Sign language, 319–320
Signatures
    in evaluation reports, 94, 105, 109, 116, 119
    in IEPs, 244–245
    in progress notes, 142
    in progress reports, 97, 130, 134, 138
    in reevaluation reports, 124, 127
Singsong voice of clinician, 326–327
Smothering the client, 296–297, 357
SOAP format for progress notes, 156–162, 357
Social and developmental history, in evaluation reports, 82–83
Sound differentiated from letter, 325–326
Special education, 357. *See also* IEPs; Public schools
Special Education/Related Services section in IEPs, 215, 251–252
Speech
    in evaluation reports, 90–91, 113–114
    in reevaluation reports, 121–122, 126

Speech and language milestones in evaluation reports, 89, 102, 111
Speech–language clinicians. *See also* Therapy
    appearing foolish during therapy, 306–307
    assessment skills of, 340
    boredom of, 312–313
    certification of, 178–187, 192
    clinician–client ratio in group therapy, 261
    continuing education for, 187, 190, 191
    definition of, 352
    developing and planning skills of, 339
    fostering dependency by, 297–299
    habits of, that may be misinterpreted, 312–313
    head nodding and forward upper body movement by, during therapy, 309–310
    interpersonal skills of, 338–339
    job market for, 350
    licensure for speech–language pathologists, 190, 191
    loquaciousness of, during therapy, 296
    nervousness of clinicians and students, 4, 195–196, 279–280, 312–313
    overpowering clients by, during therapy, 308
    personal qualities of, 340–341
    professional responsibilities of, 348–350
    professional technical skills of, 339–340
    reporting skills of, 340
    risky questions by, 305–306
    self-evaluation by, 329–344
    singsong voice of, 326–327
    smothering the client by, 296–297, 357
    stages in introductory clinical functioning, 2–8
    teaching skills of, 339
    verbal models used by, 292–296
    working too much and, 318–319
Speech–language pathologists, 190, 191, 357
Speech–language pathology assistant, 357
SSI-3 (*Stuttering Severity Instrument for Children and Adults–Third Edition*), 118
Standards, 208–209, 219, 272–274, 351
Stimulus words and materials, 318–319
Streamlining paperwork process, 167–177
Structured Photographic Expressive Language Test–Preschool, 107–108
Student Self-Appraisal, 343–344, 357
Stuttering Severity Instrument for Children and Adults–Third Edition (SSI-3), 118
Stuttering Standard Interview Procedure, 117–118
Subheadings and headings in evaluation reports, 87
Subjective observations in progress notes, 156–157
Subjective-Objective-Assessment-Plan (SOAP), 156–162, 357
Supervision of clinicians, 329–330. *See also* Self-evaluation
Support between behavioral objective and procedures, 74–77

Tactile and visual imagery, 303
Tangible reinforcement, 287–288

Teaching skills of clinicians, 339

Terminal objectives, 38–39, 357

Test for Auditory Comprehension of Language, 290, 290n

Testing. *See also* specific tests

Additional Testing section in progress reports, 96

praise and encouragement during, 290–291

reinforcement during, 290–291

results of standardized testing in progress reports, 133, 136–137

Therapeutic objectives

definition of, 358

in progress reports, 96, 129, 131, 135

Therapy

access to client for, 282, 283

appearing foolish during, 306–307

assignments and, 316–317, 318

carry-over and, 314–318

choice constancy and, 299–300

clinician's having too much work, 318–319

closing of session, 321–323

curriculum-based therapy, 272–276, 352

definition of, 358

differentiating sound from letter, 325–326

directions during, 308–309

elicitation techniques, 301–304

fostering dependency during, 297–299

game "mirage" and, 313–314

group therapy, 171–172, 261, 262–267

habits of clinician that may be misinterpreted, 312–313

head nodding and forward upper body movement by clinician during, 309–310

individual therapy, 169–171, 261

loquaciousness of clinician, 296

mirror usage during, 323–324

monitoring and, 315–316

opening of sessions, 321

overpowering clients by clinician during, 308

participation percentages and patterns in, 334–335

pause time during, 323

percentage of correct responses in, 336

play therapy, 261, 267–272, 355

reading sequence, 300–301

receptive tasks during, 309–310

record keeping during group sessions, 171–172

record keeping during individual sessions, 169–171

reinforcement during, 282–290, 336

response rate of target behaviors in, 335–336

risky questions during, 305–306

seating arrangement during, 280–282

sign language, 319–320

singsong voice of clinician, 326–327

smothering the client during, 296–297, 357

steps in, and paperwork requirements, 167–169

verbal models used by clinicians during, 292–296

videotaping and audiotaping sessions of, 296, 311, 313, 323, 332–334, 343

wrap-up of session, 322

Therapy conference reports, 198–205, 358

Therapy conferences

areas covered during, 197

definition of, 358

length of, 195–196

preparation for, 205

purpose of, 195, 196–197

reports on, 198–205

sample reports on, 199–205

Therapy in a group, 171, 262–263, 358

Therapy program, 358

Third-person writing style in evaluation reports, 85–87

Title registration for speech–language pathologists, 190

Tracking clinical hours

for CCC application after Jan. 2005, 185–187, 192

for CCC application before Dec. 2004, 178–185, 192

clinical tracking sheets, 180–185

Transition Planning section in IEPs, 254–255

Transitional objectives, 358

Treatment plan, 358

Type Token Ratio, 113

Ungrammatical utterances by clinician, 295–296

Unnatural production by clinician, 294–295

Utah Test of Language Development–Third Edition, 136–137

Verbal Language Development Scale, Revised, 111, 111n

Verbal models used by clinicians

"OK" syndrome, 292–294

ungrammatical utterances, 295–296

unnatural production, 294–295

Verbs for behavioral objectives, 13, 14

Vertical example of recording responses, 175–177

Video and audio critiques, 296, 311, 313, 323, 332–334, 343, 358

Video Critique Form, 333

Visual and tactile imagery, 303

Vocal parameters

in evaluation reports, 92–93, 104, 108, 119

in reevaluation report, 125–126

Voice

behavioral objectives for, 26–27

condition examples for, 19

definition of, 358

in evaluation reports, 114

performance examples for, 15

reevaluation report on, 120, 125–127

Voice Assessment Protocol for Children and Adults, 125–126

Wisconsin Procedure for Appraisal of Clinical Competence (W-PACC), 338–341

Word selection in evaluation reports, 84

Worksheets

observation and practicum requirements, 182

for recording clinical practicum hours in speech–language pathology, 184 for recording evaluation and diagnostic hours in speech–language pathology, 188

for recording therapy hours in speech–language pathology, 189

student worksheet for recording clinical practicum contacts in speech–language pathology, 183

Video Critique Form, 333

W-PACC (*Wisconsin Procedure for Appraisal of Clinical Competence*), 338–341

Wrap-up of therapy session, 322

Writing reports. *See* Evaluation reports; Progress reports; Reevaluation reports; Therapy conference reports

Writing style in evaluation reports, 84–87

Young children
play therapy with, 261, 267–272, 355
record keeping with, 173

About the Author

Susan Moon Meyer, PhD, is a professor of special education, speech–language pathology, at Kutztown University in Kutztown, Pennsylvania. Dr. Meyer has been extensively involved in private practice in various settings (hospitals, nursing homes, home health, etc.). She has been regularly asked to review books for the journal *Child Language Teaching and Therapy* and was an editorial consultant for *Language Speech and Hearing Services in Schools*. Dr. Meyer has been named to *Who's Who in America, Who's Who in American Women, Who's Who in America: 2000 Outstanding People of the 20th Century, Who's Who in the East, Dictionary of International Biography, Who's Who of Women, Who's Who in the World, Who's Who in American Education*, and the *National Distinguished Service Registry: Speech, Language, and Hearing.* She has served as Pennsylvania legislative councilor to the American Speech-Language-Hearing Association, Pennsylvania's Speech-Language-Hearing Association's vice president of professional preparation, and president of the Northeastern Speech-Language-Hearing Association. Dr. Meyer has received several awards recognizing her professional service, including the first Honors of the Northeastern Speech-Language-Hearing Association.